Watch videos from *Vertigo and Disequilibrium,*
Second Edition online at MediaCenter.thieme.com!

	WINDOWS	MAC	TABLET
Recommended Browser(s)**	Recent browser versions on all major platforms and any mobile operating system that supports HTML5 video playback *** all browsers should have JavaScript enabled*		
Flash Player Plug-in	Flash Player 9 or Higher* ** Mac users: ATI Rage 128 GPU does not support full-screen mode with hardware scaling*		Tablet PCs with Android OS support Flash 10.1
Recommended for optimal usage experience	Monitor resolutions: • Normal (4:3) 1024×768 or Higher • Widescreen (16:9) 1280×720 or Higher • Widescreen (16:10) 1440×900 or Higher DSL/Cable internet connection at a minimum speed of 384.0 Kbps or faster WiFi 802.11 b/g preferred.		7-inch and 10-inch tablets on maximum resolution. WiFi connection is required.

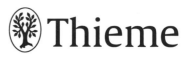

Vertigo and Disequilibrium

A Practical Guide to Diagnosis and Management

Second Edition

Peter C. Weber, MD, MBA
Director, Ear Institute
New York Eye and Ear Infirmary of Mount Sinai
Professor of Otolaryngology–Head and Neck Surgery
Icahn School of Medicine at Mount Sinai
Chief, Otology/Neurology/Skull Base
Mount Sinai System
New York, New York

167 illustrations

Thieme
New York • Stuttgart • Delhi • Rio de Janeiro

Executive Editor: Timothy Y. Hiscock
Managing Editor: J. Owen Zurhellen IV
Editorial Assistant: Mary B. Wilson
Director, Editorial Services: Mary Jo Casey
Production Editor: Kenneth L. Chumbley
International Production Director: Andreas Schabert
Vice President, Editorial and E-Product Development: Vera Spillner
International Marketing Director: Fiona Henderson
International Sales Director: Louisa Turrell
Director of Sales, North America: Mike Roseman
Senior Vice President and Chief Operating Officer: Sarah Vanderbilt
President: Brian D. Scanlan
Cover Image: Used with permission from Fotolia, Zffoto

Library of Congress Cataloging-in-Publication Data

Names: Weber, Peter C., 1961-
Title: Vertigo and disequilibrium : a practical guide to diagnosis
    and management / [edited by] Peter C. Weber.
Description: Second edition. | New York : Thieme, [2017] |
    Includes bibliographical references and index.
Identifiers: LCCN 2016035322| ISBN 9781626232044 (hardcover :
    alk. paper) | ISBN 9781626232051 (e-book)
Subjects: | MESH: Vertigo—diagnosis | Vertigo—therapy | Dizziness—
    prevention & control | Vestibule, Labyrinth—pathology
Classification: LCC RB150.V4 | NLM WV 255 | DDC 616.8/41—dc23
    LC record available at https://lccn.loc.gov/2016035322

© 2017 Thieme Medical Publishers, Inc.
Thieme Publishers New York
333 Seventh Avenue, New York, NY 10001 USA
+1 800 782 3488, customerservice@thieme.com

Thieme Publishers Stuttgart
Rüdigerstrasse 14, 70469 Stuttgart, Germany
+49 [0]711 8931 421, customerservice@thieme.de

Thieme Publishers Delhi
A-12, Second Floor, Sector-2, Noida-201301
Uttar Pradesh, India
+91 120 45 566 00, customerservice@thieme.in

Thieme Publishers Rio de Janeiro, Thieme Publicações Ltda.
Edifício Rodolpho de Paoli, 25º andar
Av. Nilo Peçanha, 50 – Sala 2508
Rio de Janeiro 20020-906, Brasil
+55 21 3172 2297

Cover design: Thieme Publishing Group
Typesetting by Prairie Papers

Printed in China by Everbest Printing Investment   5 4 3 2 1

ISBN 978-1-62623-204-4

Also available as an e-book:
eISBN 978-1-62623-205-1

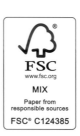

Contents

Menu of Accompanying Videos

Video 2.1 Demonstration of Romberg testing while on compliant foam. This test isolates the vestibular system by decreasing visual (eyes closed) and proprioceptive (foam pad) influences.

Video 2.2 Demonstration of the use of Frenzel goggles. This apparatus may detect vestibular nystagmus by decreasing visual fixation. The second part of the video shows nystagmus while using this instrument.

Video 2.3 Smooth pursuit with normal endpoint in left gaze position.

Video 2.4 Lateral gaze direction changing nystagmus such that left gaze is left beating and right gaze is right beating, in addition abnormal gait that is slightly wide based and right leaning. Consistent with central pathology.

Video 2.5 Normal gaze testing and facial nerve function.

Video 2.6 Classic example of downbeating nystagmus consistent with central lesion.

Video 2.7 Classic example of upbeating nystagmus consistent with central lesion.

Video 2.8 Gaze nystagmus.

Video 2.9 Demonstration of the head impulse or head thrust test. This test is mainly administered in the plane of the horizontal canal. The examiner should pay close attention to any re-fixation saccades that would be indicative of a peripheral vestibular abnormality, which can be seen in the second part of the video.

Video 5.1 Head thrust test (also called head impulse test) demonstrated in a healthy patient.

Video 7.1 Vestibular neurectomy.

Video 8.1 Left geotropic lateral semicircular canal benign paroxysmal positional video.

Video 8.2 Left apogeotropic lateral semicircular canal benign paroxysmal positional video.

Video 8.3 Right upbeat torsional nystagmus seen in right posterior semicircular canal benign paroxysmal positional vertigo eye video.

Video 8.4 Right posterior benign paroxysmal positional vertigo animation.

Video 8.5 Right posterior canalith repositioning animation.

Video 8.6 Right Dix-Hallpike video.

Video 8.7 Benign paroxysmal positional vertigo surgery.

Video 11.1 Superior canal dehiscence.

Video 12.1 Perilymph fistula.

Video 13.1 Hyperventilation induced nystagmus.

Video 15.1 Rotary exam of vestibular ocular reflex in an infant.

Video 15.2 Balance exam in a child.

Video 15.3 Balance Subtest of Bruinink-Oseretsky Test of Motor Proficiency Second Edition (BOT2).

Foreword

This second edition of *Vertigo and Disequilibrium: A Practical Guide to Diagnosis and Management*, authored and edited by Peter Weber, MD, is a must read by physicians, audiologists, and therapists challenged with the care of people with dizziness and vertigo. Dr. Weber succinctly introduces the subject in the first chapter, providing the essential information needed in taking a history from a patient with vertigo, dizziness, or disequilibrium, setting the stage for developing a decision tree for categorizing the nature of the complaint and the suspected diagnosis. This introduction is the springboard to subsequent chapters that focus on the office examination, physiology, testing of the vestibular and central nervous systems, pertinent imaging studies, and those devoted to specific pathologic processes and diseases causing problems of vertigo and disequilibrium.

The strengths and limitations of computerized testing of the vestibular patient are detailed in Ch. 3 by Drs. Judson and Galatioto. In technical yet practical description, the battery of tests available for assessing the vestibular system are described and demonstrated with figures and video clips. They emphasize that the purpose of testing is to help identify the presence or absence of a lesion. This chapter diffuses the potential anxiety of being intimidated when requesting and interpreting these diagnostic tests.

Chapter 4 provides one of the most compressive compilations of imaging studies demonstrating pathology of the temporal bone and posterior fossa and disorders of circulation. The figures are of excellent resolution, well labeled with arrows, and described with concise legends. Some of the diseases are relatively rare, making this an even more important resource for those charged with diagnosing vestibular disorders. This chapter is an excellent collection that rivals textbooks devoted to this aspect of diagnostic imaging.

The majority of the textbook concentrates on specific inner ear, central, and metabolic disorders causing vertigo and disequilibrium. They are authored by experts in the field. One of the more common vestibular disorders is benign paroxysmal positional vertigo. In Ch. 8, Dr. White addressed the pathophysiology, diagnosis, medical treatment, and efficacy of BPPV. Dr. Gacek continued the review and detailed the surgical technique he advocated for refractory BPPV with singular nerve section..

Another highlight of the textbook are the chapters devoted to vertigo and disequilibrium at the extremes of age. Though there is overlap with a number of vestibular disorders in elderly and pediatric patients, there are disease processes that are unique to these populations. (Chs. 14 and 15). It is important to recognize congenital and hereditary disorders that have associated symptoms and findings of vertigo or balance disorders. Sophisticated computerized testing may not be tolerated by very young patients. The details of pediatric clinical testing are enhanced by the video segments that accompany the chapter.

Though relatively rare, there are a number of seldom seen vestibular disorders that can challenge the clinician. Rare sources of vertigo and disequilibrium—including those from medications, ototoxicity, perilymphatic fistula, autoimmune disease, autonomic disorders, neoplasms, cervical origin, and mal de barquement—are highlighted in Chs. 12, 13, and 17. It is underestimated how often migraine is the primary or accompanying source of vertigo. Chapter 16 details the history, pathophysiology, testing, diagnosis, and medical and dietary treatment of this neurogenic source. This is very well written and organized, which provides the reader with a comprehensive understanding of how migraine can cause or confound the diagnosis.

Superior semicircular canal dehiscence became a recognized pathology entity in 1998 by Lloyd Minor, MD. Five authors provide their collective experience with this fascinating disorder, which explains some very unusual symptoms, such as hearing bodily sounds like autophony, chewing, and movement of the eyes. The vestibular components can become debilitating and incapacitating. The astute clinician should be suspicious of this disorder and focus in on the appropriate diagnostic tests and treatment options. This is comprehensively covered in Ch. 11. The contributions of physiology and stimulation of the SCC toward eye movements are explained in a clear and understandable manner. The details of the audiological, vestibular, and diagnostic tests are succinctly reviewed.

The role of vestibular rehabilitation therapy (Ch. 20) emphasizes the diagnostic tests, function of inquiry by survey, and therapeutic exercises that are supportive for recovery. The author acknowledges the requirements of using science and art toward providing effective intervention.

This second edition has a number of outstanding modifications and additions. As mentioned, the video clips in a number of the chapters enhance the readers' understanding of the issues being covered. The list of references at the end of the chapters has been expanded and updated. The role of implantable vestibular devices (Ch. 21) shares the present and future endeavors to restore vestibular function to those with diminished or absent function. Finally, the appendix compiles a list of practical and frequently asked questions from clinicians and patients. Dr. Weber provides concrete and succinct answers.

In summary, this second edition of Vertigo and Disequilibrium: A Practical Guide to Diagnosis and Management provides a comprehensive and up-to-date single source textbook covering common and unusual vestibular diseases and disorders. It is well written for clinicians, therapists, physicians, audiologists and surgeons evaluating and managing patients with vertigo and disequilibrium. This is a "must have" book that should be read and referenced.

Barry E. Hirsch, MD, FACS
Professor, Departments of Otolaryngology,
Neurosurgery, and Communication Sciences and Disorders
Director, Division of Otology, Neurotology
University of Pittsburgh Medical Center
Pittsburgh, Pennsylvania

Preface

Dizziness is one of the most common complaints patients experience and seek a physician's advice for. Typically, it is to their primary doctors and then to the ENT specialist. Many physicians are tentative when it comes to making a diagnosis or initiating treatment programs because of a lack of understanding of the vestibular system and how it can interact with other systems of the body. Indeed, many causes of disequilibrium and/or dizziness are multifactorial. For many, the vestibular system is this big black box that is poorly understood because it is not well taught in medical school and even in residency programs. Thus it seems complex when in fact it is rather straightforward. Therefore many patients don't get the care they need.

The aim of this book is to demystify the vestibular system and vestibular disorders. To examine how other systems can also cause dizziness and how they interact with the vestibular system. How to take a history and perform an examination that will often times make the diagnosis and treatment clear. This second edition adds a few new parameters to consider and updated treatment modalities. As with the first edition, this addition also has a DVD. We have expanded the videos to include some of the testing and diagnoses. It is our hope that this will prove beneficial to you.

Because physicians and other care providers from all specialties manage these patients, this book is not just for otolaryngologists. Rather, neurologists, physical therapists (especially our rehab section with video), internists, geriatricians, family practitioners, audiologists and even cardiologists will benefit from this book. Any medical professional with an interest in vestibular disorders and the system will appreciate this book.

The authors are some of the foremost experts in the field and have been able to simply explain not just the easy patients into treatment algorithms but even the complex techniques. In the final chapter of this book newer applications that are in the development stages are discussed.

Peter C. Weber, MD, MBA

Acknowledgments

I would like to formally thank all the contributing authors who gave up a significant amount of their precious time and put forth so much effort into making each and every chapter concise, easy to read, and full of pertinent knowledge. Without their dedication, this book would not have been possible. Just as in our first edition, for which Kelly Boudin and Adam Aiello made some fantastic treatment videos, Dr. Bryan Hujsak, the head of vestibular rehabilitation at the Ear Institute of Mt Sinai/New York Eye and Ear, has prepared some great teaching videos for this book.

J. Owen Zurhellen and his team at Thieme deserve special thanks for trying to herd all of us to keep on schedule, while producing an incredible book.

Finally, I want to thank my family, who are always a deep inspiration to me and who keep me happy, sane, and focused on providing great care to patients and balancing my time.

Contributors

Douglas D. Backous, MD
Center for Hearing and Skull Base Surgery
Swedish Medical Group
Seattle, Washington

Stephen P. Cass, MD, MPH
Professor
Department of Otolaryngology
University of Colorado SOM
Aurora, Colorado

Sujana S. Chandrasekhar, MD, FACS
Otology/Neurotology
President, American Academy of Otolaryngology–Head
  and Neck Surgery
Past Chair, Board of Governors, AAO-HNS
Director, New York Otology
New York Head and Neck Institute
Director, NSLIJ, LHH/MEETH Comprehensive Balance Center
Director of Neurotology
James J. Peters VA Medical Center
Clinical Professor of Otolaryngology
Hofstra-Northwell School of Medicine
Clinical Associate Professor of Otolaryngology
Icahn School of Medicine at Mount Sinai
Staff Physician
Lenox Hill Hospital and Manhattan Eye, Ear, Throat Institute
James J. Peters Bronx Veterans Administration Medical Center
Mount Sinai Hospital
New York Eye and Ear Infirmary
Saint Barnabas Medical Center
Livingston, New Jersey

Francois Cloutier, MD, FRCSC
Associated Professor
Faculty of Medicine
Montreal University
Department of Otolaryngology–Head and Neck Surgery,
  Otology/Neurotology
Pierre-Boucher Hospital
Longueuil, Quebec, Canada

Candice Colby, MD
Neurotology–Ear and Skull Base Surgery, Otolaryngology
ENT Consultants
Grand Rapids, Michigan

Colin L. W. Driscoll, MD
Professor and Chair
Mayo Clinic
Department of Otolaryngology–Head and Neck Surgery
Rochester, Minnesota

Richard R. Gacek, MD, FACS
Professor
Otolaryngology–Head and Neck Surgery
University of Massachusetts Medical School
Worcester, Massachusetts

Jessica Galatioto, AuD
Audiology Supervisor
Ear Institute–Hearing and Balance
New York Eye and Ear Infirmary of Mount Sinai
New York, New York

Michele M. Gandolfi, MD
Neurotology
House Ear Clinic
Los Angeles, California

Justin S. Golub, MD
Assistant Professor
Otology, Neurotology, and Skull Base Surgery
Department of Otolaryngology–Head and Neck Surgery
Columbia University College of Physicians and Surgeons
New York-Presbyterian/Columbia University Medical Center
New York, New York

Marcelle Groenewald, MBChB, DCH(SA), PG Dip Int Res Ethics
Medical Doctor, First Medical Officer
Allergy Service Unit
No 1 Military Hospital
Pretoria, South Africa

Samuel P. Gubbels, MD, FACS
Director
University of Colorado Health Hearing and Balance Center
Associate Professor
Department of Otolaryngology
University of Colorado School of Medicine
Aurora, Colorado

Michael E. Hoffer, MD, FACS
Professor
Department of Otolaryngology and Neurological Surgery
University of Miami, Miller School of Medicine
Miami, Florida

Louis M. Hofmeyr, MBChB, MMED
Otorhinolaryngologist
Department of Ear, Nose, Throat
University of Pretoria
Pretoria, South Africa

Tina C. Huang, MD
Department of Otolaryngology–Head and Neck Surgery
University of Minnesota
Minneapolis, Minnesota

Bryan D. Hujsak, PT, DPT, NCS
Director, Vestibular Rehabilitation
The Ear Institute, Hearing, and Balance Center
The New York Eye and Ear Infirmary of Mount Sinai
New York, New York

Randy Judson, AuD, CCC-A, F-AAA
Director, Communicative Sciences
The Ear Institute
New York Eye and Ear Infirmary of Mount Sinai
New York, New York

Ana H. Kim, MD
Associate Professor
Associate Director, Cochlear Implant Program
Director, Otologic Research
Department of Otolaryngology–Head and Neck Surgery
Columbia University Medical Center
New York, New York

John I. Lane, MD
Professor of Radiology
Department of Radiology
Mayo Clinic
Rochester, Minnesota

Kennith F. Layton, MD, MS, FAHA
Chairman
Department of Radiology
Director, Interventional Neuroradiology
Baylor University Medical Center
Dallas, Texas

Samuel C. Levine, MD
Professor
Neurotology, Otolaryngology, and Neurosurgery
University of Minnesota
Minneapolis, Minnesota

Nauman F. Manzoor, MD
Department of Otolaryngology–Head and Neck Surgery
University Hospitals Case Medical Center
Cleveland, Ohio

Jameson K. Mattingly, MD
Department of Otolaryngology
University of Colorado SOM
Aurora, Colorado

Sean O. McMenomey, MD, FACS
Center for Hearing and Skull Base Surgery
Swedish Medical Group
Seattle, Washington

Cliff A. Megerian, MD, FACS
President, University Hospitals Physician Services
Julius W. McCall Professor and Chairman
Otolaryngology–Head and Neck Surgery
Case Western Reserve University School of Medicine
Richard W. and Patricia R. Pogue Endowed Chair
Director, Ear, Nose, and Throat Institute
University Hospitals Case Medical Center
Cleveland, Ohio

Alan G. Micco, MD, FACS
Associate Professor
Otolaryngology, Neurological Surgery and Medical Education
Chief, Section of Otology, Neurotology and Skull Base Surgery
Residency Program Director
Northwestern University Feinberg School of Medicine
Chicago, Illinois

Kathryn Y. Noonan, MD
Lebanon, New Hampshire

Yael Raz, MD
ENT Specialist
University of Pittsburgh Medical Center Presbyterian
Pittsburgh, Pennsylvania

James E. Saunders, MD
Professor, Otology and Skull Base Surgery
Department of Surgery
Dartmouth-Hitchcock Medical Center
Lebanon, New Hampshire

Maroun T. Semaan, MD, FACS
Associate Professor and Director of Otology/Neurotology
Department of Otolaryngology–Head and Neck Surgery
University Hospitals Case Medical Center
Cleveland, Ohio

Mikhaylo Szczupak, MD
Department of Otolaryngology–Head and Neck Surgery
University of Miami Miller School of Medicine
Miami, Florida

Laura Wazen, DPT
Equinox Physical Therapy
Sarasota, Florida

Peter C. Weber, MD, MBA
System-wide Chief, Otology, Neurotology/Skull Base Surgery
Mount Sinai Health System
Director, Ear Institute–NYEE
Department of Otolaryngology
Mount Sinai Health System
Chief, Otology/Neurology/Skull Base
Mount Sinai System
New York, New York

Judith White, MD, PhD
Medical Director, Swedish Balance Center
Swedish Neuroscience Institute
Seattle, Washington

Cameron C. Wick, MD
Department of Otolaryngology–Head and Neck Surgery
University of Texas Southwestern Medical Center
Dallas, Texas

Robert J. Witte, MD
Associate Professor
Department of Radiology
Mayo Clinic
Rochester, Minnesota

1 Taking the History of the Vertiginous Patient

Peter C. Weber

◼ Introduction

This chapter gives an overview of what questions are to be asked during the history to assist in making the overall diagnosis. A physician who can master the three most common vestibular diagnoses—benign paroxysmal positional vertigo, vestibular neuronitis (labyrinthitis), and Meniere disease—can manage 80% of all vestibular complaints.[1,2,3,4]

Taking the time to establish a full and accurate history is the most important diagnostic endeavor in medicine. The diagnosis of a patient with vertigo or dizziness can almost always be ascertained 80% of the time by taking an accurate history without exception.[5,6] As a history is taken from a patient with complaints of vertigo, it is important to understand the various pathophysiologic and disease entities that may cause the complaint. Careful questioning about the patient's symptoms, their duration, triggering events, and what, if anything, makes them better or worse, plays an important role in defining a possible etiology for the patient's complaint and allows the physician to arrive at a provisional diagnosis to better direct the patient's care.

The etiology of true vertigo can be either central or peripheral. The history may well elucidate various factors that may affect the peripheral or central systems, such as congenital abnormalities, drugs, trauma, toxins, or infections. However, other etiologies may cause patients to think they are having vertigo when other systems, such as cardiac, metabolic, or neurologic systems, are truly the root cause. Once a history is taken, the physical examination can then assist and confirm the validity of one's suspicions about the etiology of the complaint. After the physical examination, various tests can be ordered to help pinpoint the diagnosis.

◼ History

Intake forms are utilized by many physicians and can assist in the history taking. The information on an intake form can lead the physician to follow-up questions and to arrive at a differential diagnosis relatively quickly and efficiently.[1,5] However, I tend not to use intake forms; instead, I gain more useful information from actually letting the patient describe the condition to me. The patient's description of what the patient experiences or is experiencing is paramount in my assessment. It is important to ascertain what the patient actually means by "dizziness." For some patients, dizziness actually means rotation—either the world is spinning or moving around them or they are spinning around in the world. Dizziness is in essence what we call true vertigo, and it is more typical of a peripheral disorder, although central disorders cannot be completely eliminated. The patient who complains more of just lightheadedness or that they "just don't feel quite right," is probably not describing a vestibular disorder per se, but may be suffering from a systemic disorder, such as poor circulation, arrhythmia, neurogenic disorder, anemia, thyroid disorder, orthostatic tachycardia syndrome, or other cardiac problem. Patients who have a complaint of disequilibrium, i.e., their balance is off, are more likely to have a peripheral weakness or a central disorder, such as a cerebellar lesion, unilateral vestibular weakness, mal de barquement syndrome, or fistula.[6] These disorders are all discussed in detail in this book.

If the patient describes true vertigo, one needs to know if the vertigo is episodic, the duration of the spell, the number of times it has occurred, and if there are any triggering events, such as a high-salt diet, allergies, movement, turning, recent upper respiratory tract infection, stress, headaches, loud noises, barotrauma, or other trauma. This information is important because it can help frame the types of diagnoses one must consider.

■ Episodic Vertigo

If the complaint of true vertigo is associated with episodic spells that typically last seconds to minutes and are associated with positional movements, such as rolling over in bed or turning the head quickly, the most likely diagnosis is benign paroxysmal positional vertigo (BPPV). However, if during a diving incident the patient heard a loud pop and then had significant dizziness and continued to have episodic dizziness after this, with or without some type of associated hearing loss, one might consider barotrauma/perilymphatic fistula as the diagnosis. Exposure to loud noise that causes brief vertiginous episodes could be related to a superior canal dehiscence syndrome (which may also include a low-frequency conductive hearing loss).

The most common disorder with episodic vertigo is Meniere's disease. However, Meniere's disease is not really a disease, but rather a syndrome, with signs and symptoms caused by a multitude of triggers. The key is determining the trigger, if possible, so that the treatment is individualized. Meniere's disease is also a diagnosis of exclusion; therefore, the physician must rule out all other causes of episodic vertigo before diagnosing Meniere's disease and possibly mistreating the patient. Many etiologies can mimic an episodic dizzy spell, including multiple sclerosis (ask about other episodic neural complaints), autoimmune inner ear disease (Does the patient have fatigue, arthritis, or other autoimmune complaints?), otosclerotic inner ear syndrome (Is there an associated hearing loss and does it run in the family?), migraine-induced vertigo[7] (Does the patient have headaches before or after the spell, visual complaints, difficulty with carnival rides now or as a child, history of migraines in the past?), or allergy-induced vertigo spells (typically associated with allergic breakouts/exposure).

By definition, true Meniere's consists of four separate symptoms during a spell: the vertiginous episode, hearing loss (which resolves when the attack is completed, but over time and repeated spells becomes permanent and usually starts in the low frequencies), aural fullness, and tinnitus. However, the vast majority of my patients never have all four symptoms with each spell, but rather two or three. Any of the other disorders mentioned can be associated with hearing loss as well. Therefore, just because the patient complains of episodic dizzy spells, does not mean that they have Meniere's disease. Rather, Meniere's disease is a constellation of symptoms and a diagnosis of exclusion; thus, further tests and a physical examination must be completed prior to making the diagnosis. If not, the patient will be treated for idiopathic Meniere's (diet and diuretic) instead of being treated for the specific cause of Meniere's symptoms.[8]

The most important test is MRI with gadolinium contrast enhancement (which is also necessary in labyrinthitis). As discussed, it is also important to directly question the patient about the many triggers that induce a Meniere's attack because this information will affect treatment. Allergies, autoimmune conditions, headaches, high-salt or high-sugar diet, or stress may be the underlying cause and need to be treated appropriately to gain control of the episodes. Thus, diuretics and a low-salt diet might not be the appropriate treatment for every Meniere's patient.

■ Single Vestibular Event

Most probably, the patient who inspires significant debate or consternation is the one who presents with their first true vertiginous spell. In this situation, the diagnosis could be just about anything. Possible common etiologies include virus-induced labyrinthitis, the first episode of Meniere's disease, multiple sclerosis, or vascular compromise. The key here in forming a diagnosis is the questions that need to be asked and answered. Typically, in labyrinthitis, the vertiginous episode lasts longer than 1 to 8 hours (an episode of a few hours' duration is more likely Meniere's disease). A bad dizzy spell typically lasts 1 day to 3 days.[9,10] There may have been an antecedent upper respiratory tract infection or some other condition that weakened the immune system. The residual effects of the "bad" dizzy spell consist of disequilibrium, lightheadedness, and "dizzy feeling," and they generally take 3 to 6 weeks to clear for a full recovery. Often, during this time, because the patient feels unsteady and lightheaded and has difficulty with ambulation, an otolaryngologist is asked to evaluate them. Hearing loss, tinnitus, and aural fullness may occur in labyrinthitis but are not typical. In contrast, in Meniere's disease, after the episode of vertigo, which typically lasts a few hours, the patient returns to a normal state. Note that Meniere's disease cannot be diagnosed after only one attack of vertigo, since by definition Meniere's consists of episodic spells.

■ Dizziness but Not Vertigo

Other questions can point to disorders that are not as common and do not typically involve true vertigo. Patients whose complaints of "dizziness" consist of a feeling of falling, disorientation, or disequilibrium and that occur when things are moving past them, such as when riding in a car and other cars move past them, or when going up and down the aisles of a large supermarket or store, may be experiencing vascular loop compression syndrome. In this particular etiology, a vascular loop abuts or wraps around the eighth cranial nerve complex just outside the internal auditory canal. If the vessel spasms and kinks the nerve, it may produce a type of neuronitis or other injury that causes the nerve to engage in abnormal firing, thus eliciting the "vertiginous" symptoms. Other disorders, such as a poor vestibular ocular reflex, may also induce similar symptoms.

Some patients complain of disequilibrium when walking or standing still. They feel like they are moving back and forth and may even walk with their legs spread slightly wider or they may require a cane. Although these phenomena can certainly be associated with central lesions or a hypofunctioning vestibular system, it is also important to ascertain if the patient has recently been on a boat, cruise, fun park, or long car/plane ride, all of which may cause the patient to feel that they are still swaying or rocking back and forth. This is probably mal de debarquement syndrome, which is usually self-limiting but sometimes can last years. Occasionally, an antiseizure medication like clonazepam (Klonopin) may provide benefit.

For some patients, especially the elderly, sitting or standing up too quickly is the triggering event for vertigo. When asked, the patient will actually describe a sensation more like lightheadedness. This typically is related to orthostatic hypotension, which is easily confirmed. Other patients complain of lightheadedness or dizziness when extending their neck to look up. This may occur with vertebral or basilar artery insufficiency that causes occlusion of the blood flow in these vessels, especially in patients with significant osteoarthritis. Autonomic dysfunction, another rare cause of lightheadednes or dizziness, occurs more often in younger patients; for diagnosis, tilt table testing is important.

The complaint of disequilibrium, rather than true vertigo, is usually associated with entities like acoustic neuroma, Arnold-Chiari malformation, the sequelae of vestibular neuronitis, hypoactive vestibular system, cerebellar injury, and vascular insufficiency or stroke. Certainly, other central etiologies may also cause disequilibrium. Lightheadedness, on the other hand, probably is more often associated with vascular insufficiency or syncope-type episodes. Other types of lightheadedness may be due to anemia, cardiac arrhythmias, hypo- or hyperthyroidism, leukemia, diabetes, or other autoimmune disorders. Temporal bone trauma may also induce vertigo. Other important concerns are otorrhea, history of ear infections, hearing status, venereal disease exposure, HIV or hepatitis exposure, otalgia, or tinnitus. The patient's answers to questions about these concerns could support an infectious etiology or cholesteatoma. Family history is also important, as some processes demonstrate a familial pattern.

References

1. Ruckenstein MJ. A practical approach to dizziness. Questions to bring vertigo and other causes into focus. Postgrad Med 1995;97(3):70–72, 75–78, 81
2. Post RE, Dickerson LM. Dizziness: a diagnostic approach. Am Fam Physician 2010;82(4):361–368, 369
3. Derebery MJ. The diagnosis and treatment of dizziness. Med Clin North Am 1999;83(1):163–177, x
4. Hogue JD. Office evaluation of dizziness. Prim Care 2015;42(2):249–258
5. Roland LT, Kallogjeri D, Sinks BC, et al. Utility of an Abbreviated Dizziness Questionnaire to differentiate between causes of vertigo and guide appropriate referral: a multicenter prospective blinded study. Otol Neurotol 2015;36(10):1687–1694
6. Friedland DR, Tarima S, Erbe C, Miles A. Development of a statistical model for the prediction of common vestibular diagnoses. JAMA Otolaryngol Head Neck Surg 2016;142(4):351–356
7. Furman JM, Balaban CD. Vestibular migraine. Ann N Y Acad Sci 2015;1343:90–96
8. Goebel JA. 2015 Equilibrium Committee Amendment to the 1995 AAO-HNS Guidelines for the Definition of Ménière's Disease. Otolaryngol Head Neck Surg 2016;154(3):403–404
9. Kerber KA. Acute continuous vertigo. Semin Neurol 2013;33(3):173–178
10. Jeong SH, Kim HJ, Kim JS. Vestibular neuritis. Semin Neurol 2013;33(3):185–194

2 Office Examination of the Vestibular Patient

Jameson K. Mattingly, Laura Wazen, and Stephen P. Cass

■ Introduction

The vestibular physical exam begins with a thorough history, as careful characterization of the patient's symptoms with knowledge of the various disease entities allows formulation of a differential diagnosis. The physical examination should be thorough and directed at confirming or refuting the potential etiologies of the "dizziness" complaint. Although it is tempting to jump to additional studies, such as imaging and vestibular testing, a significant amount of information can be gleaned from the office examination. The examination should include neurologic (including gait and balance), otologic, and neurotologic examinations, or aspects of each driven by the history. In many instances, a thorough physical exam can help avoid further testing that can be both expensive and uncomfortable to the patient.

■ Physical Examination

Functional balance relies upon the interaction of vestibular, visual, and proprioceptive systems, and abnormalities in any one of these can result in the sensation of dizziness, imbalance, or vertigo. A thorough physical examination, then, should include testing of these three elements, by including general otolaryngologic, neurologic, otologic, and neurotologic examinations. Specific attention should be paid to evaluating the oculomotor system in the neurologic examination, as vestibular abnormalities can alter the eye movements in a characteristic way that may provide clues to either central or peripheral etiologies.

The physical examination should begin immediately upon initial interaction with the patient. The examiner should pay close attention to the patient's gait, use of any assistive devices (e.g., walker or cane) or glasses, and any signs of central neurologic dis-orders, such as a previous stroke or brain injury.[1] Regarding assistive devices, proper use should not be overlooked, and can be assessed by asking the patient to use the device with both walking and turning. If the use appears impaired, the patient may have never been instructed in how to use the device, or they may have a delayed response reaction to prevent falling. Additionally, vital signs should be reviewed, with particular attention to orthostatic blood pressures. A decrease of greater than 20 mm Hg in systolic blood pressure after transitioning from a supine or seated position to standing is consistent with orthostatic hypotension.[1]

■ Neurologic Examination

The neurologic examination of the dizzy patient includes all of the categories of the standard neurologic examination: evaluation of mental status, cranial nerves, motor and sensory systems, coordination and other cerebellar testing, Romberg testing, and assessment of gait.[2] The cranial nerve examination should include a thorough evaluation of oculomotor function, including saccades and pursuit, and a search for nystagmus with the eyes open in the light as well as gaze-evoked nystagmus. While examination of eye movements is critical, assessment of all cranial nerves, and motor and sensory function of the extremities, should also be performed. The latter point is critical in evaluating for neuropathy, which can be the etiology of, or contribute to, vestibular symptoms. Neurologic findings, such as ataxia, dysarthria, visual disturbance, and extremity weakness, point toward a central cause of vestibular symptoms.

Romberg testing evaluates the patient's use of visual, vestibular, and proprioceptive cues to maintain balance. The test should be performed with the feet as close together as possible, and with the hands across the chest. Interpretation of the Romberg test allows the clinician to evaluate the patient's ability to use the previously mentioned cues to maintain balance. With eyes open (Romberg condition 1), the patient has all three sources of inputs. When the patient performs the test with eyes closed (Romberg condition 2), visual inputs are removed, thus leaving vestibular and somatosensory inputs to maintain balance. Patients who can maintain balance in condition 1, but fall in condition 2, are visually dependent to maintain balance, and thus would be at risk for falls if walking in darkened environments. With eyes open on a foam pad (Romberg condition 3), the patient can use visual and vestibular cues, while somatosensory cues are altered. Patients who fall in this condition are somatosensory dependent, and would be at risk for falls if walking on a compliant or uneven surface, such as grass, sand, gravel, or even very plush carpet. If the patient has sensory deficits, such as peripheral neuropathy, they may not be able to utilize the remaining sensation they have in their feet on surfaces that do not provide hard, stable somatosensory cues. With eyes closed on a foam pad (Romberg condition 4), the use of visual cues has been removed and somatosensory cues have been altered by the cushion, thus leaving vestibular inputs as the remaining set of balance information (**Video 2.1**). Therefore, falls in this condition suggest a vestibular issue, either peripheral or central.

Gait assessment is a crucial component of evaluating the vestibular patient, and it should encompass multiple key points, including evaluation of the base of support, path sway, ambulation with head turns, and overall assessment of gait quality. Base of support (BOS) is the distance between the two feet when standing or walking, and they should be ~ 4 inches apart.[3] The examiner should notice if the patient's BOS is normal, narrowed, or widened. A narrow BOS can create more instability and risk of falls for the vestibular patient. A widened BOS is commonly seen with patients suffering from bilateral vestibular loss, as it is a compensation used to create more stability.

Assessing path sway determines if the patient is walking straight or veering to one or both sides. Normally, a patient should be able to walk a straight line, staying within a 12-inch path. If sway is present, the direction should be noted, as a patient with unilateral vestibular loss can drift when walking, either pulling toward the strong side or drifting toward the weak side. Ambulation with head turns can help determine if a patient can maintain a steady and straight path when walking and turning the head to the side, looking up and down, and if they are able to maintain their walking pace during the head turn. Patients with vestibular problems may drift in the direction they are looking. Due to dizziness that head motion causes, a patient may avoid turning their head entirely and alternatively look only with their eyes. For example, the patient may turn without first using their head to look in the new direction to prevent head motion-induced symptoms (*en bloc*). Notice if the head turns cause increased sway, staggering, loss of balance, slowing of gait speed, veering, or dizziness, or if symptoms occur only with head turns in a certain direction. For example, in patients with benign paroxysmal positional vertigo (BPPV), dizziness or imbalance is elicited when the patient tips the head back.

Gait quality should also be assessed; the examiner assesses if the patient has normal step lengths, signs of foot scuffing or decreased heel strike, and the patient's posture. Foot scuffing may increase the patient's risk of tripping and falling, and those with peripheral neuropathy may be unaware it is occurring. Scuffing of the feet may be an attempt to increase proprioceptive cues in the absence of appropriate vestibular or visual inputs.

Patients with vestibular disorders often report difficulty with activities associated with postural control. These patients may complain of difficulty maintaining balance when changing positions, such as going from supine to sitting, or sitting to standing. Postural control can be assessed by standardized tests of static stability, such as the Romberg or single-leg stance tests. It can also be assessed by observing dynamic functional activities that require postural control, such as how the person goes from sitting to standing or their ability to walk unsupported. Testing static postural control is often a measure that is utilized in the office evaluation because it is quick, reproducible from one visit to the next, and quantifiable. The measure is usually a reflection of the patient's ability to maintain a set posture over time without increased sway or loss of balance, and results have been standardized by age group, with most clinicians utilizing 30 seconds as the minimal duration guideline for a normal test during Romberg testing and a minimum of 5 seconds as a normal duration for single-leg stance trials.[4,5] During dynamic postural control evaluation, care must be taken to rule out other contributing factors that could affect performance, such as orthopedic issues (e.g., joint pain, muscle weakness, limited flexibility) or neurologic issues (e.g., Parkinson's disease or neuropathy).

Oculomotor Examination

The oculomotor system should be examined to detect the presence of characteristic eye movement abnormalities suggestive of either central or peripheral vestibular system dysfunction. This is a pivotal portion of the neurologic examination, as ocular findings can help localize the lesion. The bedside eye movement examination should include an assessment of the presence of any nystagmus, alignment and range of movement of the eyes, involuntary saccades, vergence, and pursuit eye movements.[2]

The presence of nystagmus should be carefully evaluated. The most common nystagmus seen in vestibular abnormalities is jerk nystagmus. Jerk nystagmus has a slow component due to vestibular input signals and a fast component that resets the eye back to the center of the orbit. Although the direction of the slow component is more clinically useful, nystagmus is described in the direction of the fast component due to a greater ease of visualization by the examiner. Characteristics of spontaneous nystagmus of peripheral vestibular origin include the presence of nystagmus with the head still, decreased nystagmus with visual fixation, and increased when fixation is absent, such as with infrared video or Frenzel goggles (**Video 2.2**).[6] Certain characteristics of the nystagmus should also be noted, such as the timing and speed of the components, as these findings can point toward specific diagnoses.

Misalignment of the visual axes, such as with strabismus, may produce complaints similar to those of a vestibular disorder. Misalignment of the visual axis is not an abnormality of the vestibular system per se, but can certainly result in double or blurred vision, or vertiginous sensations that can mimic the presentation of a vestibular disorder. The examiner should begin with a general inspection of the patient's eyes while both eyes are open and the patient is viewing a single target; the examiner should look for misalignment of the visual axes. Any obvious misalignment of the eyes or any visual disturbances through the full range of eye movements should be noted. More subtle ocular misalignments may be detected using the cover test.[2] To perform the cover test, ask the patient to fixate on a distant target, cover one of the patient's eyes, and look for movement of the uncovered eye. If no movement is detected, remove the cover and place it on the other eye, looking for movement of the uncovered eye. If movement is noted in one eye after covering the other eye, an ocular misalignment is present. Eye movements that occur only after uncovering indicate the presence of an ocular misalignment that is present only when one eye is viewing. The finding may also indicate a restriction or weakness of an extraocular muscle, although it can point to lesions of the vestibular system. However, those with long-standing misalignment may have compensated well and report minimal diplopia.

The finding of vertical misalignment not attributed to ocular muscle palsy suggests the presence of a skew deviation.[2] Skew deviation has been reported mostly commonly in association with brainstem or cerebellar lesions, and also can be due to imbalances along peripheral or central pathways that mediate otolith-ocular reflexes.[7] Generalized limitation of range of movement may be a sign of a systemic issue, such as myasthenia gravis. Limitation of voluntary vertical gaze may indicate abnormality of the midbrain, including neurodegenerative disorders, such as progressive supranuclear palsy, mass lesions, infarction, hemorrhage, hydrocephalus, or encephalitis.[2]

Eye movements in an opposite, but coordinated, fashion characterize vergence. These movements are important with movement of a target closer to the viewer (convergence) or further from the viewer (divergence), and are typically slow and smooth. Abnormal oscillation of the eyes during vergence, called convergence spasm, suggests a functional disorder, and should not be confused with bilateral sixth nerve palsy. Nystagmus that is present in primary gaze may change during vergence. For example, congenital nystagmus is typically dampened by convergence, and central vestibular nystagmus may be exaggerated or change direction during convergence.[2]

Saccades represent rapid changes in eye position from one target to another. Asking the patient to fixate alternately between two stationary targets with the head held still can test these movements. One target, such as the examiner's nose, should be placed so that the patient can fixate upon it with the eye in primary position, with a second target, such as a finger, positioned to produce an approximate 15° saccade. The examiner should assess the velocity, accuracy, and initiation time of the saccades.[8] Slowing of the saccades suggests brainstem dysfunction, such as internuclear ophthalmoplegia, and inaccurate or dysmetric saccades point to cerebellar lesions. Abnormalities in saccadic initiation may be seen in patients with Parkinson's disease and Huntington's disease. Extraneous or corrective saccades may be noted during fixation or pursuit. Smooth pursuit is used to track slow objects and relies on the visual cortex. Smooth pursuit can decline with age, sedation, inattention, and changes in visual acuity.[1] Square-wave jerks are saccades away from and back to the fixation. Square-wave jerks are seen commonly in older individuals, and may be considered a nonspecific finding. In younger individuals, square-wave jerks are considered abnormal and are most often seen with anxiety or with abnormalities of the cerebellum or brainstem. Ocular flutter and opsoclonus are rapid saccadic to-and-fro movements of the eye without a normal intersaccadic interval in the horizontal plane and multidirectional movement, respectively.[2,6] The causes of ocular flutter and opsoclonus include structural lesions of the pons or cerebellum, viral encephalitis, paraneoplastic syndromes, or toxic agents or medications. (**Video 2.3, Video 2.4, Video 2.5, Video 2.6, Video 2.7,** and **Video 2.8**)

Otologic Examination

It is valuable to begin with a complete head and neck examination, and then to focus on the otologic portion of the exam. The ear should be examined, preferably using magnification. All obstructing debris should be removed so that complete visualization of the tympanic membrane is possible. The normal landmarks of the tympanic membrane should be identified and attention paid to the status of the middle ear and ossicular chain. If normal landmarks are obscured, infection, middle ear effusion, perforation, or cholesteatoma should be ruled out. The pneumatic otoscope should be used to confirm normal tympanic membrane mobility and to elicit signs or symptoms of vestibular sensitivity to pressure. Pressure-induced eye symptoms, such as nystagmus, may point toward a perilymph fistula or superior semicircular canal dehiscence.

Determining the status of the patient's hearing can help elicit a peripheral vestibular disorder, as peripheral etiologies are frequently associated with hearing loss and tinnitus. Although not as sophisticated as formal audiometric testing, finger rub or tuning fork examinations can help diagnose a hearing loss, with the latter having the ability to differentiate between conductive and sensorineural losses. The finger rub test is approximately the same as a 30-dB stimulus at 4000 Hz.[2] Commonly performed tuning fork exams include the Weber and Rinne tests. The Weber test is performed by placing the tuning fork on the vertex of the head while asking the patient if they hear it midline (normal response) or laterally (pathologic response). The Rinne test is performed by placing the tuning fork over the mastoid, then comparing this to the loudness of the vibrating tines near the external auditory canal. A normal response, or Rinne positive, is air conduction louder than bone conduction, while an abnormal response, or Rinne negative, is bone conduction louder than air conduction. Rinne negative is usually indicative of a conductive hearing loss. For example, a Weber test that lateralizes to an ear that also has a Rinne negative (bone conduction greater than air conduction) may be indicative of a conductive hearing loss. Conductive hearing loss might be associated with otosclerosis, superior semicircular canal dehiscence, cholesteatoma, or fluid within the middle ear space.[2] The tuning fork tests can also detect a unilateral sensorineural loss, if, for example, the Rinne test demonstrates air conduction greater than bone conduction bilaterally, but the Weber test lateralizes to the good ear. It is not unusual for vestibular schwannomas or other processes that affect the inner ear to cause sensorineural hearing loss in addition to vestibular symptoms.

The tuning fork can also help point to superior semicircular canal dehiscence. A 128-Hz tuning fork placed on the ankle that is heard by the patient indicates a third-window phenomenon, as in superior semicircular canal dehiscence. This finding may also be associated with additional auditory symptoms (e.g., ear fullness, autophony, or pulsatile tinnitus) in superior semicircular canal dehiscence.[9] Despite this, the reliability of the tuning fork is limited, and any abnormal response should be confirmed and further elaborated on by using comprehensive audiometry.

Neurotologic Examination

The neurotologic examination includes several tests that are particularly useful when evaluating patients with dizziness. Tests considered to be essential for a full examination include search for spontaneous nystagmus with eyes open in the dark, post-head-shaking nystagmus, bedside vestibulo-ocular reflex (VOR) tests, including the head thrust/impulse test and dynamic visual acuity, Dix-Hallpike test, and Romberg testing with eyes closed on a foam pad.[2] These physical examination tools should be used on all patients presenting with vestibular issues. Many of these tests are facilitated by use of infrared video goggles or Frenzel glasses (**Video 2.2**). Frenzel glasses enable a reduction of visual fixation while allowing the examiner to view the patient's illuminated and magnified eyes, while infrared video goggles allow examination of the eyes while they are open in the dark. In this way, vestibular nystagmus not present during visual fixation may be seen. Nystagmus that increases in intensity or that is seen only when the eyes are open in the dark point toward a peripheral etiology.[2]

A search for spontaneous vestibular nystagmus can be performed with the head upright, and positional nystagmus can be assessed in the supine and head right and left lateral positions. The Dix-Hallpike maneuver is used to elicit BPPV and should be performed on all patients presenting with vestibular issues, even if the symptoms appear to be nonpositional. This test is performed by rotating the patient's head 30° to 45° to the testing side followed by a rapid placement into a supine position (**Fig. 2.1**).

The characteristic nystagmus with BPPV has a short latency followed by an upbeat and torsional nystagmus that generally lasts less than 1 minute. A search for post-head-shaking nystagmus (rapid horizontal head movements for 30 seconds followed by an abrupt stop) can also be performed and can help detect unilateral vestibular weakness. Despite its usefulness in detecting asymmetric central function, this test is not reliable for central vestibular

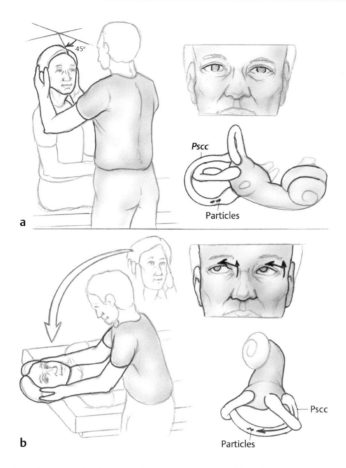

Fig. 2.1 **(a,b)** Demonstration of the Dix-Hallpike maneuver in the right head-hanging position. The characteristic nystagmus is vertical (upbeating) torsional, consistent with origin in the posterior canal. The vertical direction of nystagmus can change if the origin is in a canal other than the posterior one, such as with anterior canal BPPV. Used with permission from Pensak ML, Choo DI, eds. Clinical Otology, 4th ed. New York, NY: Thieme; 2015:436.

abnormalities.[2] Nystagmus can also be induced with vibratory stimuli to the skull and neck. Vibration stimulates the labyrinths bilaterally, with the asymmetry in those with unilateral vestibular damage resulting in nystagmus with the slow phase directed toward the side of the lesion.[10] Vibratory stimulation is a reliable and easily administered bedside test for asymmetric peripheral vestibular damage.

The head thrust or head impulse test is used to determine whether the VOR is adequate to maintain gaze stabilization during brisk head movements (**Video 2.3**). These high-frequency and high-acceleration motions allow testing of the VOR that is above the range of the smooth pursuit system.[11] In the normal condition, patients will not have difficulty keeping the eyes fixated on a point during motion.[12] Although testing can be performed in the plane of all canals, testing of the superior and posterior canals

is much more difficult than testing of the horizontal canal. To perform the test, begin by rotating the patient's head ~ 30° to the left or right, and then return it quickly to the center while examining the ability of the eyes to stay fixated on the target (e.g., examiner's nose). In patients with normal vestibular function, the movement of the eye with the head thrust is negligible, while those with unilateral vestibular loss will have a re-fixation saccade to the target (**Video 2.9**).

Dynamic visual acuity or "illegible E" testing is also another useful modality for evaluating the VOR. After visual acuity has been established, such as with a Snellen chart, the patient rotates the head 60° in both directions at a frequency of 1 to 2 Hz. This frequency is above the frequency for the smooth pursuit system, and thus is primarily a test of the VOR.[13] Patients with normal vestibular function will have a decrease in visual acuity around 1 line, those with unilateral weakness will have a decrease in 3 to 4 lines, and those with bilateral weakness, a decrease of 5 to 6 lines.[14]

■ Conclusion

The physical exam is a crucial part of the evaluation of the vestibular patient and should be focused on confirming or refuting potential etiologies of the "dizziness" complaint. The examination should include neurologic, otologic, and neurotologic examinations, or aspects of each driven by the history to evaluate the interaction of the vestibular, visual, and proprioceptive systems. Specific attention should be directed at the oculomotor system, gait, and posture, as well as otologic and neurotologic exams, with the latter especially important for lesion localization. A thorough physical exam can help avoid further testing that can be both expensive and uncomfortable for the patient.

Questions
Q1: Rinne testing with AC greater than BC, and Weber testing lateralizing to the contralateral side, suggest what type of hearing loss?
Q2: Left-sided vestibular hypofunction will result in nystagmus beating in which direction?
Q3: Dynamic illegible E testing reveals a decrease in visual acuity of five lines on a Snellen chart. On which side does the patient have vestibular hypofunction?
Q4: How does Romberg testing on a compliant foam pad isolate the vestibular influence on postural control?

Answers

A1: Sensorineural hearing loss of the test ear.

A2: Right.

A3: Likely bilateral weakness.

A4: With Romberg eyes closed testing on a foam pad, the use of visual cues has been removed and somatosensory cues have been altered by the cushion, thus leaving vestibular inputs as the remaining set of balance information.

References

1. Kutz JW Jr. The dizzy patient. Med Clin North Am 2010;94(5):989–1002

2. Furman J, Cass S, Whitney S, eds. Vestibular Disorders: A Case-Study Approach to Diagnosis and Treatment. 3rd ed. New York, NY: Oxford University Press, Inc.; 2010

3. Kuo AD, Donelan JM. Dynamic principles of gait and their clinical implications. Phys Ther 2010; 90(2):157–174

4. McCaslin D, Dundas A, Jacobson G. The bedside assessment of the vestibular system. In: Jacobson G, Shepard N, eds. Balance Function Assessment and Management. UK: Plural Publishing; 2008:87

5. Vellas BJ, Wayne SJ, Romero L, Baumgartner RN, Rubenstein LZ, Garry PJ. One-leg balance is an important predictor of injurious falls in older persons. J Am Geriatr Soc 1997;45(6):735–738

6. Hullar T, Zee D, Minor L. Evaluation of the patient with dizziness. In: Flint P, et al, eds. Cummings Otolaryngology Head and Neck Surgery. 6th ed. Philadelphia, PA: Saunders Elsevier Inc.; 2015:2525–2547

7. Brandt T, Dieterich M. Pathological eye-head coordination in roll: tonic ocular tilt reaction in mesencephalic and medullary lesions. Brain 1987;110(Pt 3):649–666

8. Robinson DA, Keller EL. The behavior of eye movement motoneurons in the alert monkey. Bibl Ophthalmol 1972;82:7–16

9. Benamira LZ, Maniakas A, Alzahrani M, Saliba I. Common features in patients with superior canal dehiscence declining surgical treatment. J Clin Med Res 2015;7(5):308–314

10. Ohki M, Murofushi T, Nakahara H, Sugasawa K. Vibration-induced nystagmus in patients with vestibular disorders. Otolaryngol Head Neck Surg 2003;129(3):255–258

11. Halmagyi GM, Curthoys IS. A clinical sign of canal paresis. Arch Neurol 1988;45(7):737–739

12. Tabak S, Collewijn H, Boumans LJ, van der Steen J. Gain and delay of human vestibulo-ocular reflexes to oscillation and steps of the head by a reactive torque helmet. I. Normal subjects. Acta Otolaryngol 1997; 117(6):785–795

13. Baloh RW. Approach to the evaluation of the dizzy patient. Otolaryngol Head Neck Surg 1995;112(1):3–7

14. Dannenbaum E, Paquet N, Chilingaryan G, Fung J. Clinical evaluation of dynamic visual acuity in subjects with unilateral vestibular hypofunction. Otol Neurotol 2009;30(3):368–372

3 Computerized Testing of the Vestibular Patient

Randy Judson and Jessica Galatioto

■ Introduction

A careful and thorough history is the most important part of the differential diagnosis of a vestibular disorder. The clinical history and comprehensive neurotologic examination provide the diagnosis for a large number of patients who report dizziness or imbalance. After the patient's symptoms have been reviewed, the clinician can determine the appropriate computerized testing to be ordered to confirm and quantify the presence or absence of a vestibular disorder.

There is no single diagnostic test that will definitively determine the source of a patient's complaints of dizziness.[1] Often, a battery of tests is ordered to help render a diagnosis. Computerized testing of the dizzy patient may not be indicated for all patients, but should be used for patients whose diagnosis is not evident from history or bedside testing alone. An appropriate diagnostic work-up of the dizzy patient will allow the clinician to document any abnormalities, as well as guide the physician to the proper medical or rehabilitative treatment for the patient.

The primary purpose of computerized vestibular testing is to determine the presence or absence of a lesion. If abnormal test results are obtained, the examination then must determine if the origin is peripheral or central, if the lesion is unilateral (and which side) or bilateral, and whether the results indicate which end-organ (site of pathology) may be contributing to the symptoms. The interpretation of vestibular test results depends on integrating the findings from examinations specific to all six semicircular canals and four otoliths.[2]

The structures of the vestibular system that are assessed during computerized testing include the following: horizontal semicircular canal (HSCC), posterior semicircular canal (PSCC), anterior semicircular canal (ASCC), otoliths (saccule and utricle), and the vestibular nerve (inferior and superior portions).

Before 1990, assessment of peripheral vestibular structures was limited to only the HSCCs and the superior portion of the vestibular nerve.[3] Currently, computerized testing can assess the function of each of the structures mentioned. Each test assesses a different part of the vestibular system and also examines various frequencies of movement (**Fig. 3.1**). Computerized vestibular tests include videonystagmography (VNG) with bithermal caloric testing (BCT), sinusoidal harmonic acceleration (SHA) testing and step testing via the rotational chair test (RCT), vestibular evoked myogenic potential (VEMP) testing, video head impulse testing (vHIT), and computerized dynamic platform posturography (CDP). It must also be remembered that not all patients with vestibular signs and symptoms have abnormal electrophysiologic test results.

Balance disorders are often accompanied by otologic symptoms, including changes in hearing, tinni-

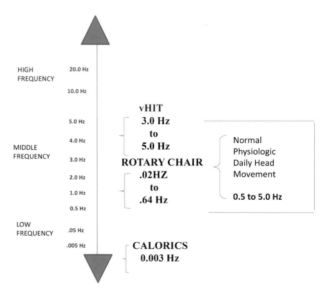

VOR frequency range and corresponding electrophysiologic testing

Fig. 3.1 Frequency progression of computerized vestibular tests.

tus, or aural fullness. A comprehensive evaluation of hearing should accompany and, if possible, precede any additional testing.

Similar to the bedside evaluation, some computerized vestibular tests use eye movement as a method of assessing vestibular function. The vestibulo-ocular reflex (VOR) is one of three vestibular reflexes, along with the vestibulospinal reflex (VSR) and the vestibulocolic reflex (VCR), that can be assessed with computerized testing. We evaluate the VOR with VNG, RCT, and the vHIT. The VSR is assessed with platform posturography. Vestibular evoked myogenic potential (VEMP) will evaluate the VCR.

A large number of medications may affect the results of many computerized tests. Any central nervous system (CNS) depressant may result in abnormal eye movements, decreased alertness, and findings that may mimic vestibular hypofunction. CNS stimulants may increase vestibular responses. Apparently, the VEMP is the only computerized vestibular test whose results are not influenced by medication or hearing loss.[4] No medication should be stopped or started without the permission of the patient's physician.

■ Computerized Tests of Vestibular Function

Videonystagmography with Bithermal Caloric Testing

The VOR functions to create compensatory eye movements that are equal to, but opposite to, head movement, to maintain a steady visual image. Videonystagmography is a direct measure of VOR function. The VOR is directly measured via infrared goggles during VNG testing. Historically, electronystagmography (ENG) was used to record eye movements; surface electrodes recorded changes in the corneoretinal potential, assessing the eyes' movement. VNG is now the preferred method.

Videonystagmography uses digital and infrared recording technology to record eye movements and allows for both subjective and objective analysis of changes in eye position.[5] Because of its many clinical advantages over ENG, VNG yields a more accurate analysis and interpretation of eye movements.[5,6] Both ENG and VNG consist of a series of subtests that may vary from center to center, but generally fall into three categories: oculomotor testing, positional testing, and BCT.

Oculomotor Testing

Oculomotor testing helps differentiate between peripheral vestibular end-organ and the central vestibular system. Oculomotor testing includes gaze stability testing, saccadic tracking, smooth pursuit tracking, and optokinetic tracking.

Gaze Stability

Gaze stability testing is accomplished under two conditions—with vision, and with vision denied—for at least 20 to 30 seconds in each eye gaze direction. The patient is asked to fixate on a target, typically displayed on a light bar located 4 feet from the patient. Based on center gaze, left gaze, and right gaze, the clinician will determine if nystagmus is present. If nystagmus is present with vision denied, the examiner will have the patient fixate on the target to determine if the nystagmus diminishes or abates with vision. Nystagmus is defined as rapid movement of the eyes, with two distinct phases: the slow phase, which results from vestibular input, and the quick, corrective phase, in which the eyes move in the opposite direction. The direction of the nystagmus is defined by the direction of the quick component, but is usually measured by the slow phase (slow phase velocity).

Horizontal nystagmus that is diminished by at least 50% with vision is considered peripheral, whereas nystagmus that is not reduced or abolished with vision may be indicative of a central pathology.[7] Peripheral nystagmus should follow Alexander's law,[7,8] which states that the slow phase of nystagmus caused by a unilateral peripheral vestibular pathology increases when the patient stares in the direction of the fast phase.[8] Vertical nystagmus may occur in a normal patient, but it can indicate central pathology.

Saccadic Tracking

Saccadic tracking measures the ability of the patient to coordinate eye movement with visual target movement. In the VNG test battery, eye velocity, latency, and accuracy are measured. An abnormal finding in saccadic tracking may be due to an oculomotor pathology or a central dysfunction once technical error (drowsiness, inattentiveness, drugs, anticonvulsants, sedatives, antidepressants, etc.) has been ruled out. Abnormal results in both directions are of lesser clinical value and may be due to an oculomotor/visual acuity problem.[9] Significant asymmetric smooth pursuit (between rightward and leftward) may be due to a structural disorder, degenerative disorders, or medication or alcohol intake.[10] Test results may also be affected by a strong spontaneous nystagmus.

Smooth Pursuit (Pendular Tracking)

Pendular tracking is assessed by having the patient follow a target as it moves smoothly, rightward and leftward, on the light bar. The speed of the target gets progressively faster making the task more difficult over the duration of the evaluation. Disturbances of smooth pursuit are usually nonspecific. The test is highly affected by attention and cooperation. Asymmetric pursuit may indicate a CNS abnormality or an acute peripheral lesion (if peripheral, it must be accompanied by a strong spontaneous nystagmus). If there are no other central signs, abnormal pendular tracking may indicate oculomotor problems (or, in the elderly, may be indicative of age-related oculomotor slowing). Norms are age and gender dependent.

Optokinetic Tracking (OPK)

Optokinetic testing, as assessed on the VNG, is not a true test of the entire optokinetic system, which requires full field visual stimuli (these results could be obtained if OPK is assessed using the RC). In the VNG, OPK measures the eye movement elicited by the tracking of a moving field leftward and rightward on a light bar; a normal response is symmetric. Optokinetic asymmetry, if noted, may be a sign of a nonlocalizing CNS dysfunction.[9] Patients who demonstrate normal smooth pursuit should also demonstrate normal and symmetric OPK. For an optokinetic test to be judged abnormal, drugs, inattentiveness, poor vision, uncooperativeness, and congenital nystagmus must also be ruled out.

Positional Testing

Static Positional Testing

Nystagmus provoked by head or body position is assessed as part of the VNG battery. Positional testing is performed with vision and with vision denied (mental alerting tasks are used whenever the patient is denied vision). The patient is tested in at least four head positions (head left, head right, supine flat, supine head ventroflexed 30°).[9] Nystagmus observed in the head right or head left position may be caused by neck rotation. This can be ruled out by testing the patient in the body left or body right position. If body rotations do not elicit nystagmus, the nystagmus may be cervicogenic in origin.[11]

In each position, eye movements are observed for at least 20 to 30 seconds with vision denied to determine the presence of nystagmus. If nystagmus is observed, it will be described by the direction of the fast phase, the degree of the slow phase, and whether or not it can be fatigued with visual fixation. If the observed nystagmus is diminished with fixation, the nystagmus is identified as peripheral in nature, possibly indicating a unilateral peripheral pathology; this will often be corroborated by periph-

eral findings on other subtests of the VNG.[11] Nystagmus that cannot be fatigued with fixation, whether direction fixed or direction changing in any position or in multiple head positions, may be indicative of CNS pathology (usually in the cerebellar system).[11]

If the slow phase velocity of horizontal nystagmus is equal to or exceeds 6° per second in any single head position with ENG and is equal to or exceeds 4° per second in any single head position with VNG, it is considered a significant finding.[11] Vertical nystagmus without visual fixation may be considered abnormal if it is equal to or exceeds 6° per second in any single head position. Vertical nystagmus that is not fatigued with visual fixation is a central finding.

Dynamic Positional Testing: Dix-Hallpike Diagnostic Maneuver

Following tests of static positioning, where nystagmus is recorded while the patient's head remains in various positions, as a subtest of VNG, a Dix-Hallpike diagnostic maneuver is performed to determine if there is any nystagmus during the actual positioning of the head. During the maneuver, the patient's eyes are observed and recorded and the patient is asked to report any vertiginous symptoms.

Hallpike is performed to document the presence of benign paroxysmal positional vertigo (BPPV). In some centers, in the presence of a positive Hallpike, the clinician will immediately perform the maneuver to treat the BPPV.

By far the most common location of the BPPV is the PSCC, followed by HSCC BPPV; however, BPPV may be present in the ASCC or concurrently in multiple canals.[12] Patients with PSCC BPPV display the normal few beats of nystagmus during the movement followed by a burst of intense nystagmus after the movement is completed. The nystagmus rapidly builds up in intensity, reaches a crescendo, slowly diminishes, and finally disappears, usually within 10 to 15 seconds, while the head is held in position. The nystagmus has a primarily upward component with a torsional component toward the lower ear.[13]

Subjective vertigo is the absence of recordable nystagmus during the diagnostic positioning maneuvers. It does not preclude a diagnosis of BPPV, especially in the presence of a very suggestive history.[12] The reported subjective vertigo should follow a pattern similar to expected nystagmus: latency, a transient crescendo-decrescendo nature, and fatigability.

Head-Shake Nystagmus (HSN)

A head-shake test, performed with the VNG goggles, with vision denied, may also be included (and recorded) as part of the VNG battery to determine the presence or absence of post-HSN. Eye movement is recorded prior to, during, and after the head-shake stimulus, with the head tilted 30° forward. HSN may be the result of peripheral as well as central vestibular lesions.[14] The recording of three or more beats of horizontal nystagmus after horizontal head shake, if contralesional, may suggest a (unilateral) peripheral vestibular imbalance.[14.] Typically, if the origin is peripheral, other subtests of the VNG will support this diagnosis. A diagnosis of peripheral vestibular dysfunction cannot be ruled out based solely on a negative head-shake test.[15]

Post-HSN may also be due to central pathology and patterns may vary. It may be purely vertical, purely horizontal, mixed horizontal–vertical, or mixed horizontal–vertical–torsional.[16] Post-HSN may be the result of a central velocity storage abnormality.

Bithermal Caloric Testing

Bithermal caloric testing (BCT) is used to stimulate the HSCC of both the right and left ear. Each ear is stimulated separately with water or air, allowing the examiner to assess the function of the right and left systems independently. Bithermal caloric testing is a very useful computerized test and has many advantages, including the ability to aid in identifying the site of dysfunction and lateralizing a lesion. The equipment for BCT is also readily available in most areas, which makes the test readily accessible for evaluation of the dizzy patient. However, BCT does not examine the entire right and left peripheral system. During BCT, only low-frequency (0.003 Hz) stimulation is presented to the HSCC (innervated by the superior portion of the vestibular nerve). This leaves the functioning of other neural structures of the vestibular system, such as the PSCC, ASCC, utricle, saccule, and inferior vestibular nerve, unknown.

Bithermal caloric testing also takes a relatively long time to perform when compared with the rest of the VNG battery. It requires a minimum of four stimulations: right cool (RC), right warm (RW), left cool (LC), and left warm (LW). Four stimulations can take ~ 30 minutes to complete. The process may be longer depending on the patient. Lastly, BCT does not give any information about vestibular compensation; therefore, BCT is best used as part of a battery of tests to aid a physician in diagnosis.

During BCT, the patient is supine with the head ventroflexed 30° while the ear canal is stimulated (via air or water) to create a temperature gradient across the HSCC, which causes a change in the density of endolymph.[17] (It should be noted that the nystagmus created is measured via the slow phase, but it is named by the fast phase.) Warm stimulation causes the endolymph to become lighter, creating ampullopetal deflection of the cupula, generating nystagmus, with a fast phase beating toward the stimulated ear.[17] The opposite occurs with cool stimulation. Cool stimulation causes the endolymph to

increase in density and become heavier, creating an inhibitory response, causing nystagmus that beats away from the stimulated ear.[17]

The acronym COWS (cool opposite and warm same) is used for the above response pattern. For example, cool air stimulation of the right ear will create a left-beating nystagmus, and warm stimulation of the right ear will create a right-beating nystagmus. The nystagmus is recorded via infrared VNG goggles that deny vision, while the patient is alerted. Mental alerting is needed to ensure that central suppression does not occur, reducing the obtained nystagmus (**Fig. 3.2**).[18]

The peak response of nystagmus is recorded from all four stimulations and is then analyzed. The sum total of both right stimulations and both left stimulations is compared using Jongkee's formula (first described in 1962), to determine if a significant reduced vestibular response (RVR) is present.[19] RVR may also be referred to as a unilateral weakness (UW). UW of 20% or 25% (depending on the laboratory) is generally judged to be a significant finding and can be calculated using the following formula[19]:

$$UW = (RC + RW) - (LC + LW)/(RW + RC + LW + LC)$$

A UW of 20 to 25% is judged to be significant for peripheral dysfunction on the ipsilateral side of the reduced response, indicating significant horizontal canal dysfunction on that side. For example, a 37% UW in the right ear would be reported as a significant right UW, suggestive of right peripheral vestibular dysfunction.

Directional preponderance (DP) is computed to determine if caloric responses create more right-beating nystagmus than left-beating nystagmus. A value of 30% to 35% is typically judged to be a significant DP, but the value may vary by laboratory. The following formula is used[19]:

$$DP = (RW + LC) - (LW + RC)/(RW + RC + LW + LC)$$

A DP is typically seen in the presence of a spontaneous nystagmus. In this scenario, the eyes are already moving prior to caloric stimulation; hence, there is a tendency for the eyes to move farther in one direction. A significant DP is typically indicative of an acute peripheral vestibular disorder. DP is sometimes found in isolation (without spontaneous nystagmus or UW). An isolated significant DP is generally due to a benign transient disorder, which 50% of the time is BPPV or Meniere's disease.[20] Approximately 5% of patients with an isolated significant DP will have a central nervous system (CNS) lesion. If present, the CNS lesion should be apparent to the clinician during physical examination.[20]

In addition to calculation of UW and DP, all four calorics are evaluated to determine if hypoactive or hyperactive responses are present. Responses are considered hypoactive if the sum of both irrigations on each side is less than 12° per second.[17] The authors of this chapter recommend that the pres-

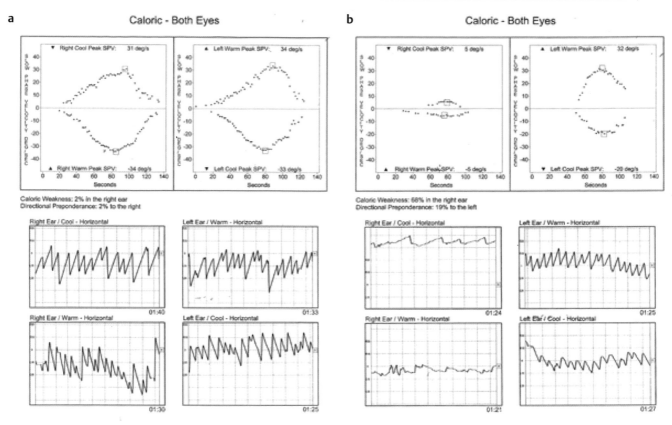

Fig. 3.2 This graphic representation is commonly referred to as "pods" and is used to display results obtained during bithermal caloric testing (BCT). **(a)** Results of BCT exhibiting normal responses. The peak slow phase velocity was identified during each stimulation and used for calculation of unilateral weakness (UW) and directional preponderance (DP); both are nonsignificant. The four small boxes below are a visual representation of the obtained nystagmus for each stimulation. **(b)** Results of BCT exhibiting a significant right UW. Peak slow phase velocities of nystagmus were identified during each stimulation and used to calculate UW and DP; UW is 68% in the right ear, indicating dysfunction on the right side. The graphic representation of obtained responses shows an obvious difference between right and left stimulations.

ence of bilateral weakness be confirmed with a RCT, as RCT is not dependent on the stimulus travelling through the outer and middle ear.

There are two methods of identifying hyperactive caloric responses. Calorics may be considered hyperactive if both of the cool stimulations produce a response of greater than 50° per second, or both warm stimulations produce a response of greater than 80° per second.[21] Alternatively, responses may be considered hyperactive if they exceed 99° per second for combined cool stimulations and 146° per second for combined warm irrigations, and a total caloric response exceeding 221° per second.[22] Once technical error has been ruled out, in the presence of hyperactive caloric responses, CNS involvement cannot be ruled out.

When interpreting BCT, it is important to remember that the BCT is completely dependent on the presumption that the right ear and left ear receive equal stimulation to the HSCC. To validly compare the caloric response of the right ear and left ear, the examiner must consider the effect of inter-ear ana-

tomic differences, surgical ears, middle ear pathology, and occluding cerumen, as they can alter true caloric responses.

Monothermal Caloric Testing

The monothermal warm screening test (MWST) or the monothermal cool screening test (MCST) may sometimes be used in place of a four-irrigation protocol. Instead of a UW calculation, an inter-ear difference (IED) calculation is performed[23]:

$$\text{For MWST: IED (\%)} = 100 \times (RW - LW)/(RW + LW)$$

$$\text{For MCST: IED (\%)} = 100 \times (RC - LC)/(RC + LC)$$

Both the MWST and the MCST perform better than chance; however, the MWST is a better screening tool for identifying caloric abnormalities.[23] When an IED of 10% is used as the criterion, the false-negative rate for the MWST is low, at 1% to 3%.[23] Monothermal caloric testing can be used as a screening tool when a patient cannot tolerate all four calorics, but it should not be used in place of the preferred four-stimulation protocol to assess vestibular function.[24] The authors of this chapter recommend a four-stimulation protocol when possible to minimize false negatives and missed bilateral hypofunction, and also to gain a better understanding of vestibular function.

Performing only a VNG is not a comprehensive vestibular evaluation, nor does VNG assess all parts of the vestibular system. Although much useful information is obtained from BCT, comprehensive testing of the vestibular mechanism requires that tests evaluate the system over a larger part of its operational range. Other computerized vestibular tests will need to be performed to assess otolith function, VSR and VCR function, inferior vestibular nerve function, vestibular compensation, and vestibular function at higher frequencies. If only a VNG were performed, 68% of patients with abnormal findings on other vestibular tests would be missed.[25]

Rotational Chair Testing

Rotational chair testing (RCT) objectively assesses VOR function at frequencies higher than those tested with BCT. Rotational chair testing does not require the stimulus to pass through the outer and middle ear and is thus more precisely controlled. This allows the examiner to effectively assess the vestibular system in patients with tympanic membrane perforations, current ear pathology, and/or a history of ear surgery. Rotational chair testing is a full-body passive rotational evaluation (the patient does not actively move the head/body, but instead the whole body is

rotated at various frequencies), while eye movement is observed and recorded with infrared video goggles.

According to the American Academy of Otolaryngology/Head and Neck Surgery, there are four types of RCT: (1) rotational chair step velocity testing (SVT); (2) rotational chair sinusoidal harmonic acceleration testing (SHA); (3) rotational chair high-frequency or high-velocity sinusoidal rotation; and (4) chair rotation with visual fixation (VFX).[26]

Sinusoidal harmonic acceleration testing is typically performed in most vestibular laboratories. The patient is subjected to a series of rightward and leftward rotations, at octave frequencies from 0.01 Hz to 0.64 Hz. The patient is seated in a chair, with the head immobilized, while wearing infrared goggles. The chair is rotated via a servo-controlled torque motor. The patient's eyes must remain open for evaluation and recording of the VOR response. The entire system may be enclosed in a light-proof enclosure; however, there are newer systems commercially available, without an enclosure and, instead, vision and light are blocked out by goggles (**Fig. 3.3**).

In SHA rotational testing, VOR function is obtained and named by the slow phase of the response. The gain (amount of eye movement) of the VOR is measured. The symmetry and the phase of the gain are analyzed. Gain is the ratio of slow phase eye velocity to chair velocity.[27] Phase is the timing difference between the peak amplitude of the chair movement (stimulus) and the eye movement.[27] Symmetry of the gain is assessed by a comparison of the responses from leftward and rightward rotations.

Normal gain, phase, and symmetry indicate normal horizontal canal functioning for the frequencies tested. This pattern may also indicate a compensated vestibular system, when accompanied by a UW

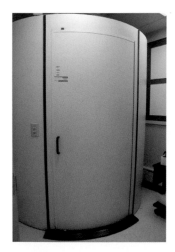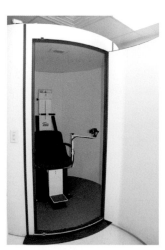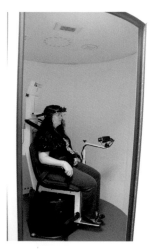

Fig. 3.3 From left to right: rotational chair enclosure; rotational chair inside enclosure; subject seated in chair wearing goggles and safety harness (note that testing is completed with door closed).

identified during BCT. A phase lead with normal gain symmetry may also indicate a compensated unilateral vestibular dysfunction.

An uncompensated unilateral vestibular dysfunction will manifest as an asymmetry at two or more consecutive frequencies (usually in the low frequencies), with a possible increase in phase lead.[28] Bilateral vestibular dysfunction will typically show reduced gain for both rightward and leftward rotations and should match caloric findings (**Fig. 3.4**).[28]

Rotational chair testing does not allow the examiner to determine the side of the lesion, and RCT should not be used by itself to identify a uni-lateral vestibular dysfunction. Rotational chair testing should be used to complement caloric testing.[29] Rotational testing (including SHA, VFX, OPK) was found to be more sensitive than calorics for identifying a vestibular dysfunction (71% sensitivity, compared with 31% sensitivity for calorics); however, because of lack of an independent ear evaluation, RCT's specificity is less than that for calorics (54%, compared with 86% for calorics).[29] A combination of BCT and SHA testing has been found to have stronger predictive capabilities than either test alone for identifying peripheral vestibular pathology.[30]

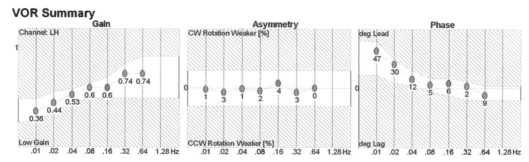

Normal gain for all rotations, normal phase for all rotations, and normal symmetry; seen in patients with compensated unilateral weakness and normal subjects.

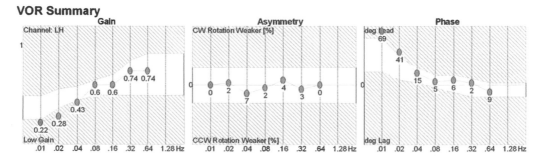

Low gain and phase lead for slow rotations; seen in patients with a non-localizing unilateral peripheral vestibular pathology.

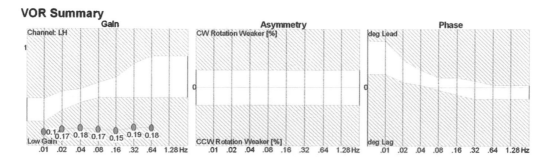

Low gain for all rotations; seen in patients with a bilateral weakness.

Fig. 3.4 Three common response patterns obtained during sinusoidal harmonic acceleration testing (SHA) in rotational chair testing (RCT).

Video Head Impulse Test (vHIT)

The vHIT is a test of high-frequency vestibular functioning that better approximates typical head movement. The vHIT is a comprehensive assessment of the system that cannot be achieved with the BCT and/or the SHA. The vHIT is a computerized adaptation of the bedside head impulse test that Halmagyi and Curthoys developed in 1988, using observed corrective saccades to identify a peripheral vestibular lesion.[31] To differentiate superior neuritis from inferior neuritis, all six semicircular canals (SCC) should be evaluated. The vHIT evaluates the function of the semicircular canals (lateral, anterior, posterior) in coplanar pairs, depending on the direction of the head thrust.

The vHIT measures the compensatory eye movements made when the examiner moves the patient's head in high-velocity head rotations while the patient maintains fixation on a target. Prior to the vHIT, magnetic-field coil systems were used as the gold standard to measure and record eye movement during head impulse testing.[32] The vHIT is more clinically accessible, because it uses an infrared video recording system attached to lightweight goggles that record the eye movements. The vHIT responses give the examiner diagnostic accuracy equivalent to the search coil recordings.[33]

The assumption of the vHIT is that the patient will successfully maintain visual fixation on the target when the head is moved if the VOR system is intact. In the presence of vestibular pathology, the patient will generate a catch-up saccade to regain the target when the head is moved. This will generally occur when the head is rotated toward the impaired semicircular canal.[3]

When the head is moved and the eyes successfully maintain focus on the target, there should be a gain of 1.0 or close to 1.0 (gain is expected to be 1.0 in

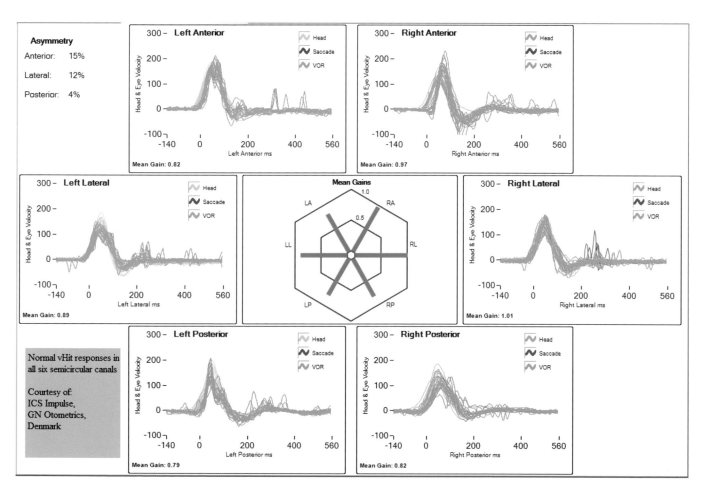

Fig. 3.5 A hex plot is used to display the responses obtained for all six semicircular canals during the video head impulse test (vHIT). The vestibulo-ocular reflex (VOR) gain is displayed as a bar originating in the center of the hexagon with the outermost hexagon equal to a gain of 1.0.[34] Results obtained for each canal are represented in each of the boxes around the hexagon. Courtesy of ICS Impulse, GN Otometrics, Denmark.

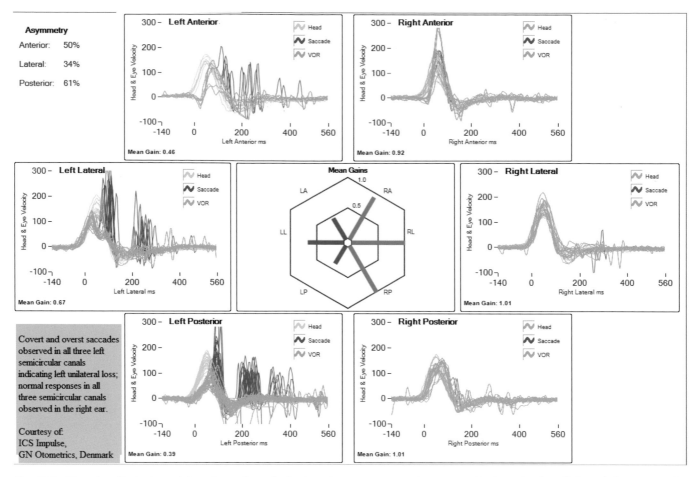

Fig. 3.6 Hex plot displaying a left unilateral vestibular loss. Lower gains can be seen in the hex plot for all three left semicircular canals. Courtesy of ICS Impulse, GN Otometrics, Denmark.

a healthy patient; however, the range of normal gains can be 0.79 to 1.20).[34] If that is not possible, the eye must correct with a saccade. There are two types of saccades: covert and overt saccades. Covert saccades are involuntary and occur while the head is moving. Overt saccades are voluntary and occur ~ 200 milliseconds or later after the head movement. The overt saccades are identifiable by a trained observer; however, covert saccades cannot be identified without computerized equipment. During a bedside evaluation, the tester might assume that the patient's vestibular system is unimpaired if an overt saccade was not observed. The vHIT, however, can provide an objective measurement of the covert saccades that could not be identified by observation alone. The vHIT records the gain of the VOR plus overt and/or covert catch-up saccades (**Fig. 3.5**).[32]

The head impulse has a frequency that is 400 times faster than the caloric test and the duration of head turn is ~ 200 milliseconds.[35] The vHIT will measure responses at latency intervals from zero up to 400–600 milliseconds. After each head turn, the head velocity and the eye velocity are displayed simultaneously. There should be ~ 10 to 20 head turns to assess each canal (in each direction).

Eza-Nunez et al classified vHIT responses into four groups: (1) normal gain without catch-up saccades; (2) normal gain with overt catch-up saccades; (3) low gain without catch-up saccades; and (4) low gain with catch-up saccades.[36] In evaluation of the semicircular canals with vHIT, both low gain and catch-up saccades must be demonstrated to identify a peripheral vestibular disorder[36]

There are common eye-velocity response patterns for patients with various pathologies. With bilateral loss of vestibular function, the gain will be low for head turns in both directions, with overt and covert corrective saccades present. Further diagnostic information can be obtained when measuring the gain and the configuration of the saccades. Testing the vertical semicircular canals (left anterior/right posterior and right anterior/left posterior) gives additional information on the status of the whole vestibular nerve.[37]

Adding the vHIT to the vestibular testing battery provides information that other computerized evaluations do not provide. Because of differences in the temporal frequencies of each electrophysiologic test, however, the results of the vHIT and the results of caloric and rotational testing do not always coincide. If a caloric weakness is greater than 39.5%, the vHIT gains are more likely to be reduced on the same side.[3] A slightly reduced gain may also be recorded in the contralateral side (**Fig. 3.6**).

Recent research reports that, in a population of patients with Meniere's disease, ipsilesional abnormal caloric testing, in the presence of normal head impulse testing, was found.[38] This study further supports the notion that vHIT and caloric testing should both be incorporated into a comprehensive vestibular function battery. Conversely, the vHIT should not be used alone or as a substitute for other tests.

As with other procedures, the vHIT evaluation is only as good as the tester and the impact of other physical technical parameters of the recording. Mantokoudis et al did a prospective study of 1,358 vHIT tracings and found that 44% had at least one artifact and 43% were uninterpretable. About 72% demonstrated disruptive eye movements. Only ~ 42% of the tracings that they reviewed were free of artifacts and did not have eye movements that interfered with the analysis.[39]

Vestibular Evoked Myogenic Potentials (VEMP)

Clinically, VEMP testing is used to assess the function of the otoliths and CN VIII, and it is also sensitive for the diagnosis of superior semicircular canal dehiscience (SSCD). Currently, in many vestibular laboratories, the vHIT combined with ocular and cervical VEMPs (oVEMP and cVEMP) is being used to evaluate the three semicircular canals and the two otoliths in each ear.

In the two modes of VEMP testing, cVEMP and oVEMP, VEMPs are recorded by delivering sound to the inner ear while asking the patient to contract a muscle: the sternocleidomastoid muscle (SCM) for cVEMP testing and the inferior oblique ocular muscles for oVEMP. The change in electromyographic (EMG) activity is recordable via surface electrodes and gives information about otolith function. VEMP testing is noninvasive, is generally tolerated well by patients, and is relatively quick to perform. In addition, hearing is not necessary for the patient to successfully participate in VEMP testing. Due to the relative ease of VEMP testing, it also can be successfully applied to pediatric patients (**Fig. 3.7**).

VEMP testing should be part of a complete vestibular evaluation. The testing gives the examiner information about the saccule and utricle, information not obtained with any other computerized vestibular evaluation. The origin of the cVEMP response is the saccule and inferior vestibular nerve, while the origin of the oVEMP is the utricle and the superior vestibular nerve.[40]

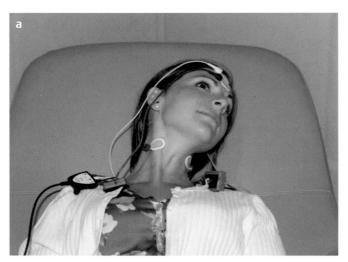
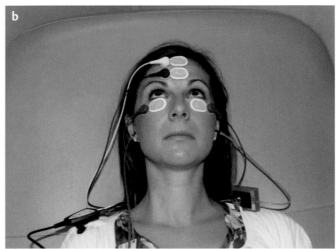

Fig. 3.7 Patient undergoing vestibular evoked myogenic potentials (VEMP) testing with air-conduction stimuli via inserts. **(a)** Patient undergoing cervical VEMP (cVEMP) testing. Sound is presented to the right ear with patient in the semi-reclined position while the sternocleidomastoid muscle (SCM) is contracted. The peripheral end-organ tested is the right saccule. **(b)** The same patient undergoing ocular VEMP (oVEMP) testing. Sound is presented to the right ear while the patient gazes upward; responses are recorded from the contralateral inferior oblique eye muscle. The peripheral end-organ tested is the left utricle.

cVEMP

The cVEMP response is present ipsilateral to auditory stimulation and represents function of the vestibulo-colic reflex (VCR).[40] The VCR originates in the saccule and terminates in the motor neurons of the SCM.[40] Sound is presented to the ear via an inserted ear-phone. The patient is positioned semi-reclined and instructed to turn away from the stimulated ear and to maintain the contraction during the recording. Adequate muscle contraction is necessary to record a cVEMP. During the cVEMP, the saccular afferents are activated and the response is recorded as an inhibitory response from the SCM.[41]

A repeatable cVEMP, in response to a 500-Hz air-conducted sound, should be present with stimuli between 75 dBnHL and 90 dBnHL.[42] The cVEMP response is expected to occur at a latency P13 and N23 milliseconds (**Fig. 3.8**). The amplitude of a positive and negative peak is measured on each side. An asymmetry ratio between the ears is calculated using the following formula (VEMP asymmetry ratio)[42]:

$$100 \times [(\text{Amplitude of right} - \text{Amplitude of left})/(\text{Amplitude of right} + \text{Amplitude of left})]$$

An asymmetry of greater than ~ 33% to 47% (age dependent) is considered to be significant.[42] If an asymmetry is obtained, the lower amplitude is generally the affected side, except in the presence of SSCD.[42]

oVEMP

The oVEMP response is present bilaterally (larger on the contralateral side) to auditory stimulation and represents function of the utricle. It originates in the utricle and superior vestibular nerve and is recorded from the contralateral inferior oblique eye muscle. There is also a response from the ipsilateral inferior rectus.[40] Sound (500 Hz best response) is presented to the ear via an inserted earphone or via bone conduction (placement of galvanic stimulator is typically on the forehead).

The patient is instructed to gaze upward and to maintain the position during the recording. A 30° upward gaze has been found to elicit the maximal amplitude.[42] During oVEMP testing, the utricle afferents are activated and the response is recorded as excitatory activity from the contralateral inferior oblique eye muscle.[43] The oVEMP response is expected to occur at a latency of N10 and P15 milliseconds.

The amplitude of the oVEMP response will vary greatly from patient to patient; therefore, the valuable information gained by testing comes from comparing the relative asymmetry between right and left.[2] A significant oVEMP asymmetry would be ≥ 34%.[44] (The formula is identical to that for cVEMP asymmetry.)[3]

When they are used together, vHIT and VEMP testing provide more diagnostic information than either test alone. Catch-up saccades in the lateral or

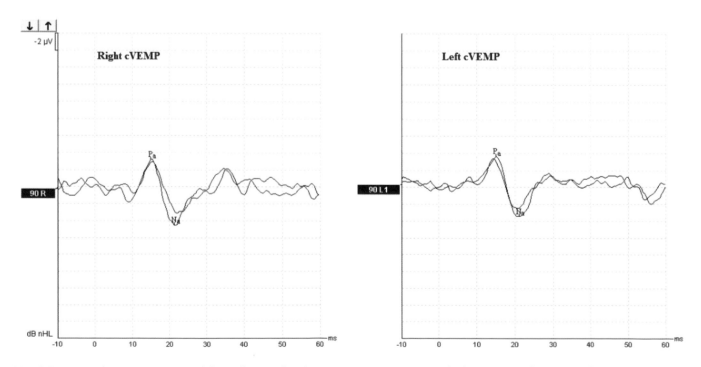

Fig. 3.8 Normal cVEMP responses bilaterally. Amplitude asymmetry ratio is 5%, which is nonsignificant. Results suggest normal saccular function bilaterally.

anterior canals, identified with the vHIT, combined with abnormal oVEMP responses, indicate superior vestibular neuritis. Catch-up saccades in the posterior canals on vHIT and abnormal cVEMP responses indicate inferior vestibular neuritis.

Superior Semicircular Canal Dehiscence and VEMP

A VEMP that is elicited by stimulation below 75 dBnHL may suggest SSCD. In the normal population there should be no recordable VEMP thresholds below 75 dBnHL. In addition, when comparing the amplitude symmetry, the VEMP response from the affected ear will be larger, as opposed to VEMP asymmetries demonstrated in other pathologies. An oVEMP amplitude equal to or greater than 17.1 µV is consistent with SSCD. The amplitude of the oVEMP has been shown to be superior to the threshold of the cVEMP in the diagnosis of SSCD.[45]

Central Neurologic Disorders and VEMP

Abnormalities in VEMP testing results may indicate central neurologic disorders; however, they are not disease specific and do not give information on etiology. In brainstem and cerebellar pathologies, prolonged response latencies and decreased response amplitudes are found. Some central pathologies will show normal cVEMP responses and an absent oVEMP response, with the abnormal oVEMP response contralateral to the central lesion.[46]

Computerized Dynamic Posturography

Computerized dynamic posturography (CDP) is a part of the comprehensive assessment protocol for patients with balance and equilibrium disorders. It provides a method for clinically assessing the patient's ability to use visual, somatosensory, and vestibular cues to maintain balance. Computerized dynamic posturography is a systemic balance function test rather than a vestibular function test. It is the only measure in the vestibular test battery that tests the vestibulospinal reflex (VSR). Patients who are candidates for CDP include[47]:

1. Patients being monitored while taking potential vestibulotoxic medication

2. Patients with vestibular symptoms who have not shown any abnormality on other evaluations (including normal caloric findings)

3. Patients who have a history of brain or vestibular trauma

4. Patients receiving vestibular rehabilitation, in order to monitor progress or change

5. Patients with a history of falls, or a potential for future falls

6. Patients with aphysiologic or exaggerated symptoms of disbalance

In order for a patient to undergo CDP, they must be able to stand without support. A harness is used to secure the patient to the platform, eliminating the risk of falling. The patient's feet are properly placed on the footplate to ensure accurate scoring. A complete CDP examination consists of three subtests: (1) the sensory organization test (SOT), (2) amplitude scaling (AS), and (3) motor control testing (MCT). Patient responses are scored based on a comparison with responses of age-equivalent persons with no vestibular symptoms.

There are six conditions in the SOT. The patient has three trials in each condition. For condition 1, the platform and the surround are fixed and the patient's eyes are open. In condition 2, the support surface remains fixed but vision is denied. The patient's vision is sway referenced (moving visual surround) but the platform remains fixed in condition 3. In condition 4, the platform moves but the patient can use vision to help maintain balance. Vision is denied while the platform support surface moves in condition 5. Vision is conflicted and the platform moves in the final condition 6.

A sensory analysis is performed by forming ratio pairs of specific conditions.[48] For a SOT to be considered abnormal, the values of the composite score and at least one equilibrium score must be less than those achieved by 95% of the age-matched normal persons. Based on low scores on these test condition ratio pairs, inferences can be made regarding poor use of visual, somatosensory, and vestibular input cues and the implications of their dysfunction. Specific sensory dysfunction patterns describe the functional status of the patient's use of sensory information and are not intended to provide a specific diagnosis.[48]

In addition, a "visual preference" may be revealed, in which the patient may demonstrate the ability to ignore input from the visual system when it is functionally inaccurate. Vision preference would indicate a normal strategy to maintain balance and for postural control.[49] If the patient performs better on the "harder" conditions than on the "easier" conditions (aphysiologic patterns), a diagnosis of symptom amplification or an aphysiologic disorder can be made.[50] A composite equilibrium score is provided that represents the patient's overall performance on the SOT subtest. In addition, the center of gravity is plotted to determine the degree of sway or alignment around the patient's center of gravity.

Motor control testing (MCT) evaluates the patient's ability to maintain balance after unexpected movements of the footplate. Sequences of small, medium, or large platform changes, in forward and backward directions, trigger automatic postural responses.[48] The onset latency, strength, and symmetry of responses is calculated for each leg.[48] The examiner will review the data to determine if certain patterns of MCT latencies obtained can provide further information regarding the site of the lesion.[48]

The final part of a comprehensive CDP evaluation is the adaptation test, which evaluates the patient's ability to maintain balance and decrease sway when the footplate support moves, changing from a toes-up to a toes-down direction. There is a sequence of five trials in which response time is measured. Poor adaptation abilities and range-of-motion deficiencies may be identified.

Honiker et al investigated CDP with a modified head shake added to SOT condition 2 and condition 5 (vision denied conditions).[51] They determined that a head-shake protocol may assist in identifying peripheral vestibular system hypofunction when used in conjunction with VNG and RCT.[51]

Computerized dynamic posturography can detect abnormalities with high specificity (90%).[52] When combined with the VNG and RCT, the sensitivity of CDP is 61% to 89%.[52] In addition to describing the functional impact of the dysfunction, the interpretation also indicates the implication for treatment. Computerized dynamic posturography offers information that cannot be obtained with other laboratory tests, so its results are complementary, not redundant, when used in conjunction with the other tests discussed in this chapter.[47,50]

Other Tests

Electrocochleography (ECoG) has been used for many years to demonstrate the presence of endolymphatic hydrops. Electrocochleography measures the ratio between the summating potential (SP) and the whole nerve action potential (AP) in response to a high-intensity sound. An elevated ratio (50% or greater using gold tiptrode insert phones) is consistent with endolymphatic hydrops. Over the years, studies have both supported and repudiated the clinical usefulness of ECoG in the diagnosis of Meniere's disease.[53] In a study in which members of American Neurotology Society/American Otological Society were questioned, 50% reported that they did not have "confidence" in the test and did not use the ECoG to diagnose Meniere's disease.[53]

■ Conclusion

Computerized testing for vestibular disorders has been available for over 25 years. Using the old gold standards, VNG with calorics and RCT, the examiner would fail to adequately diagnosis ~ 60% of patients with symptoms.[54] Currently, according to Barin and Jurado, a combination of vHIT, cVEMP, and oVEMP test results will provide a comprehensive assessment of the labyrinth and both branches of the vestibular nerve. Performing caloric testing in addition will add low-frequency information on the functioning of the lateral canals and their afferent neural pathways.[54] Furthermore, RCT remains useful for assessing vestibular function (especially bilateral dysfunction) and compensation. Performing these tests will help guide the physician to the proper medical or rehabilitative treatment for the patient, help the physician determine if additional testing is needed, and can assist vestibular therapists in creating a personalized vestibular rehabilitation program for each patient (**Table 3.1**).

Table 3.1 Common vestibular pathologies with computerized vestibular test findings

Test	Unilateral Vestibular Neuritis	Vestibular Migraines	Superior Semicircular Canal Dehiscence	Meniere's Disease	Central Lesion
Calorics	UW 20°–25° or greater; possible DP 30° or greater.	Most consistent finding is a unilateral caloric weakness.	Bithermal caloric responses robust and symmetric.	Unilateral, early, or mild disease shows normal caloric responses; late disease may have abnormalities ranging from mild to severe UW with or without DP.	No way of separating end-organ peripheral from central disorders on the basis of the caloric responses.
Oculomotor	In acute phases, possible oculomotor abnormalities; later stages may be unremarkable.	Central oculomotor deficits may be present; smooth pursuit tests often give abnormal results.	Unremarkable oculomotor testing.	Unremarkable oculomotor testing.	Asymmetric pursuit; abnormal saccadic tracking.
Positionals	Direction-fixed nystagmus 4° or greater. Nystagmus reduced or abolished with vision.	Some show central signs in the form of positional direction-changing nystagmus.	Negative Dix-Hallpike maneuver/negative positional nystagmus.	Negative Dix-Hallpike maneuver/negative positional nystagmus.	Nystagmus not reduced or abolished with vision. Direction-changing nystagmus.
Gaze	Possible spontaneous nystagmus. Gaze-evoked nystagmus follows Alexander's law.	Unilateral or bilateral gaze-induced horizontal nystagmus is common.	No spontaneous or gaze-evoked nystagmus.	No spontaneous or gaze-evoked nystagmus.	Nystagmus not reduced or abolished with vision. Vertical or torsional nystagmus.
Rotational chair	If unilateral: may be normal if compensation has occurred or asymmetric if not. If bilateral, low gain at all frequencies with phase lag.	High gain value with accompanying phase shift is usually demonstrated.	Results are within normal limits.	Little or no reduction in and possible enhancement of VOR gain/possible asymmetric gain	Usually does not provide localized findings.
vHIT	Low gain with overt and covert saccades in acute stage. May recover over time.	Saccadic eye-motion testing is usually normal, but a rebound nystagmus may be present with hyperresponsive neural findings.	All semicircular canals show normal function.	Relatively normal vHIT gain in early stages. Slightly enhanced VOR gain at later stages.	If cerebellar damage exists, there may be the presence of catch-up saccades to head movement at slow velocities.
cVEMP	Attenuated or absent in a percentage of patients. Asymmetry on the ipsilesional side.	Generally, hyperactive VEMP responses are found, but they may also be reduced.	Lower than normal threshold.	Increased thresholds, or absent responses.	Most commonly, either decreased or abolished responses.
oVEMP	Bilateral abnormal response. Asymmetry on the ipsilesional side.	Lower response rates, smaller amplitude, and higher threshold.	Amplitudes larger than normal and thresholds lower than normal. Asymmetric N10.	Lower response rates, smaller amplitude, and higher threshold. Bilateral response with lesional ear more affected.	Increased latency is the most prevalent abnormality, followed by absent oVEMPs.

Abbreviations: cVEMP, cervical VEMP; DP, directional preponderance; oVEMP, ocular VEMP; UW, unilateral weakness; VEMP, vestibular evoked myogenic potentials; vHIT, video head impulse test; VOR, vestibulo-ocular reflex.

References

1. Gandolfi MM, Reilly EK, Galatioto J, Judson RB, Kim AH. Cost-effective analysis of unilateral vestibular weakness investigation. Otol Neurotol 2015;36(2):277–281

2. Curthoys IS. The interpretation of clinical tests of peripheral vestibular function. Laryngoscope 2012; 122(6):1342–1352

3. McCaslin DL, Jacobson GP, Bennett ML, Gruenwald JM, Green AP. Predictive properties of the video head impulse test: measures of caloric symmetry and self-report dizziness handicap. Ear Hear 2014;35(5):e185–e191

4. Vanspauwen R, Weerts A, Hendrickx M, et al. No effects of anti-motion sickness drugs on vestibular evoked myogenic potentials outcome parameters. Otol Neurotol 2011;32(3):497–503

5. Ganança MM, Caovilla HH, Ganança FF. Electronystagmography versus videonystagmography. Braz J Otorhinolaryngol 2010;76(3):399–403

6. Kang S, Kim US. Normative data of videonystagmography in young healthy adults under 40 years old. Korean J Ophthalmol 2015;29(2):126–130

7. Snow JB, Wackym PA. Evaluation of the vestibular system. In: Ballenger's Otorhinolaryngology Head and Neck Surgery. 17th ed. Shelton, CT: People's Medical Publishing House; 2009:137

8. Jeffcoat B, Shelukhin A, Fong A, Mustain W, Zhou W. Alexander's law revisited. J Neurophysiol 2008; 100(1):154–159

9. Mekki S. The role of videonystagmography (VNG) in assessment of dizzy patient. Egypt J Otolaryngol 2014; 30(2):69–72

10. Brandt T, Strupp M. General vestibular testing. Clin Neurophysiol 2005;116(2):406–426

11. McCaslin DL. Electronystagmography/Videonystagmography. San Diego, CA: Plural Publishing; 2012: 107–110

12. Bhattacharyya N, Baugh RF, Orvidas L, et al; American Academy of Otolaryngology-Head and Neck Surgery Foundation. Clinical practice guideline: benign paroxysmal positional vertigo. Otolaryngol Head Neck Surg 2008;139(5, Suppl 4):S47–S81

13. Büttner U, Helmchen C, Brandt T. Diagnostic criteria for central versus peripheral positioning nystagmus and vertigo: a review. Acta Otolaryngol 1999;119(1):1–5

14. Hain TC. Head-shaking nystagmus and new technology. Neurology 2007;68(17):1333–1334

15. Angeli SI, Velandia S, Snapp H. Head-shaking nystagmus predicts greater disability in unilateral peripheral vestibulopathy. Am J Otolaryngol 2011;32(6):522–527

16. Huh YE, Kim JS. Patterns of spontaneous and head-shaking nystagmus in cerebellar infarction: imaging correlations. Brain 2011;134(Pt 12):3662–3671

17. Barin K. Background and technique of caloric testing. In: Jacobson GP, Shepard NT, eds. Balance Function Assessment and Management. 2nd ed. San Diego, CA: Plural Publishing; 2016:283–318

18. McGovern TN, Fitzgerald JE. The effect of mental alerting on peripheral vestibular nystagmus during spontaneous, gaze (30 degrees left, 30 degrees right) and body positional (left & right lateral lying) testing using electronystagmography (ENG). Int J Audiol 2008;47(10):601–606

19. Jongkees LB, Maas JP, Philipszoon AJ. Clinical nystagmography. A detailed study of electro-nystagmography in 341 patients with vertigo. Pract Otorhinolaryngol (Basel) 1962;24:65–93

20. Halmagyi GM, Cremer PD, Anderson J, Murofushi T, Curthoys IS. Isolated directional preponderance of caloric nystagmus: I. Clinical significance. Am J Otol 2000;21(4):559–567

21. Barber HO, Stockwell CW. Manual of Electronystagmography. Mosby; 1980.

22. Jacobson GP, Newman CW, Peterson EL. In: Jacobson GP, Newman CW, Kartush JM, eds. Handbook of Balance Function Testing. Clifton Park, NY: Thomson Delmar Learning; 1997:193–233

23. Murnane OD, Akin FW, Lynn SG, Cyr DG. Monothermal caloric screening test performance: a relative operating characteristic curve analysis. Ear Hear 2009;30(3):313–319

24. Bush ML, Bingcang CM, Chang ET, et al. Hot or cold? Is monothermal caloric testing useful and cost-effective? Ann Otol Rhinol Laryngol 2013;122(6):412–416

25. Chung W, Chu H. Clinical role of rotary chair test, ENG and CDP. Otolaryngol Head Neck Surg 2010;143(2):226

26. Rotational (Rotary) Chair Testing, American Academy of Otolaryngology-Head and Neck Surgery: Position Statement,http://www.entnet.org/content/rotational-rotary-chair-testing. Adopted September 2014. Accessed on June 1, 2015

27. Bahner C, Petrak M, Beck DL, Smith A. In the trenches, Part 3: caloric and rotational chair tests. Hearing Review 2013;20(4):42–48

28. Worthington D, Davis L, Zelowski C, Burrows H. Understanding rotary chair data in vestibular diagnosis. Presentation at American Academy of Audiology AudiologyNOW 2009

29. Arriaga MA, Chen DA, Cenci KA. Rotational chair (ROTO) instead of electronystagmography (ENG) as the primary vestibular test. Otolaryngol Head Neck Surg 2005;133(3):329–333

30. Ahmed MF, Goebel JA, Sinks BC. Caloric test versus rotational sinusoidal harmonic acceleration and step-velocity tests in patients with and without suspected peripheral vestibulopathy. Otol Neurotol 2009;30(6):800–805

31. Halmagyi GM, Curthoys IS. A clinical sign of canal paresis. Arch Neurol 1988;45(7):737–739

32. Petrak MR, Bahner C, Beck D. Video head impulse testing (vHIT): VOR analysis of high frequency vestibular activity. The Hearing Review Website, http://www.hearingreview.com/2013/08/video-head-impulse-testing-vhit-vor-analysis-of-high-frequency-vestibular-activity. Published on August 27, 2013. Accessed June 5, 2015

33. MacDougall HG, Weber KP, McGarvie LA, Halmagyi GM, Curthoys IS. The video head impulse test: diagnostic accuracy in peripheral vestibulopathy. Neurology 2009;73(14):1134–1141

34. Curthoys IS, MacDougall HG, McGarvie LA, et al. The video head impulse test (vHIT). In: Jacobson GP, Shepard NT, eds. Balance Function Assessment and Management. 2nd ed. San Diego, CA: Plural Publishing; 2016:391–430

35. McGarvie LA, Curthoys IS, MacDougall HG, Halmagyi GM. What does the head impulse test versus caloric dissociation reveal about vestibular dysfunction in Ménière's disease? Ann N Y Acad Sci 2015;1343:58–62

36. Eza-Nunez P, Farinas-Alvarez C, Perez-Fernandez N. The caloric test and the video head impulse test in patients with vertigo. International Adv Otol 2014; 10(2):144–149

37. Macdougall HG, McGarvie LA, Halmagyi GM, Curthoys IS, Weber KP. The video head impulse test (vHIT) detects vertical semicircular canal dysfunction. PLoS ONE 2013;8(4):e61488

38. McCaslin DL, Rivas A, Jacobson GP, Bennett ML. The dissociation of video head impulse test (vHIT) and bithermal caloric test results provides topological localization of vestibular system impairment in patients with "definite" Ménière's disease. Am J Audiol 2015;24(1):1–10

39. Mantokoudis G, Saber Tehrani AS, Kattah JC, et al. Quantifying the vestibulo-ocular reflex with video-oculography: nature and frequency of artifacts. Audiol Neurootol 2015;20(1):39–50

40. Jacobson GP, McCaslin DL, Piker EG, Gruenwald J, Grantham SL, Tegel L. Patterns of abnormality in cVEMP, oVEMP, and caloric tests may provide topological information about vestibular impairment. J Am Acad Audiol 2011;22(9):601–611

41. Curthoys IS. A critical review of the neurophysiological evidence underlying clinical vestibular testing using sound, vibration and galvanic stimuli. Clin Neurophysiol 2010;121(2):132–144

42. McCaslin DL, Jacobson GP. Vestibular evoked myogenic potentials (VEMPS), In: Jacobson GP, Shepard NT, eds. Balance Function Assessment and Management. 2nd ed. San Diego, CA: Plural Publishing; 2016:533–579

43. Kantner C, Gürkov R. Characteristics and clinical applications of ocular vestibular evoked myogenic potentials. Hear Res 2012;294(1-2):55–63

44. Piker EG, Jacobson GP, McCaslin DL, Hood LJ. Normal characteristics of the ocular vestibular evoked myogenic potential. J Am Acad Audiol 2011;22(4):222–230

45. Zuniga MG, Janky KL, Nguyen KD, Welgampola MS, Carey JP. Ocular versus cervical VEMPs in the diagnosis of superior semicircular canal dehiscence syndrome. Otol Neurotol 2013;34(1):121–126

46. Venhovens J, Meulstee J, Verhagen WI. Vestibular evoked myogenic potentials (VEMPs) in central neurological disorders. Clin Neurophysiol 2015

47. Monsell EM, Furman JM, Herdman SJ, Konrad HR, Shepard NT. Computerized dynamic platform posturography. Otolaryngol Head Neck Surg 1997; 117(4):394–398

48. Nashner LM. Computerized dynamic posturography. In: Jacobson GP, Newman CW, Kartush JM, eds. Handbook of Balance Function Testing. Clifton Park, NY: Thomson Delmar Learning; 1997:280–307

49. Perez NI, Rama JI, Martinez Vila E. Vision preference in dynamic posturography analysed according to vestibular impairment and handicap. Rev Laryngol Otol Rhinol (Bord) 2004;125(4):215–221

50. Black FO. What can posturography tell us about vestibular function? Ann N Y Acad Sci 2001;942:446–464

51. Honaker JA, Converse CM, Shepard NT. Modified head shake computerized dynamic posturography. Am J Audiol 2009;18(2):108–113

52. Di Fabio RP. Sensitivity and specificity of platform posturography for identifying patients with vestibular dysfunction. Phys Ther 1995;75(4):290–305

53. Nguyen LT, Harris JP, Nguyen QT. Clinical utility of electrocochleography in the diagnosis and management of Ménière's disease: AOS and ANS membership survey data. Otol Neurotol 2010;31(3):455–459

54. Barin K, Jurado M. What is being tested in different vestibular function tests. Presented at American Academy of Audiology AudiologyNOW 2014

4 Radiological Studies for the Vestibular Patient

Kennith F. Layton, John I. Lane, Robert J. Witte, and Colin L. W. Driscoll

■ Introduction

Imaging plays an important role in the diagnosis and treatment of patients with vestibular abnormalities. There are multiple imaging tools available for evaluation of patients with vestibular and temporal bone abnormalities. Among the imaging modalities available today, computed tomography (CT), magnetic resonance imaging (MRI), magnetic resonance angiography (MRA), magnetic resonance venography (MRV), and digital subtraction angiography (DSA) are the most commonly used. Each imaging modality has inherent strengths and weaknesses that will depend on the anatomic location and pathology studied. Often, multiple imaging modalities are complementary and add information not available from a single technique. Communication with the radiologist prior to testing ensures that the most appropriate modality is employed for the clinical situation. Certain implanted devices, such as cardiac pacemakers and cochlear implants, are relative contraindications to MRI, but some patients with certain types of these devices can be scanned safely under carefully controlled circumstances[1,2] Older intracranial aneurysm clips and other metallic devices may also preclude MRI examination.

■ Imaging Modalities

Computed Tomography

Computed tomography is especially well suited for evaluation of the osseous structures of the middle and inner ear. Computed tomography provides excellent anatomic detail in areas where bone and air are closely apposed. A complete temporal bone CT study consists of one axial acquisition with the patient supine and an additional coronal acquisition with the patient prone and the neck extended. The advent of slip-ring technology and multidetector CT (MDCT) scanners has dramatically improved the utility of CT in vestibular disease. Advancements in detector technology have resulted in excellent multiplanar reformatting from a single axial acquisition, reducing imaging times and motion artifacts. Temporal bone imaging on current MDCT scanners uses a helical acquisition and 0.3 to 0.6 mm collimation. The data are then reformatted in the axial, coronal, and potentially other planes if needed (**Fig. 4.1**).

Using such a protocol, high-resolution images of both temporal bones can be obtained in 8 to 10 seconds. Small structures, such as the ossicles, cochlea, semicircular canals, facial nerve canal, and vestibular aqueduct, can be confidently identified on modern CT studies. With the current technology, structures as small as 0.4 mm can be depicted accurately. Normal CT anatomy of the temporal bone is illustrated in **Fig. 4.2, Fig. 4.3,** and **Fig. 4.4**.

Magnetic Resonance Imaging

The improved soft tissue contrast of MRI complements the bone detail of CT when imaging the temporal bone. Magnetic resonance imaging provides exquisite imaging of fluid-filled structures, fat, cranial nerves, and the central nervous system. Labyrinthine anatomy is best depicted on T2-weighted sequences, which accentuate bright signal from perilymphatic, endolymphatic, and cerebrospinal fluid. Commonly employed three-dimensional (3D) T2-weighted MR cisternogram sequences include fast spin-echo (FSE), constructive interference in the steady state (CISS), and true fast imaging with steady-state precession (FISP) (**Fig. 4.5**).

Each has its inherent advantages. T1-weighted sequences with gadolinium contrast agents are used for detecting enhancement due to infection, inflammation, or tumors. In certain situations, fat-saturation techniques can be useful in nulling inherent bright signal from fat or bone marrow and improving the conspicuity of abnormal contrast enhancement. Magnetic resonance imaging also provides the abil-

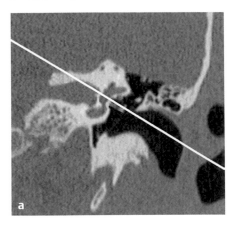
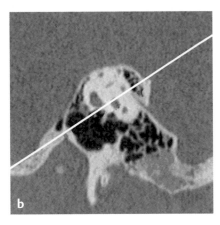
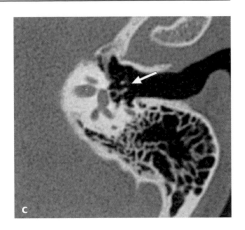

Fig. 4.1 **(a)** Volumetric CT with isotropic voxels (0.6 cubic mm) permits reconstructions in any plane without loss of resolution. **(b)** Orthogonal coronal and sagittal reconstructions from axial acquisition demonstrate degrees of obliquity (*white lines*) required to produce **(c)** double oblique axial reconstruction profiling of the stapes in its entirety (*arrow*).

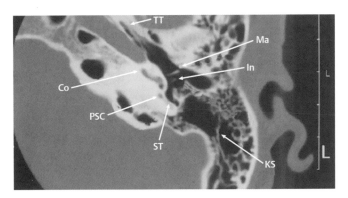

Fig. 4.2 Normal anatomy depicted on axial high-resolution CT. TT, tensor tympani; Ma, malleus; Co, cochlea; In, incus; PSC, posterior semicircular canal; ST, sinus tympani; KS, Koerner septum.

Fig. 4.3 Axial CT demonstrates normal anatomy. Co, basal turn cochlea; Ma, head of malleus; In, short process incus; KS, Koerner septum; HSC, horizontal semicircular canal; Ve, vestibule; IAC, internal auditory canal.

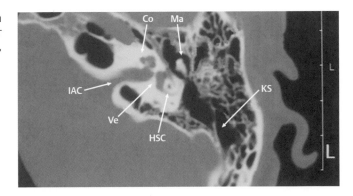

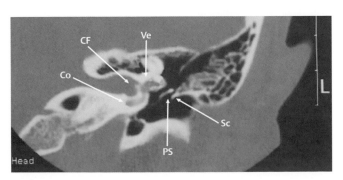

Fig. 4.4 High-resolution coronal CT demonstrates normal anatomy. CF, crista falciformis; Ve, vestibule; Co, basal turn cochlea; Sc, scutum; PS, Prussak space.

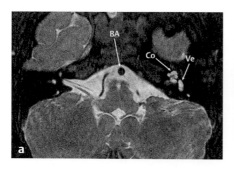
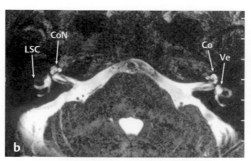
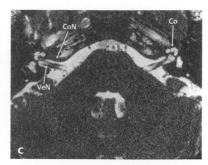

Fig. 4.5 Three Tesla (3T) magnetic resonance images demonstrate normal anatomy with **(a)** 3D FSE, **(b)** CISS, and **(c)** true FISP techniques. BA, basilar artery; Co, cochlea; Ve, vestibule; LSC, lateral semicircular canal; CoN, cochlear nerve; VeN, vestibular nerve.

ity to image in any plane without repositioning the patient. By changing the scan parameters, coronal, axial, and sagittal images in any obliquity can be easily obtained.

It is imperative to optimize resolution when imaging the small structures of the temporal bone. The field of MRI is constantly changing and several recent hardware and software advances have been particularly useful. Higher-field-strength imaging systems of 3 Teslas (3T) have more recently become available for routine clinical imaging and allow higher spatial resolution than systems operating at a field strength of 1.5 T or lower. Spatial resolution can also be improved with 3D (volume) pulse sequences that provide spatial resolution of less than 1 mm.[3] Bilateral surface coils placed over the ears can be used alone or in combination with a head coil to provide

more signal and improved resolution when imaging the temporal bone (**Fig. 4.6**).[4] Normal MRI anatomy of the temporal bone is illustrated in **Fig. 4.7, Fig. 4.8, Fig. 4.9,** and **Fig. 4.10**.

Perilymphatic opacification with gadolinium agents has recently been investigated as a means of visualizing the endolymphatic structures of the inner ear that remain unopacified on 3D FLAIR sequences. This can be achieved by transtympanic injection with unilateral transmission across the round window into the perilymphatic space or by delayed imaging (4 to 8 hours) after intravenous administration to acquire bilateral perilymphatic opacification (**Fig. 4.11**). This technique has been employed successfully to confirm the diagnosis of inner ear pathologies, such as endolymphatic hydrops in the setting of Meniere's disease and vestibular migraine.[5,6]

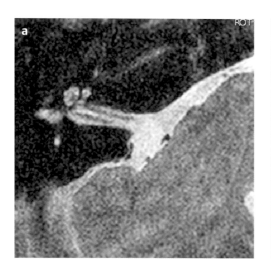
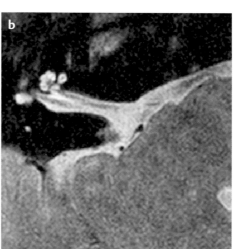

Fig. 4.6 Comparison of volume head coil only versus hybrid phased-array combination head and surface coils at 3T. **(a)** Volume head coil only provides inferior signal-to-noise within the labyrinth compared with **(b)** combination head and surface coil device.

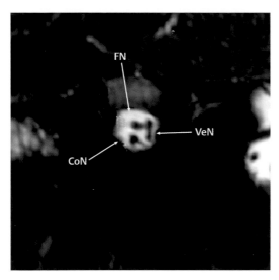

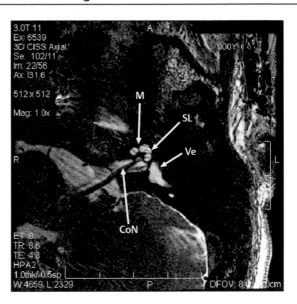

Fig. 4.7 Three Tesla 3D T2-weighted MRI through the internal auditory canal in the oblique sagittal plane demonstrates the normal nerves. FN, facial nerve; CoN, cochlear nerve; VeN, vestibular nerve.

Fig. 4.8 Three Tesla 3D CISS MRI demonstrates exquisite anatomy of the inner ear and internal auditory canal. M, modiolus; SL, spiral lamina; Ve, vestibule; CoN, cochlear nerve.

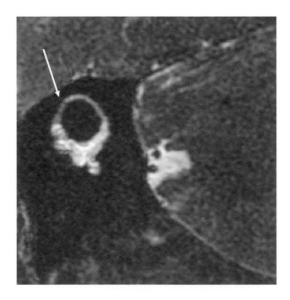

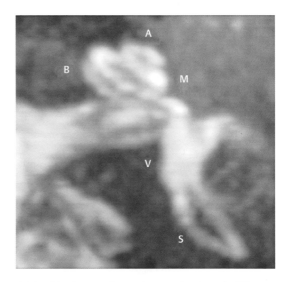

Fig. 4.9 Oblique sagittal 3T 3D CISS MRI demonstrates the normal superior semicircular canal (*arrow*).

Fig. 4.10 Maximum intensity projection (MIP) magnetic resonance image demonstrates the normal inner ear anatomy. B, basal turn cochlea; M, middle turn cochlea; A, apical turn cochlea; V, vestibule; S, semicircular canal.

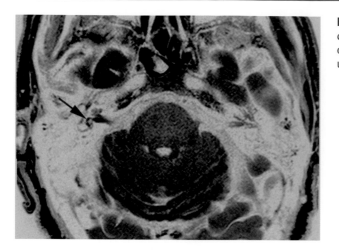

Fig. 4.11 REAL IR sequence obtained 4 hours after gadolinium demonstrates hypointense signal in the right labyrinth representing opacified perilymph outlining unopacified endolymph in a normal utricle (*arrow*).

Magnetic Resonance Angiography

The development of MRA techniques now allows noninvasive imaging of central nervous system (CNS) vascular lesions. Although uncommon, a vascular lesion can present as a vestibular abnormality. Common MRA techniques in use include noncontrast multiple overlapping thin slab acquisition (MOTSA), three-dimensional time-of-flight (3D TOF), and contrast-enhanced MRA (**Fig. 4.12**). These techniques provide a detailed depiction of the major intracranial arteries, especially near the circle of Willis. Abnormalities identified on MRA are often investigated further with conventional DSA.

Magnetic Resonance Venography

In contrast to MRA, MRV evaluates the intracranial venous structures. MRV techniques in common use include phase-contrast, two-dimensional time-of-flight (2D TOF), and gadolinium bolus imaging. Phase-contrast imaging allows for venous imaging without superimposed arterial structures, but contrast-enhanced MRV provides much higher spatial resolution (**Fig. 4.13**). The dural venous sinuses, large cortical veins, jugular bulbs, internal jugular veins, and deep cerebral veins are well visualized with MRV. As with MRA, abnormalities on MRV often require definitive evaluation with conventional DSA.

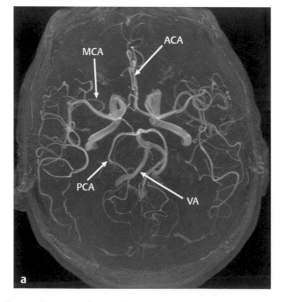
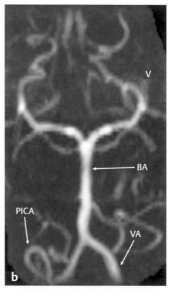

Fig. 4.12 **(a)** Multiple overlapping thin slab acquisition (MOTSA) intracranial MRA clearly depicts the major intracranial arteries on the collapsed whole-head image and **(b)** an anterior maximum intensity projection image of the posterior fossa. MCA, middle cerebral artery; ACA, anterior cerebral artery; PCA, posterior cerebral artery; VA, vertebral artery; BA, basilar artery; PICA, posterior inferior cerebellar artery; V, vein.

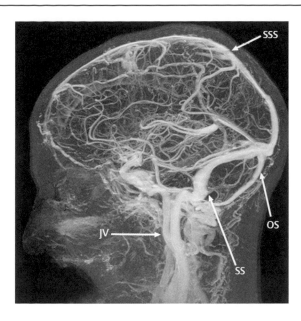

Fig. 4.13 Contrast-enhanced MRV in the lateral projection clearly depicts the venous structures. SSS, superior sagittal sinus; OS, occipital sinus; SS, sigmoid sinus; JV, jugular vein.

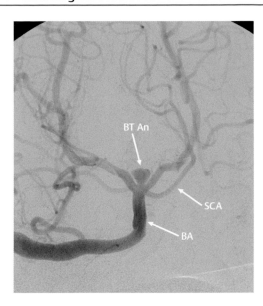

Fig. 4.14 Anteroposterior DSA image from a right vertebral artery injection clearly demonstrates an aneurysm at the basilar tip. The arterial lumen is seen with better resolution than with MRA techniques. BT An, basilar tip aneurysm; BA, basilar artery; SCA, superior cerebellar artery.

Digital Subtraction Angiography

Digital subtraction angiography is a minimally invasive procedure that directly images the lumen of arteries and veins. Digital subtraction angiography requires the intra-arterial placement of a catheter into the vascular territory of interest and injection of iodinated contrast. Although it is a very safe procedure, it does carry a small risk of bleeding or infection at the vascular access site, as well as a risk of stroke. However, these risks are small and occur in less than 1% of cases. With the advent of modern noninvasive imaging, the initial evaluation and screening of patients with suspected vascular abnormalities is generally performed with MRI or CT. Digital subtraction angiography is now relegated to further defining abnormalities depicted on MRA and MRV studies. Digital subtraction angiography can provide additional information about vascular lesions that cannot be obtained from MRA and MRV. Specifically, the flow dynamics of vascular lesions are best depicted with DSA, which precisely delineates the arterial and venous components of a lesion. Additionally, the spatial resolution of DSA is much higher than MRA and can be important in the evaluation of vascular abnormalities (**Fig. 4.14**). Furthermore, certain lesions may be treated with endovascular techniques performed at the time of diagnostic cerebral angiography.

■ Imaging Findings for Various Pathologic Entities in the Vestibular Patient

Dizziness can be the result of a large number of different pathologies. It is important to understand the strengths and weaknesses of the different imaging modalities so the appropriate testing can be pursued based on the differential diagnosis. In general, if the problem is thought to be in the temporal bone (e.g., cholesteatoma), imaging begins with a CT scan, and if it is thought to be an intracranial process (e.g., vestibular schwannoma), MRI is the initial test ordered.

The remainder of this chapter reviews the imaging findings in various pathologic conditions. Dizziness is often not the primary symptom in many of these disorders, but all of the pathologies should be considered when a patient complains of dizziness.

Trauma

Patients with temporal bone trauma are generally imaged with high-resolution CT.[7] Axial and coronal imaging at 1 mm thickness or less is preferred. As mentioned previously, isotropic imaging with axial

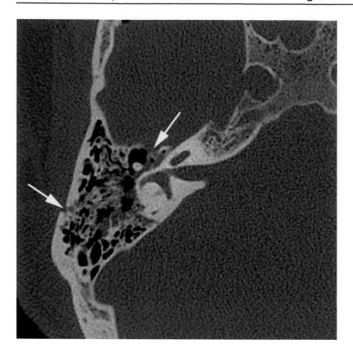

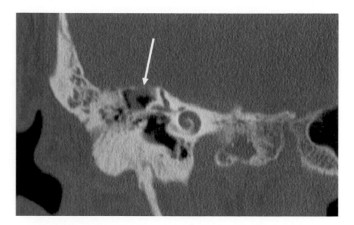

Fig. 4.16 High-resolution CT coronal reformat showing a defect in the tegmen tympani (*arrow*) with fluid in the mastoids and middle ear.

Fig. 4.15 Axial CT demonstrates a longitudinal fracture (*arrows*) through the right temporal bone and middle ear cavity.

and coronal reformats may supplant direct coronal imaging in trauma patients. It may be useful to delay high-resolution CT examinations until there is adequate resorption of any associated hemotympanum that could obscure traumatic ossicular injuries. Magnetic resonance imaging is generally considered only in the face of a normal high-resolution CT in patients with continued clinical symptoms. Entities like labyrinthine hemorrhage, facial nerve injury, and brainstem injury are best seen with MRI.[8]

Temporal bone fractures are usually the result of blunt trauma to the temporoparietal calvaria. Longitudinal fractures extend obliquely through the long axis of the temporal bone and are the most common variety, occurring in 70 to 90% of cases (**Fig. 4.15**). These fractures often involve the squamous portion of the temporal bone, external auditory canal (EAC), middle ear, petrous apex, and tegmen tympani. Longitudinal fractures tend to extend around the labyrinthine structures due to their dense bony capsule. They can result in disruption of the ossicles and tympanic membrane and often present with a conductive hearing loss. Recent reports indicate that classifying temporal bone fractures as petrous (violation of otic capsule) and nonpetrous (otic capsule intact) may be more useful clinically than the traditional longitudinal, transverse, and mixed descriptions.[9] Injury of the seventh nerve usually involves the first genu or proximal tympanic segment.[10] Fractures extending through the roof of the tegmen tympani or posterior mastoid air cells can result in a cerebrospinal fluid (CSF) leak or fistula (**Fig. 4.16**).

High-resolution CT imaging after the instillation of intrathecal contrast can be used to detect such an injury. Transverse fractures of the temporal bone are less common but more severe than longitudinal fractures (**Fig. 4.17**). These fractures occur along the short axis of the temporal bone, extending through the foramen magnum, occipital bone, jugular fossa, petrous bone, and body of the sphenoid bone. Transverse fractures often spare the middle ear but disrupt the vestibule, vestibular nerve, cochlear nerve, and facial nerve. This can cause severe impairment, including complete loss of cochlear and vestibular function. Air within the inner ear can result from fractures through the mastoid air cells or middle ear. Extension into the carotid canal is not uncommon and can result in injury to the internal carotid artery. Facial nerve injury occurs in 50% of transverse fractures and generally involves the labyrinthine segment proximal to the geniculate ganglion.[11] A perilymphatic fistula can result from disruption of the ossicles with stapes mobilization or fractures

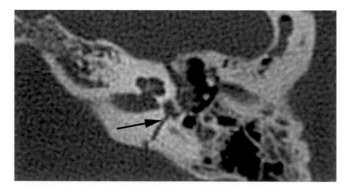

Fig. 4.17 Axial CT demonstrates a transverse fracture (*arrow*) through the left temporal bone and vestibule.

extending into the footplate of the stapes or through the round or oval windows. Explosive injuries or barotrauma may result in oval or round window membrane rupture.

Magnetic resonance imaging should be used to evaluate traumatic CNS lesions, such as brainstem contusion or temporal lobe encephalocele (**Fig. 4.18**).[12] T2-weighted images of the posterior fossa reveal contusions as areas of abnormal increased signal, with hemorrhagic components demonstrating areas of increased T1 and heterogeneous T2 signal.

Inflammatory Disorders

Inflammatory disorders causing dizziness include a diverse range of etiologies with varied imaging findings. Inflammatory disorders with imaging abnormalities include otitis media, mastoiditis, cholesteatoma, cholesterol granuloma, sarcoidosis, Wegener granulomatosis, pachymeningitis, neuronitis, and labyrinthitis.

Acute mastoiditis and its complications are well visualized with CT or MRI.[13,14] Typically, there is fluid within the mastoid air cells and middle ear cavity. In severe cases, destruction of the bony mastoid septations can occur (**Fig. 4.19**). The diagnosis of mastoiditis is often made clinically, with imaging reserved for complications, such as venous sinus thrombosis, petrous apicitis, and epidural or brain abscess. Computed tomography is generally better suited for observing air–fluid levels as well as bony destruction. Magnetic resonance imaging should be used to evaluate brain and epidural abscesses (**Fig. 4.20**).

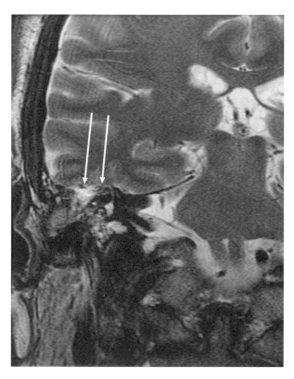

Fig. 4.18 High-resolution coronal T2-weighted image shows a traumatic defect of the right tegmen tympani (*arrows*) with CSF in the mastoid air cells. A small temporal lobe cephalocele was found at surgery.

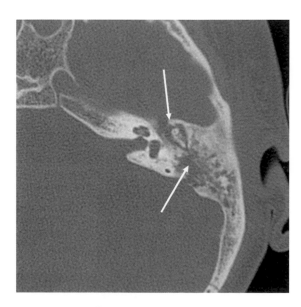

Fig. 4.19 Axial high-resolution CT shows fluid in the middle ear cavity (*upper arrow*) in this patient with acute mastoiditis and facial nerve palsy. Fluid in the mastoid air cells with destruction of the bony septa is noted (*lower arrow*).

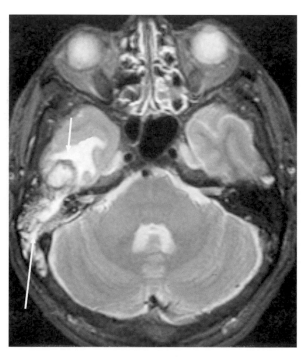

Fig. 4.20 Axial T2-weighted MRI shows fluid in the right mastoids (*upper arrow*) and an associated right temporal lobe abscess (*lower arrow*) in this patient with mastoiditis.

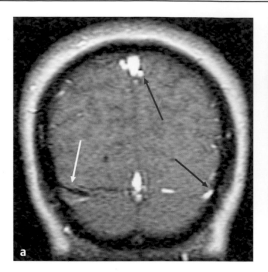
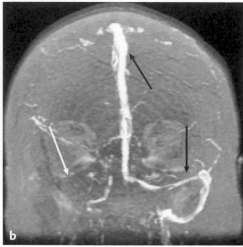

Fig. 4.21 **(a)** A source image and **(b)** collapsed MIP image from 2D TOF MRV in a patient with mastoiditis shows absence of flow in the thrombosed right transverse sinus (*white arrows*). Normal flow-related signal is seen in the superior sagittal and left transverse sinuses (*black arrows*).

Although *dural sinus thrombosis* secondary to acute mastoiditis can be suggested on CT, this entity is best demonstrated with MRI (**Fig. 4.21**). Direct extension of infection to the sigmoid sinus can result in thrombophlebitis. Aseptic propagation of venous thrombosis can involve the sigmoid, transverse, and petrosal sinuses, as well as the internal jugular vein. On contrast-enhanced CT, dural sinus thrombosis is manifested as incomplete or absent enhance-ment, and noncontrast CT demonstrates increased attenuation in the involved dural sinus (**Fig. 4.22**). T2-weighted MRI shows lack of a normal flow void in the dural sinus, and T1-weighted MRI reveals isoin-tense or hyperintense thrombus within the sinus. However, MRV provides the best evaluation of the dural venous sinuses. Contrast-enhanced MRV dem-onstrates lack of flow in the occluded dural sinus, confirming the diagnosis.

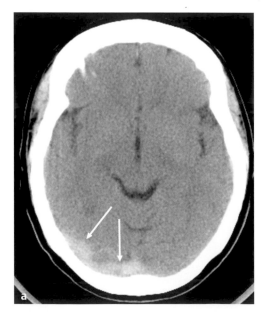
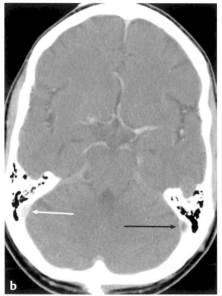

Fig. 4.22 **(a)** Noncontrast axial CT reveals increased density in the right transverse sinus (*arrows*) from right dural sinus thrombo-sis. **(b)** Contrast-enhanced head CT in another patient shows thrombosis of the left sigmoid sinus with lack of sinus enhancement (*black arrow*). Normal enhancement of the right sigmoid sinus is noted (*white arrow*).

Chronic mastoiditis produces varying amounts of fluid in the middle ear cavity and mastoid air cells. Ossicular erosion of the incus and stapes can be seen with high-resolution CT, as well as sclerosis of the mastoids. Fibrous tissue may be noted in the middle ear but is difficult to differentiate from fluid in the setting of complete opacification.

Cholesteatomas can be evaluated with CT or MRI, although CT is the preferred modality. Cholesteatomas can arise from both the pars tensa and the pars flaccida. Cholesteatomas are generally associated with a retracted and thickened tympanic membrane. The acquired cholesteatoma originates from the pars flaccida in the Prussak space and classically produces erosion of the scutum. As it enlarges, the soft tissue extends superiorly into the epitympanum or attic and displaces the malleus and incus medially. These findings are especially well depicted on high-resolution coronal CT images.[15] Cholesteatomas of the pars tensa tend to involve the sinus tympani and facial nerve recess. These lesions are best visualized on axial CT images and often displace the ossicles laterally. Both types of cholesteatoma can produce erosion of the ossicles. With MRI, cholesteatomas have nonspecific signal intensities with decreased T1 and increased T2 signal.[3] Cholesteatomas generally do not enhance after intravenous (IV) contrast administration, which can help differentiate them from other lesions, such as tumors or granulation tissue.

Recently, diffusion-weighted imaging has been suggested as a possible method to differentiate between recurrent or residual cholesteatoma and granulation tissue in the postoperative patient.[16] This technique can be useful as an alternative to "second look" operations to exclude recurrent disease after canal wall up procedures in which the postoperative clinical exam is limited[17,18] Cholesteatomas will demonstrate bright signal on diffusion-weighted images, whereas granulation tissue does not (**Fig. 4.23**). However, the best indicator that a lesion in the middle ear is a cholesteatoma is the presence of secondary findings, such as erosions of the ossicles and scutum. Labyrinthine fistulae can result from cholesteatomas eroding through the lateral semicircular canal or, very rarely, the cochlear promontory. High-resolution CT clearly depicts the bony defect, and this is an important finding to be aware of at the time of surgery (**Fig. 4.23**).[19]

Cholesterol granuloma is a lesion particularly well suited to evaluation by MRI, although CT can provide important information (**Fig. 4.24**).[20] Cholesterol granuloma results from an inflammatory response involving the deposition of cholesterol crystals in the middle ear, mastoid, or aerated petrous apex. As a part of this inflammatory response, hemorrhagic products including methemoglobin are produced. These products appear as increased signal intensity

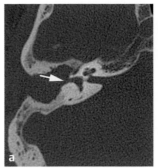
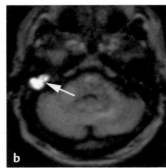

Fig. 4.23 **(a)** Axial CT image in a patient with a cholesteatoma. Opacified postoperative mastoid bowl with erosion of the lateral semicircular canal is clearly depicted (*arrow*). **(b)** HASTE DWI diffusion sequence demonstrates hyperintense signal within the opacified mastoid bowl consistent with recurrent cholesteatoma (*arrow*).

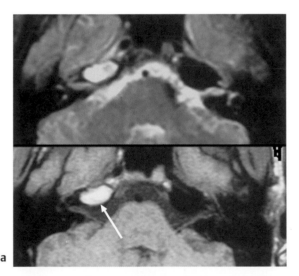
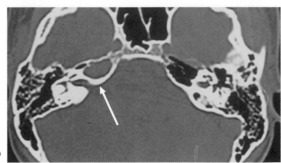

Fig. 4.24 **(a)** Axial T1- and T2-weighted MRI demonstrates increased signal in a cholesterol granuloma (*arrow*) of the right petrous apex. **(b)** Computed tomography demonstrates the smoothly marginated cholesterol granuloma (*arrow*) in the right petrous apex.

on T1- and T2-weighted sequences. Occasionally, the appearance can be confounded by the presence of hemosiderin, which produces heterogeneity and regions of decreased T1 and T2 signal. Cholesterol granulomata tend to be smoothly marginated, with little associated mass effect. Computed tomography shows a well-circumscribed, expansile mass with bony remodeling in the petrous apex or middle ear.

Sarcoidosis of the CNS often involves the meninges around the skull base, including those of the internal auditory canal (IAC), and is best imaged with MRI.[21] There is typically intense linear enhancement of the thickened meninges of the basal cisterns. The enhancing meninges can mimic a schwannoma within the IAC when there is formation of a pseudomass. The presence of additional meningeal enhancement outside the IAC, coupled with improvement after steroid treatment, usually allows for discrimination.

Acute labyrinthitis can be caused by infectious and noninfectious etiologies and can be seen with MRI as enhancement of the cochlea, vestibule, or semicircular canals.[22] Although viruses are probably the most common cause of labyrinthitis, the exact cause of labyrinthine enhancement is usually not determined, unless it is associated with meningitis. Early in the course of the disease, only mild enhancement on postcontrast T1-weighted images is noted, especially in viral infections. T2-weighted MRI will reveal abnormal decreased signal in the labyrinth in cases of fibrosing labyrinthitis (**Fig. 4.25**). Hemorrhagic labyrinthitis is common when caused by bacteria and can be seen as increased T1 signal with noncontrast MRI. As the disease progresses to the chronic stage, high-resolution CT can demonstrate calcification and sclerosis of the membranous labyrinth (**Fig. 4.26**).[23]

Congenital Anomalies

There are numerous congenital abnormalities that can be imaged in patients complaining of dizziness. These include vascular anomalies and congenital lesions of the inner ear and CNS. It can be difficult to know if the pathologies identified are related to the complaint of dizziness. Some of the examples of pathologies described in the following section only rarely would cause dizziness. However, identification of the abnormality gives the clinician the opportunity to consider its role in the patient's symptoms.

An *absent or aberrant internal carotid artery* is occasionally encountered. Absence of the internal carotid artery is a rare finding. Computed tomography of the skull base will demonstrate an absent bony carotid canal, and MRI and MRA reveal absent signal in the carotid artery (**Fig. 4.27**). In an aberrant internal carotid artery, the vessel projects more lat-

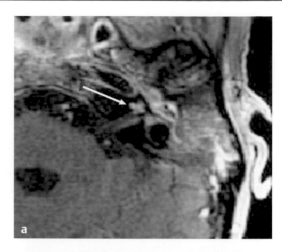

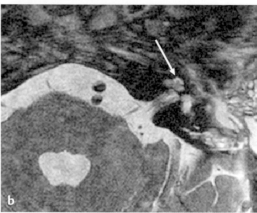

Fig. 4.25 **(a)** Axial T1-weighted MRI with contrast reveals abnormal enhancement of the cochlea (*arrow*). **(b)** Axial T2-weighted MRI demonstrates replacement of the normal fluid in the cochlea with abnormal decreased signal (*arrow*) in this patient with fibrosing labyrinthitis.

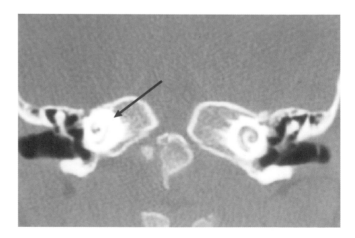

Fig. 4.26 Coronal CT demonstrates increased density of the right cochlea (*arrow*) consistent with labyrinthitis ossificans.

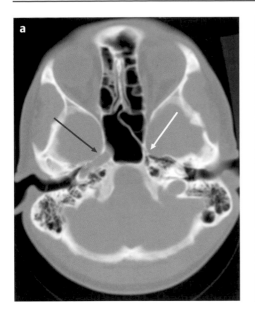 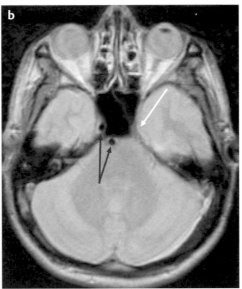

Fig. 4.27 **(a)** Axial CT and **(b)** proton-density MRI images demonstrate absence of the left carotid canal (*white arrows*) with normal flow voids in the right carotid canal and basilar artery (*black arrows*).

erally than usual.[24] Magnetic resonance imaging and CT demonstrate a soft tissue mass in the hypotympanum with lateral displacement of the tympanic membrane and remodeling of the cochlear promontory (**Fig. 4.28**).

Abnormalities of the *jugular bulb* are commonly encountered on temporal bone imaging. If there is a dehiscence in the floor of the middle ear, the jugular bulb can protrude into the hypotympanum. The clinical presentation is usually pulsatile tinnitus or hearing loss from mass effect on the middle ear structures.[25] The abnormality is best seen on CT, where a defect in the anterolateral jugular canal is present in the floor of the hypotympanum (**Fig. 4.29**). Contrast-enhanced CT or MRI may show an enhancing mass protruding into the middle ear. Close scrutiny of the jugular bulb and vein reveal the contiguous nature of the mass.

There are multiple *inner ear malformations and dysplasias,* which are well studied with CT and MRI.[26,27] Cochlear hypoplasia and dysplasia and absence of the semicircular canals, cochlea, and vestibule are sometimes encountered (**Fig. 4.30, Fig. 4.31, Fig. 4.32,** and **Fig. 4.33**).

Fusion of the middle and apical turns of the cochlea can occur, as well as abnormalities in the size of the common sac. The semicircular canals can be dysplastic and fused, with an abnormal vestibule. A dilated vestibular aqueduct can be encountered in patients with hearing loss. The patient is considered to have an *enlarged vestibular aqueduct* if it measures larger than 1.5 mm or is larger than the normal adjacent posterior semicircular canal (**Fig. 4.34**).[28] An enlarged vestibular aqueduct may be seen in association with other vestibular and cochlear abnormalities.

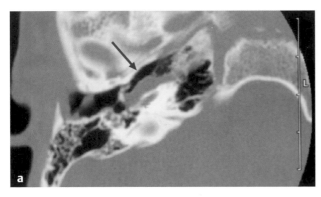 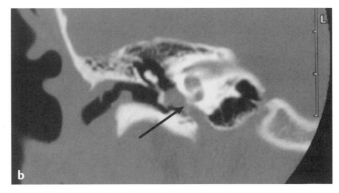

Fig. 4.28 **(a)** Axial and **(b)** coronal CT images show an aberrant right internal carotid artery (*arrows*), which must be differentiated from a middle ear mass.

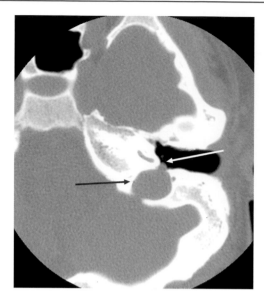

Fig. 4.29 Axial CT of the left temporal bone demonstrates a large jugular bulb (*black arrow*). Soft tissue in the floor of the hypotympanum (*white arrow*) represents the dehiscent jugular bulb.

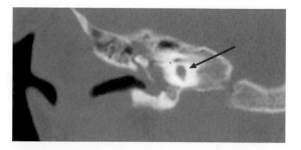

Fig. 4.30 Coronal CT demonstrates a dysplastic cochlea (*arrow*).

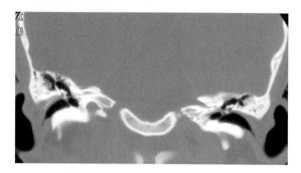

Fig. 4.31 High-resolution coronal CT in Michel aplasia. There is bilateral absence of the cochlea and atretic internal auditory canals.

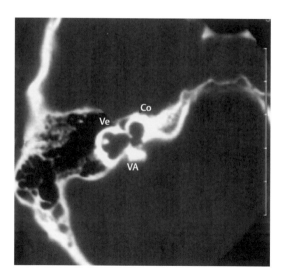

Fig. 4.32 Axial CT demonstrates Mondini dysplasia. There is confluence of the vestibule and semicircular canals with a large vestibular aqueduct and dysplastic cochlea. VA, vestibular aqueduct; Co, cochlea; Ve, vestibule.

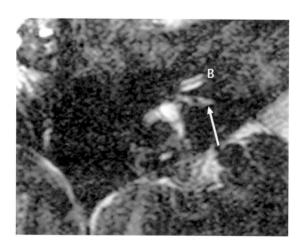

Fig. 4.33 Axial 3D CISS magnetic resonance image demonstrates atresia of the internal auditory canal (*arrow*). B, basal turn of the cochlea.

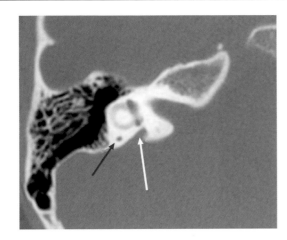

Fig. 4.34 High-resolution axial CT demonstrates a dilated vestibular aqueduct (*white arrow*), which is obviously larger than the adjacent posterior semicircular canal (*black arrow*).

Endolymphatic hydrops is the presence of dilated endolymphatic spaces. Congenital, idiopathic, and acquired causes of endolymphatic hydrops exist.[29] Any inflammatory, congenital, or traumatic lesion can ultimately result in enlargement of the endolymphatic spaces (**Fig. 4.35**). One of the more common idiopathic causes is Meniere's disease. This idiopathic condition can be occult on imaging with CT and MRI. However, there are reports of endolymphatic sac enhancement in the acute phases of Meniere's disease, which can be assessed with high-resolution contrast-enhanced MRI.[30] As previously mentioned, delayed imaging after transtympanic or intravenous administration of gadolinium using 3D

FLAIR sequences has recently been advocated for direct visualization of the endolymphatic structures of the inner ear (see **Fig. 4.11**) and, more specifically, endolymphatic hydrops.[5,6] Hypoplasia or absence of the vestibulocochlear and facial nerves can be demonstrated with high-resolution MRI through the IAC (**Fig. 4.36**).

Chiari I malformations usually present in adults with dizziness and gait difficulties. The disorder is characterized by low-lying cerebellar tonsils, which protrude through the foramen magnum (**Fig. 4.37**). The disorder is best characterized with MRI, where sagittal sections reveal the precise degree of tonsillar descent and associated abnormalities, such as hydrocephalus or syrinx formation.

Benign and Malignant Tumors

Benign and malignant tumors affecting the ear, temporal bone, and cerebellopontine angles can be exquisitely imaged with CT and MRI. A complete review of tumors is beyond the scope of this chapter, but the most common pathologies are presented (paraganglioma, hemangioma, vestibular schwannoma, meningioma, epidermoid, squamous cell carcinoma, rhabdomyosarcoma, and metastasis). Tumors can cause dizziness by involving the labyrinth, vestibular nerve, or central nervous system.

Benign Tumors

Paragangliomas involving the temporal bone typically originate from the promontory of the cochlea (glomus tympanicum) or the jugular bulb (glomus

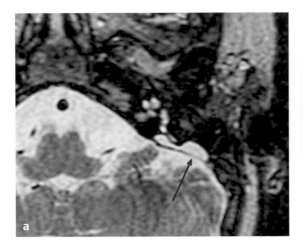
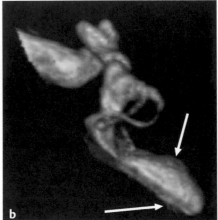

Fig. 4.35 **(a)** Axial T2-weighted image demonstrates an enlarged endolymphatic sac (*arrow*) and duct. **(b)** A maximum intensity projection image clearly demonstrates the enlarged endolymphatic sac (*arrows*).

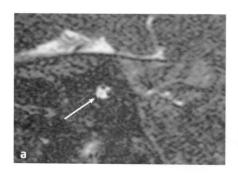
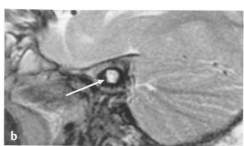
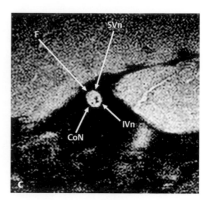

Fig. 4.36 **(a)** Sagittal 3D CISS MRI reveals a hypoplastic cochlear nerve (*arrow*). **(b)** Sagittal FSE T2-weighted MRI demonstrates an absent cochlear nerve (*arrow*). **(c)** Sagittal MRI demonstrates absence of the facial nerve. CoN, cochlear nerve; SVn, superior division vestibular nerve; IVn, inferior division vestibular nerve; F, expected location of facial nerve.

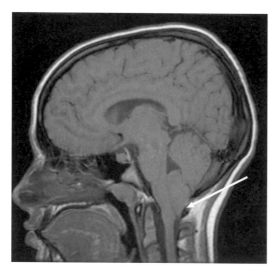

Fig. 4.37 Sagittal T1-weighted MRI in a patient with a Chiari I malformation. The low-lying cerebellar tonsils are clearly seen (*arrow*) to extend below the level of C1.

jugulare). A glomus tympanicum is usually diagnosed and treated before it erodes into the inner ear. The endochondral bone of the inner ear provides an effective barrier. Glomus jugulare tumors are often not diagnosed as early, and consequently, it is more common for them to erode into the lateral or posterior semicircular canal or the internal auditory canal and cause balance dysfunction. Computed tomography and MRI are both useful in evaluating these lesions. If the middle ear examination suggests a tumor, then a CT is the first imaging test obtained. If CT clearly shows the tumor to be limited to the middle ear (glomus tympanicum), then the MRI is not needed (**Fig. 4.38**). If the middle ear tumor might represent an extension from a glomus jugulare, then an MRI is obtained, including MRA and MRV sequences.

Computed tomography is particularly well suited for evaluation of the bony destruction and demineralization associated with paraganglioma, and MRI provides a nice evaluation of the soft tissue mass itself (**Fig. 4.39**). Contrast enhancement often provides additional value in detecting and defining the extent of the tumors. On MRI, the lesions demonstrate a heterogeneous signal pattern, with predominately low T1 and high T2 signal. Glomus tumors often demonstrate a "salt-and-pepper" appearance related to their increased vascularity and flow voids. Although MRA is not sensitive enough to demonstrate the vascularity of these tumors, DSA demonstrates a highly vascular lesion with tumor blush (**Fig. 4.40**).

Glomus tumors can be bilateral and associated with carotid body tumors as well. In this regard, close scrutiny of the middle ears and jugular foramina should be undertaken in any patient with a carotid body tumor to evaluate for synchronous lesions.

Hemangiomas can affect the facial nerve, middle ear, and IAC. They typically cause balance problems by eroding into the inner ear in the region of the geniculate ganglion or by involving the vestibular nerves in the IAC. Hemangiomas tend to be small at the time of diagnosis. Magnetic resonance imaging with contrast provides the best evaluation of the tumor itself, although CT can be useful in assessing secondary findings of "honeycomb" bony erosion and expansion.[31] As with most hemangiomas in the body, they generally demonstrate markedly increased T2 signal and enhancement. It can be difficult to differentiate a hemangioma from a facial nerve schwannoma, but it is absolutely critical from a treatment standpoint. High-quality CT and MRI studies in conjunction with history and physical examination findings will almost always result in the correct diagnosis, allowing surgery to be performed only on those in whom it is indicated.

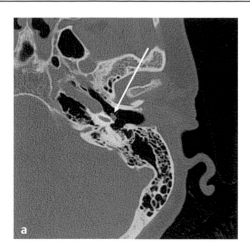

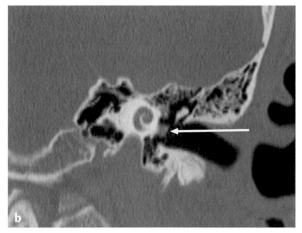

Fig. 4.38 **(a)** High-resolution axial and **(b)** coronal CT images demonstrate a small soft tissue mass (*arrows*) abutting the left cochlear promontory in this patient with a glomus tympanicum tumor.

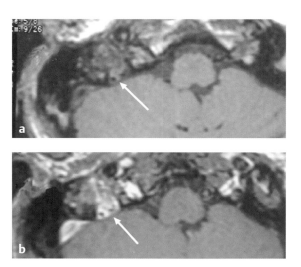

Fig. 4.39 **(a)** Axial precontrast and **(b)** postcontrast T1-weighted images demonstrate heterogeneous signal and enhancement of a right glomus jugulare tumor (*arrows*).

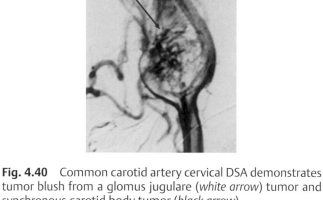

Fig. 4.40 Common carotid artery cervical DSA demonstrates tumor blush from a glomus jugulare (*white arrow*) tumor and synchronous carotid body tumor (*black arrow*).

Labyrinthine schwannomas (true "vestibular schwannomas") are the most common benign neoplasms of the labyrinth.[32] These tumors can involve the cochlea or vestibule and can occur in isolation or with an associated schwannoma of the IAC. High-resolution T2-weighted and contrast-enhanced MRI is much more sensitive to early labyrinthine schwannomas than CT (**Fig. 4.41**).[32,33] Labyrinthine schwannomas can be differentiated from labyrinthitis based on clinical findings and follow-up imaging, which demonstrates tumor growth.

Benign tumors of the cerebellopontine angle (CPA) include vestibular schwannomas, meningiomas, and epidermoid cysts. Magnetic resonance imaging is the study of choice for CPA tumors, and although CT may more clearly demonstrate expansion of the IAC or hyperostosis of the temporal bone, these findings can also be recognized on MRI. The tumors can cause dizziness or balance problems through injury to the vestibular nerves, interruption of the blood supply to the inner ear, or compression of the brainstem and cerebellum.

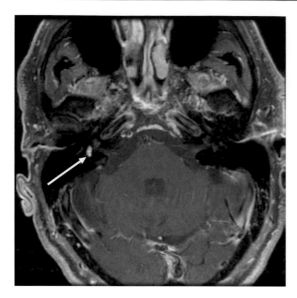

Fig. 4.41 Three Tesla axial postcontrast MRI examination in a patient with a right intralabyrinthine schwannoma. Notice the abnormal enhancement within the right vestibule (*arrow*) compared with the normal left side.

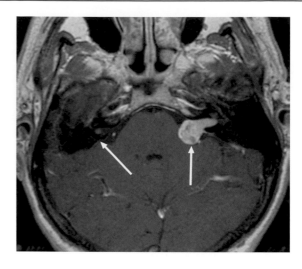

Fig. 4.42 Postcontrast axial T1-weighted MRI shows a vestibular schwannoma on the left filling the internal auditory canal and cerebellopontine angle (*right arrow*). A tiny contralateral intracanalicular schwannoma (*left arrow*) is seen on the right in this patient with neurofibromatosis (NF2).

Schwannomas arise from the vestibular, acoustic, facial, and trigeminal nerves, with at least 90% affecting the vestibular nerve. *Vestibular schwannomas* generally begin in the IAC and subsequently enlarge and extend into the CPA (**Fig. 4.42**). They are characterized by intense contrast enhancement and increased T2 signal. Larger schwannomas can have non-enhancing cystic areas within them (**Fig. 4.43**).

High-resolution heavily T2-weighted images of the IAC often allow determination of the exact nerve of origin in small lesions and can be used as a screening exam for vestibular schwannomas. How-

ever, as the tumor enlarges to fill the IAC, the nerve of origin can no longer be determined.[3] T2-weighted sequences can also depict the presence of fluid between the tumor and the fundus of the IAC. The presence of fluid between the tumor and the fundus of the IAC has prognostic implications and allows for appropriate surgical planning.[34]

The imaging appearance of *meningiomas* can overlap with schwannomas (**Fig. 4.44**). Meningiomas can involve the IAC and CPA and have intense enhancement. However, the presence of a "dural tail" and hyperostosis, along with the lack of IAC expansion,

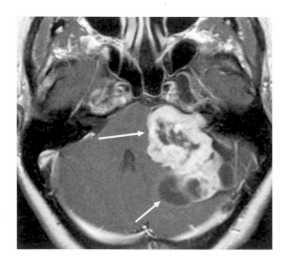

Fig. 4.43 Postcontrast axial T1-weighted MRI shows a large left vestibular schwannoma with cystic non-enhancing areas (*arrows*).

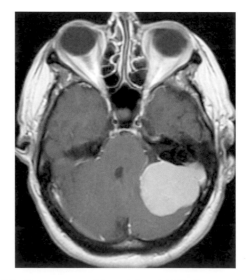

Fig. 4.44 Postcontrast T1-weighted MRI shows a homogeneously enhancing meningioma in the left CPA.

often allows discrimination between the lesions. Calcification of the tumor is also a feature strongly suggestive of meningioma rather than schwannoma. Whereas vestibular schwannomas do not demonstrate increased vascularity on catheter angiography, meningiomas typically have enlarged dural arterial feeders and prominent tumor blush at angiography.

Epidermoids of the CPA are best characterized with MRI.[35] With CT, these lesions are generally hypodense, similar to CSF density. They tend to slowly enlarge the CPA and displace or encompass the traversing cranial nerves and vessels. With MRI, epidermoids are generally isointense to CSF on T1- and T2-weighted sequences. This characteristic makes it easy to miss smaller tumors. The tumor's presence is essentially inferred, due to the compression and distortion of adjacent structures. Fortunately, FLAIR and proton-density sequences reveal the epidermoid to have slightly different signal intensity than CSF. Epidermoids do not enhance but do show a characteristically marked increase in signal on diffusion-weighted sequences (**Fig. 4.45**). This marked diffusion restriction helps differentiate epidermoids from the similar-appearing arachnoid cyst of the CPA.

Malignant Tumors

Malignant tumors of the ear and temporal bone include squamous cell carcinoma (SCC), rhabdomyosarcoma, metastases, and lymphoma. *Squamous cell carcinoma* is the most common malignant tumor affecting the ear and temporal bone and would most typically affect balance through erosion into the inner ear. Involvement of the middle ear by SCC portends a very poor prognosis and is a late finding.[36] Squamous cell carcinoma demonstrates heterogeneous soft tissue enlargement and enhancement with CT and MRI, with bony destruction seen in advanced cases on CT. Choosing the appropriate treatment requires precise knowledge about the extent of the tumor. Computed tomography and MRI are complementary in providing this information. Both modalities are commonly used with extensive lesions.

Whereas SCC tends to affect older patients, *rhabdomyosarcoma* usually occurs in children and young adults. Heterogeneous signal intensity and enhancement are seen on MRI, with frequent destruction of the skull base.

Metastases to the middle ear and temporal bone most commonly occur from breast, renal, lung, gastric, and prostate carcinomas. Metastatic disease causing dizziness and balance problems presents either as diffuse leptomeningeal spread with involvement of the IACs and vestibular nerve or as direct metastasis to the petrous apex (**Fig. 4.46**). Metastases to the petrous apex result in a heterogeneous destructive lesion with bony fragmentation on CT. Contrast-enhanced MRI often shows an irregular tumor with heterogeneous signal intensity and enhancement. Metastatic disease can produce abnormal enhancement and signal in the leptomeninges and along the cranial nerves. Leptomeningeal metastases are best evaluated with contrast-enhanced MRI, where abnormal linear or nodular enhancement of the basal meninges and cranial nerves occurs. Carcinomatous meningitis must be differentiated from infectious meningitis.

Lymphoma of the temporal bone is rare; however, involvement of the cranial nerves and meninges is not uncommon (**Fig. 4.47**). Leptomeningeal lymphoma can occur, along with parenchymal lymphoma of

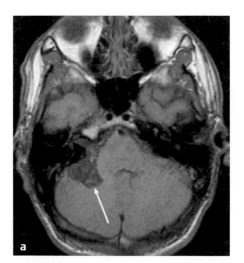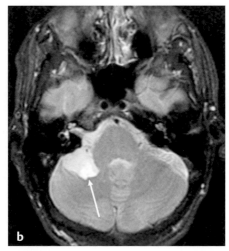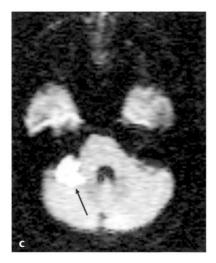

Fig. 4.45 **(a)** Axial T1-weighted MRI without contrast shows a hypointense mass (*arrow*) in the right cerebellopontine angle (CPA). **(b)** T2-weighted MRI demonstrates the mass to be hyperintense (*arrow*). **(c)** Restricted diffusion within the lesion confirms the diagnosis of a CPA epidermoid (*arrow*).

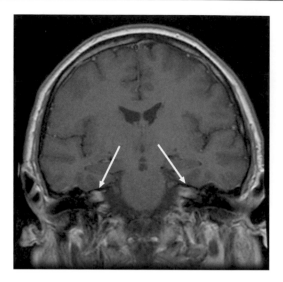

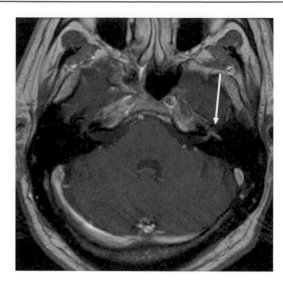

Fig. 4.46 Contrast-enhanced coronal MRI in a patient with metastatic chondrosarcoma demonstrates metastases involving the bilateral internal auditory canals (*arrows*).

Fig. 4.47 Axial postcontrast T1-weighted MRI image shows abnormal enhancement of the distal left internal auditory canal and facial nerve (*arrow*) in this patient with lymphoma.

the brain and brainstem. Lymphoma can demonstrate any density or signal intensity with CT and MRI, respectively. A clue to the diagnosis is increased density with noncontrast CT and decreased T2 signal with MRI. Lymphoma typically shows robust contrast enhancement.

Endolymphatic sac tumors are rare lesions that occur most commonly in patients with von Hippel-Lindau (VHL) disease. Endolymphatic sac tumor is a papillary cystic tumor and is generally a low-grade malignancy but variable in its presentation. It is relatively unique to patients with VHL disease. The tumor can be subtle or occult on imaging. Contrast-enhancing lesions in the endolymphatic duct/sac with or without labyrinthine hemorrhage may be seen with MRI, and high-resolution CT can show osseous erosions near the endolymphatic duct (**Fig. 4.48**).[37] If the tumor is identified when very small, it can be surgically removed to preserve hearing; therefore, early recognition is critical.

Malignant lesions of the CNS can present with vestibular symptoms. Intra-axial posterior fossa neoplasms can present with vertigo, ataxia, and disequilibrium. *Brainstem gliomas* demonstrate decreased T1 and increased T2 signal with variable enhancement (**Fig. 4.49**). Higher-grade gliomas tend to produce more contrast enhancement, although histologic grading of the tumor based on imaging findings is somewhat imprecise. Typically, an ill-defined lesion with increased T2 signal and expansion of the brainstem will be seen. Tumors of the posterior fossa, such as medulloblastoma, choroid plexus papilloma, ependymoma, and teratoma, can also be seen.

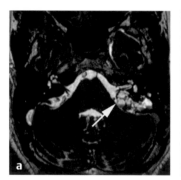

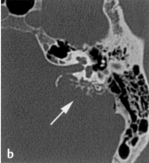

Fig. 4.48 **(a)** FSE 3D T2-weighted image demonstrates retrolabyrinthine multiloculated cystic mass with blood–fluid levels (*arrow*) characteristic of endolymphatic sac tumor. **(b)** High-resolution axial CT through the left temporal bone demonstrates associated bony destruction (*arrow*).

Medulloblastomas occur in children, arise near the midline, and invade or obstruct the fourth ventricle. The lesions typically enhance avidly and are sometimes increased in density with noncontrast CT. *Choroid plexus papillomas* of the fourth ventricle are more common in adults and result in overproduction of CSF, with resultant hydrocephalus. The tumor is often heterogeneous on MRI, with predominantly increased T2 signal. *Ependymomas* arise from the ependymal surface of the fourth ventricle (**Fig. 4.50**). This lesion can calcify and often extends through the foramina of Luschka and Magendie. Ependymomas enhance dramatically and often contain areas of

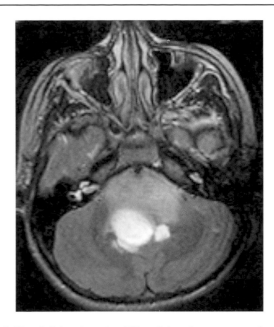

Fig. 4.49 Axial spin-echo T2-weighted sequence demonstrates a heterogeneous lesion in the pons corresponding to a brainstem glioblastoma multiforme.

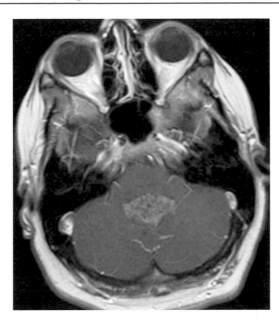

Fig. 4.50 A heterogeneous mass centered in the fourth ventricle demonstrates enhancement on postcontrast T1-weighted images in this patient with an ependymoma.

hemorrhage. *Teratomas* have characteristic imaging features, such as the inclusion of fat, bone, and soft tissue, which can be identified with CT and/or MRI.

Vascular Diseases

Posterior fossa infarction can involve the brainstem and cerebellum. Magnetic resonance imaging is recommended in evaluation of posterior fossa infarction because of the skull-base artifacts present on CT. Acute and subacute infarction is best seen with diffusion-weighted imaging as areas of restricted diffusion (**Fig. 4.51**). As an infarct progresses, MRI can also be used to evaluate for complications related to herniation or mass effect. In young patients with acute onset of symptoms, *vertebral artery dissection* should be entertained. Dissections can be evaluated with MRI, MRA, and computed tomography angiography (CTA) of the neck and posterior fossa (**Fig. 4.52**). With newer multislice scanning techniques, CTA is proving useful in the triage of patients with suspected vertebral artery dissection. It is essential that CTA include multiplanar reformatted images that can be processed on a 3D workstation for added sensitivity. In the chronic stages, infarcts demonstrate atrophy and increased T2 signal in the affected distribution (**Fig. 4.53**).

The *lateral medullary infarct* produces a classic set of findings, including ipsilateral Horner syndrome, loss of contralateral body pain and temperature sensation, loss of ipsilateral facial pain and temperature

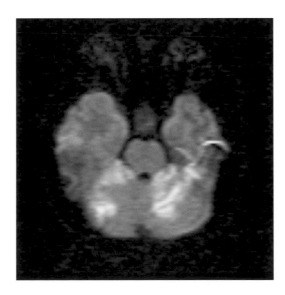

Fig. 4.51 Diffusion-weighted MRI shows bilateral cerebellar infarcts in this patient with an acute vertebral artery dissection.

sensation, paralysis of the ipsilateral palate, ipsilateral facial weakness, vertigo, nausea, hiccupping, diplopia, dysphagia, and facial pain. Occlusion of the ipsilateral vertebral artery or posterior inferior cerebellar artery is the cause. Infarction involving the *anterior inferior cerebellar artery* (AICA) can also occur. The *labyrinthine artery* usually arises from the AICA and, as a result, can result in infarct of the

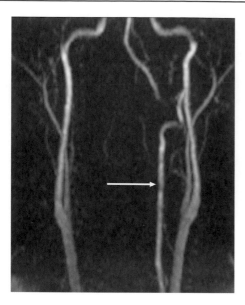

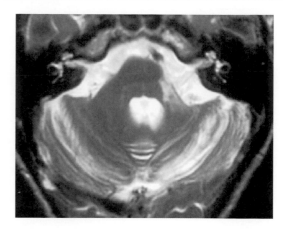

Fig. 4.53 Increased T2 signal and atrophy are seen in the left pons and brachium pontis in this patient with a remote infarct.

Fig. 4.52 Two-dimensional TOF MRI shows no flow-related signal in the right vertebral artery. Normal signal is seen in the left vertebral artery (*arrow*).

membranous labyrinth. The AICA infarct pattern can produce symptoms similar to those of a lateral medullary infarct but can also include ipsilateral hearing loss due to infarction of the cochlear nuclei and cochlear nerve entry zone.

Vertebrobasilar insufficiency (VBI) and transient ischemic attacks (TIAs) can cause vertigo or vestibular symptoms. Atherosclerotic disease is the most common cause of VBI, with other causes including hypercoagulation, dissection, arteritides, and central emboli. Atherosclerotic narrowing of the subclavian, vertebral, and basilar arteries is often discovered.[38] Magnetic resonance angiography is now the most common modality initially used to evaluate suspected VBI. With the recent advances in CTA, this modality is increasingly used to investigate posterior fossa vascular stenoses (**Fig. 4.54**).

Although the risk of catheter angiography is quite low, noninvasive techniques, such as MRI and CTA, have generally replaced this technique as first-line imaging of VBI. However, catheter angiography remains the gold standard and is still used for evaluation of difficult or ambiguous cases. Furthermore, stenotic lesions of the vertebrobasilar system are often amenable to percutaneous angioplasty or stenting, which can be performed at the time of angiography.

Posterior fossa hemorrhages can occur for many reasons. Hypertension, bleeding diatheses, vascular malformations, and anticoagulant therapy are the most common causes. Hemorrhage into the posterior fossa typically produces acute onset of signifi-

cant symptoms, including vertigo, nausea, vomiting, ataxia, and headache. Posterior fossa hemorrhage can progress rapidly to coma and death; therefore, fast and accurate diagnosis is necessary. Surgical posterior fossa decompression is often a lifesaving intervention. Cases of suspected posterior fossa hemorrhage initially should be imaged with noncontrast CT. Magnetic resonance imaging can also be used to identify the hemorrhage but often takes more time and is not readily available after hours.

Vascular malformations can affect the posterior fossa and result in vestibular symptoms or intracranial hemorrhage. *Dural arteriovenous fistulae* (dAVFs) are relatively common and can result in hemorrhage, headache, and pulsatile tinnitus. These lesions result from multiple arteriovenous shunts within the dura of the dural venous sinuses. Often, coexistent stenosis or thrombosis of the involved dural venous sinus is noted. The most common location is in the region of the transverse and sigmoid sinuses. These lesions can have a benign course without significant

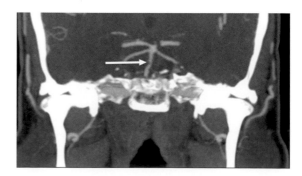

Fig. 4.54 Coronal reformat from a CTA of the head demonstrates a stenosis in the mid basilar artery (*arrow*).

sequelae. However, cortical venous drainage and venous hypertension increase the risk for subsequent intracranial hemorrhage. The arterial supply to the dAVF is primarily from external carotid artery vessels that supply the dura, although feeders from the internal carotid and vertebral arteries can be encountered (**Fig. 4.55**).

Magnetic resonance imaging and MRA often demonstrate abnormal prominent vessels leading to the abnormal dural sinus. However, catheter angiography is critical to accurately define the extent of dural sinus involvement, presence of cortical venous drainage, and arterial supply to the fistula. Catheter angiography is often performed prior to endovascular treatment of the lesions. Packing the involved dural sinus with coils often results in a cure of the lesion and halts the ominous cortical venous drainage. In cases where stereotactic radiosurgery is performed, arterial embolization of the feeding arterial vessels can supply short-term relief from tinnitus until the permanent effects of radiosurgery take place. *Brainstem cavernous malformations* are not uncommon and can present with symptoms of mass effect or acute hemorrhage. Gradient-echo MRI sequences demonstrate areas of markedly decreased signal related to hemosiderin deposition (**Fig. 4.56**).

Patients with sensorineural hearing loss (SNHL) and vertigo may have *neurovascular conflicts.* Symptomatic neurovascular conflicts result from compression of the vestibulocochlear nerve at its root entry zone by arteries or veins. Because asymptomatic patients often have small vessels in the region of the CPA and IAC, clinical and imaging correlation is

necessary to prove causation prior to surgical intervention. The presence of an artery traversing the nerve perpendicularly, with associated mass effect, increases the likelihood that it is the cause of symptoms. The presence of such lesions is best demonstrated on MRI and MRA, where both nerves and vessels can be depicted on the same images.[3]

Acquired Central Nervous System Lesions

Several acquired lesions of the CNS can present with vestibular symptoms. Multiple sclerosis, superficial siderosis, intracranial hypotension, and cerebellar degeneration can all be accurately evaluated with MRI. The cause and appearance of these lesions are quite varied, but each entity has characteristic imaging findings that often lead to the appropriate diagnosis.

Multiple sclerosis is characterized by demyelination of the CNS and is best evaluated with MRI. Demyelinating plaques can occur in the brainstem, cerebellum, and cerebral hemispheres, and at the root entry zone of cranial nerves. Magnetic resonance imaging typically shows foci of abnormal increased T2 and FLAIR signal in the periventricular white matter, brachium pontis, and brainstem (**Fig. 4.57**). Acute plaques often demonstrate contrast enhancement, and chronic plaques can show foci of decreased T1 signal. Multiple sclerosis also commonly affects the optic nerves and cervical spinal cord; therefore, evaluation of these structures is important in suspected cases of multiple sclerosis.

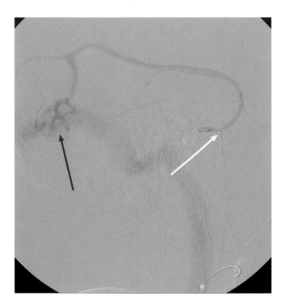

Fig. 4.55 Lateral projection superselective angiogram through a microcatheter in the middle meningeal artery (*black arrow*). A dural arteriovenous fistula (dAVF) (*white arrow*) involving the transverse sinus is clearly seen.

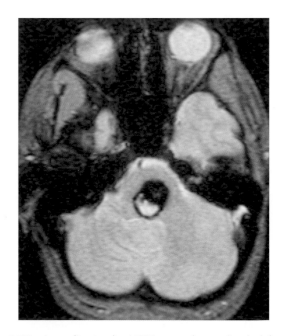

Fig. 4.56 A gradient-echo MRI image shows the dark hemosiderin rim, which is characteristic of cavernous angiomas.

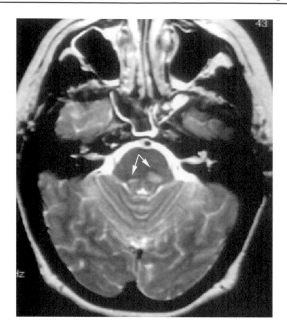

Fig. 4.57 Axial FSE T2-weighted sequence shows two foci of abnormal increased signal (*arrows*) in the brainstem due to multiple sclerosis.

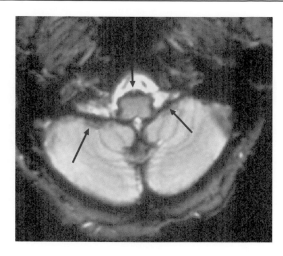

Fig. 4.58 Gradient-echo magnetic resonance image demonstrates the smooth outline of decreased signal (*arrows*) along the medulla and cerebellum in this patient with superficial siderosis.

Superficial siderosis results from the deposition of hemosiderin along the pial surface of the spinal cord, brainstem, cerebellum, and basal cisterns. Magnetic resonance imaging depicts this entity nicely with a thin, smooth coating of the pial surfaces by a band of marked hypointensity on T2 and gradient-echo images (**Fig. 4.58**).[39] Hemosiderin deposition along the nerves traversing the IAC and exiting the brainstem can result in hearing loss and vestibular symptoms. There are several causes of superficial siderosis, including trauma, surgery, aneurysm, and tumors. Subarachnoid hemorrhage from multiple episodes of bleeding is the usual cause. This can be due to an intracranial aneurysm or hemorrhagic tumor of the spinal cord. Consequently, imaging of the entire neuraxis is indicated when there is unexplained superficial siderosis.

Intracranial hypotension can present with vestibular symptoms that are accompanied by severe positional headaches. Patients often have CSF leaks, which result in "sagging" of the brain and brainstem. Associated enhancement of the dura is often encountered on contrast-enhanced MRI, along with crowding of the foramen magnum and descent of the brainstem (**Fig. 4.59**). The cause is usually iatrogenic, although spontaneous and traumatic causes are not unusual. Diagnosis of the site of CSF leak is important because blood patch or other reconstructive procedures in the sinuses or temporal bone can provide substantial relief or cure. Detection of the

CSF leak can be performed with myelography, MRI, or radioisotope myelocisternography.[40]

The *cerebellar degeneration syndromes* are a diverse group of disorders that include chronic alcohol abuse and familial ataxia syndromes. Cerebellar degeneration related to chronic alcohol ingestion typically produces marked anterior vermian atrophy. The typical vermian atrophy is evident on CT, although MRI allows for much more exquisite anatomic detail, due to the multiplanar capabilities. The familial cerebellar degeneration syndromes can present with vestibular symptoms, although ataxia is a more common finding. The presence of a positive family history, combined with cerebellar and brainstem atrophy on MRI, usually clinches the diagnosis.

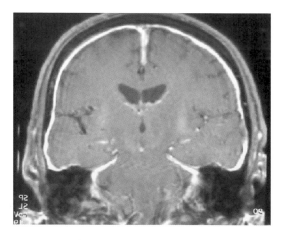

Fig. 4.59 Coronal postcontrast T1-weighted magnetic resonance image reveals thickening and enhancement of the dura in a patient with intracranial hypotension.

Osseous Lesions of the Temporal Bone

Fibrous dysplasia, otosclerosis, superior semicircular canal dehiscence, and Paget disease can involve the temporal bone and result in middle and inner ear abnormalities. These lesions are generally best characterized with CT, where the bony matrix can be evaluated. *Fibrous dysplasia* is often unilateral and produces a classic expanded bone with a ground-glass appearance on CT imaging (**Fig. 4.60**). There is wide variation in the degree of enhancement depending on the vascularity of the tumor. The bony expansion seen in fibrous dysplasia can result in narrowing of the IAC and membranous labyrinth.

Otosclerosis can be fenestral or retrofenestral (cochlear otosclerosis). Endochondral bone is replaced by less dense, spongy irregular bone, often bilaterally.[41] As the disease progresses, vascular spongy bone is replaced with more dense and sclerotic bone. The fenestral subtype involves the lateral wall of the labyrinth and results in only a conductive hearing loss, due to fixation of the footplate of the stapes. Cochlear otosclerosis, on the other hand, involves the otic capsule and results in SNHL and vestibular symptoms. Computed tomography is the imaging modality of choice and demonstrates decreased density of the demineralized bone early in the course of the disease. With MRI, the vascular demineralized bone generally shows avid contrast enhancement.[42] As the disease progresses and the bone becomes more sclerotic, contrast enhancement on MRI will cease, and CT is required to depict the areas of increased density (**Fig. 4.61**).

Dehiscence of the superior semicircular canal (SSC) is a relatively recently discovered, and important to recognize, entity. The diagnosis is suggested by the patient's history and is confirmed with vestibular testing and imaging. The Tullio phenomenon is the presence of dizziness caused by sound and is often associated with dehiscence of the SSC.[43] Computed tomography reveals absence of the bony covering of the SSC (**Figs. 4.62**). Identifying a true dehiscence from a very thin layer of bone can be an imaging challenge. Being able to reorient the volumetric images obtained on the 64-slice CT scanner to show the SSC in its entirety is quite helpful (**Fig. 4.63**).

It is important to remember that what appears to be a true dehiscence may simply represent the limits of our resolution abilities and be misleading. Computed tomography scans can lead to false-positive findings but not false-negative. Lastly, there are also cases of posterior semicircular canal dehiscence.

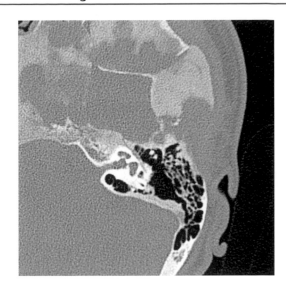

Fig. 4.60 Computed tomography of the left temporal bone shows expansion of bone with a ground-glass matrix in this patient with fibrous dysplasia.

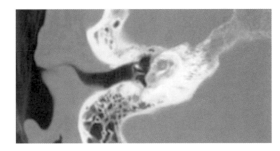

Fig. 4.61 Axial CT demonstrates abnormal otospongiosis of the cochlea in this patient with retrofenestral (cochlear) otosclerosis.

Paget disease can affect the skull base and temporal bone. There is generally expansion of the involved bone. When imaged with MRI, areas of increased T1 signal corresponding with areas of focal fat may be seen. Fibrovascular marrow may manifest as areas of increased T2 signal. Although generally best imaged with CT, basilar invagination is nicely depicted on MRI, and it can be associated with Paget disease of the skull base.[44] Dizziness most often results from progressive IAC stenosis. Surgical decompression of the IAC is beneficial in preserving cochlear and vestibular function and needs to be performed prior to loss of function.

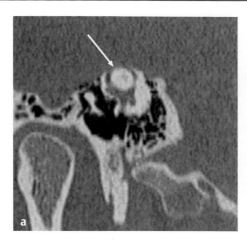
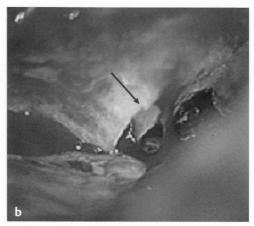

Fig. 4.62 **(a)** High-resolution oblique CT reformat shows absence of the bony covering of the superior semicircular canal (*arrow*). **(b)** Intraoperative image of the floor of the middle cranial fossa after elevation of the dura over the arcuate eminence shows a widely patent superior semicircular canal (*arrow*).

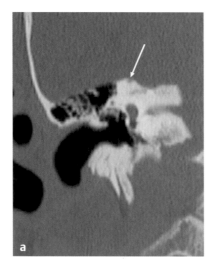
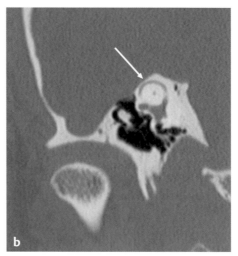

Fig. 4.63 **(a)** A routine coronal CT image reveals a possible superior semicircular canal (SSC) dehiscence (*arrow*). **(b)** However, an oblique reconstruction in the plane of the SSC in the same patient demonstrates a thin bony plate (*arrow*) over the canal without a dehiscence.

References

1. Carlson ML, Neff BA, Link MJ, et al. Magnetic resonance imaging with cochlear implant magnet in place: safety and imaging quality. Otol Neurotol 2015; 36(6):965–971

2. Martin ET, Coman JA, Shellock FG, Pulling CC, Fair R, Jenkins K. Magnetic resonance imaging and cardiac pacemaker safety at 1.5-Tesla. J Am Coll Cardiol 2004;43(7):1315–1324

3. Mark A, Casselman J. Anatomy and diseases of the temporal bone. In: Atlas SW, ed. Magnetic Resonance Imaging of the Brain and Spine. Philadelphia, PA: Lippincott Williams & Wilkins; 2002:1363–1342

4. Kocharian A, Lane JI, Bernstein MA, et al. Hybrid phased array for improved internal auditory canal imaging at 3.0-T MR. J Magn Reson Imaging 2002;16(3):300–304

5. Baráth K, Schuknecht B, Naldi AM, Schrepfer T, Bockisch CJ, Hegemann SC. Detection and grading of endolymphatic hydrops in Ménière disease using MR imaging. AJNR Am J Neuroradiol 2014;35(7):1387–1392

6. Nakada T, Yoshida T, Suga K, et al. Endolymphatic space size in patients with vestibular migraine and Ménière's disease. J Neurol 2014;261(11):2079–2084

7. Schubiger O, Valavanis A, Stuckmann G, Antonucci F. Temporal bone fractures and their complications. Examination with high resolution CT. Neuroradiology 1986;28(2):93–99

8. Zimmerman RA, Bilaniuk LT, Hackney DB, Goldberg HI, Grossman RI. Magnetic resonance imaging in temporal bone fracture. Neuroradiology 1987;29(3):246–251

9. Ishman SL, Friedland DR. Temporal bone fractures: traditional classification and clinical relevance. Laryngoscope 2004;114(10):1734–1741

10. Fisch U. Facial paralysis in fractures of the petrous bone. Laryngoscope 1974;84(12):2141–2154

11. Aguilar EA III, Yeakley JW, Ghorayeb BY, Hauser M, Cabrera J, Jahrsdoerfer RA. High resolution CT scan of temporal bone fractures: association of facial nerve paralysis with temporal bone fractures. Head Neck Surg 1987;9(3):162–166

12. Gentry LR. Temporal bone trauma: current perspective for diagnostic evaluation. Neuroimaging Clin N Am 1991;1:319–340

13. Holliday RA, Reede DL. MRI of mastoid and middle ear disease. Radiol Clin North Am 1989;27(2):283–299

14. Mafee MF, Singleton EL, Valvassori GE, Espinosa GA, Kumar A, Aimi K. Acute otomastoiditis and its complications: role of CT. Radiology 1985;155(2):391–397

15. Garber LZ, Dort JC. Cholesteatoma: diagnosis and staging by CT scan. J Otolaryngol 1994;23(2):121–124

16. Stasolla A, Magliulo G, Parrotto D, Luppi G, Marini M. Detection of postoperative relapsing/residual cholesteatomas with diffusion-weighted echo-planar magnetic resonance imaging. Otol Neurotol 2004;25(6):879–884

17. Más-Estellés F, Mateos-Fernández M, Carrascosa-Bisquert B, Facal de Castro F, Puchades-Román I, Morera-Pérez C. Contemporary non-echo-planar diffusion-weighted imaging of middle ear cholesteatomas. Radiographics 2012;32(4):1197–1213

18. Schwartz KM, Lane JI, Bolster BD Jr, Neff BA. The utility of diffusion-weighted imaging for cholesteatoma evaluation. AJNR Am J Neuroradiol 2011;32(3):430–436

19. Silver AJ, Janecka I, Wazen J, Hilal SK, Rutledge JN. Complicated cholesteatomas: CT findings in inner ear complications of middle ear cholesteatomas. Radiology 1987;164(1):47–51

20. Chang P, Fagan PA, Atlas MD, Roche J. Imaging destructive lesions of the petrous apex. Laryngoscope 1998;108(4 Pt 1):599–604

21. Seltzer S, Mark AS, Atlas SW. CNS sarcoidosis: evaluation with contrast-enhanced MR imaging. AJNR Am J Neuroradiol 1991;12(6):1227–1233

22. Seltzer S, Mark AS. Contrast enhancement of the labyrinth on MR scans in patients with sudden hearing loss and vertigo: evidence of labyrinthine disease. AJNR Am J Neuroradiol 1991;12(1):13–16

23. Schuknecht H. Infections of the inner ear. In: Schuknecht H, ed. Pathology of the Ear. Philadelphia, PA: Lea and Febiger; 1993:248–253

24. Anderson JM, Stevens JC, Sundt TM Jr, Stockard JJ, Pearson BW. Ectopic internal carotid artery seen initially as middle ear tumor. JAMA 1983;249(16):2228–2230

25. Ford KL III. Aunt Minnie's corner. High-riding jugular bulb. J Comput Assist Tomogr 1998;22(3):508

26. Jackler RK, Luxford WM, House WF. Congenital malformations of the inner ear: a classification based on embryogenesis. Laryngoscope 1987;97(3 Pt 2, Suppl 40): 2–14

27. Hasso AN, Broadwell RE. The temporal bone: congenital anomalies. In: Som P, Bergerton R, eds. Head and Neck Imaging. St Louis, MO: Mosby-Year Book; 1991:960–992

28. Valvassori GE, Clemis JD. The large vestibular aqueduct syndrome. Laryngoscope 1978;88(5):723–728

29. Schuknecht HF, Gulya AJ. Endolymphatic hydrops. An overview and classification. Ann Otol Rhinol Laryngol Suppl 1983;106:1–20

30. Fitzgerald DC, Mark AS. Endolymphatic duct/sac enhancement on gadolinium magnetic resonance imaging of the inner ear: preliminary observations and case reports. Am J Otol 1996;17(4):603–606

31. Lo WW, Shelton C, Waluch V, et al. Intratemporal vascular tumors: detection with CT and MR imaging. Radiology 1989;171(2):445–448

32. Green JD Jr, McKenzie JD. Diagnosis and management of intralabyrinthine schwannomas. Laryngoscope 1999;109(10):1626–1631

33. Mafee MF, Lachenauer CS, Kumar A, Arnold PM, Buckingham RA, Valvassori GECT. CT and MR imaging of intralabyrinthine schwannoma: report of two cases and review of the literature. Radiology 1990;174(2):395–400

34. Somers T, Casselman J, de Ceulaer G, Govaerts P, Offeciers E. Prognostic value of magnetic resonance imaging findings in hearing preservation surgery for vestibular schwannoma. Otol Neurotol 2001;22(1):87–94

35. Dutt SN, Mirza S, Chavda SV, Irving RM. Radiologic differentiation of intracranial epidermoids from arachnoid cysts. Otol Neurotol 2002;23(1):84–92

36. Stell PM, McCormick MS. Carcinoma of the external auditory meatus and middle ear. Prognostic factors and a suggested staging system. J Laryngol Otol 1985;99(9):847–850

37. Lonser RR, Kim HJ, Butman JA, Vortmeyer AO, Choo DI, Oldfield EH. Tumors of the endolymphatic sac in von Hippel-Lindau disease. N Engl J Med 2004; 350(24):2481–2486

38. Caplan LR. Brain embolism, revisited. Neurology 1993;43(7):1281–1287

39. Kobayashi T, Watanabe F, Gyo K, Miki H. Superficial siderosis of the central nervous system. Otol Neurotol 2004;25(2):193–194

40. Chiapparini L, Ciceri E, Nappini S, et al. Headache and intracranial hypotension: neuroradiological findings. Neurol Sci 2004;25(Suppl 3):S138–S141

41. Wiet RJ, Raslan W, Shambaugh GE Jr. Otosclerosis 1981 to 1985. Our four-year review and current perspective. Am J Otol 1986;7(3):221–228

42. Mark AS, Seltzer S, Harnsberger HR. Sensorineural hearing loss: more than meets the eye? AJNR Am J Neuroradiol 1993;14(1):37–45

43. Ostrowski VB, Byskosh A, Hain TC. Tullio phenomenon with dehiscence of the superior semicircular canal. Otol Neurotol 2001;22(1):61–65

44. Harnsberger H. Handbook of Head and Neck Imaging, 2nd ed. St Louis, MO: Mosby-Year Book; 1995

5 Surgical Anatomy and Physiology of the Vestibular System

Douglas D. Backous and Francois Cloutier

■ Introduction

The central and peripheral vestibular organs, in conjunction with the visual and somatosensory systems, are responsible for balance, equilibrium, and orientation in space. The vestibular apparatus of each inner ear has the three orthogonally related semicircular canals (SCCs), as well as the utricle and the saccule (together known as the otolithic organs). The SCCs sense rotational or angular acceleration of the head, while the otolithic organs are responsible for sensing linear motion of the head in the anterior-posterior, superior-inferior, and side-to-side planes. The three main vestibular reflexes are the vestibulospinal reflex, the vestibulocolic reflex, and the vestibulo-ocular reflex (VOR). The VOR is the most well studied of the three and is discussed most thoroughly in this chapter. Our goal is to provide the reader with a practical review of the surgical anatomy and physiology of the vestibular system to provide a framework for clinical examination and understanding disease processes affecting balance.

■ Anatomy

The Peripheral Vestibular Organs

The vestibular end-organs are located within the confines of the bony labyrinth in the petrous portion of the temporal bone. The utricle and the saccule, contained within the vestibule, are located lateral to the fundus of the internal auditory canal. The SCCs are located posterior to the vestibule, roughly medial to the aditus ad antrum and the mastoid air cells. The bony labyrinth contains the endolymph-containing membranous portion (scala tympani and scala vestibuli), which is surrounded by perilymph. The endolymphatic space of the membranous labyrinth is in continuity with the endolymph-containing scala media of the cochlea via the ductus reuniens (**Fig. 5.1**).

The Semicircular Canals (SCCs)

The three SCCs, situated posterior to the vestibule, are arranged orthogonally (at right angles to each other). Thus a plane drawn through the long axis of the horizontal (lateral) canal lies nearly perpendicular to a plane through both the superior (anterior) and the posterior canals. The posterior and superior canals unite in their posteromedial aspect to form the crus commune.

The ampullated end of each canal is where the neurophysiologically active structures are located. The crista ampullaris is a ridge within the ampulla of each canal that contains the vestibular hair cells, supporting cells, nerve endings, and the blood supply to these structures. The crista is oriented perpendicular to the axis of the canal, which is important physiologically (details below). The cilia of the vestibular hair cells of the crista are suspended in a gelatinous matrix known as the cupula, which stretches to the opposite wall of the ampulla, creating a sealed-off chamber in each canal. The hair cells are polarized in such a fashion that all the kinocilia are oriented in the same direction (**Fig. 5.2**). The gelatinous matrix of the cupula has a specific gravity of ~ 1, close to the specific gravity of the endolymph.[1]

In relation to the contralateral inner ear, the canals are arranged in functional pairs, so that motion that activates one canal will inhibit the contralateral member of the functional pair (**Fig. 5.3**). The two horizontal canals, which are oriented ~ 30° off the Frankfort horizontal, comprise one functional pair. The arrangement of the superior and posterior canals is somewhat more complex. The superior canal of one side is paired functionally with the posterior canal of the contralateral side. Thus these functional pairs are often referred to as the left anterior right posterior (LARP) and the right anterior left posterior (RALP) functional pairs. Each of these functional pairs is oriented roughly 45° off the midsagittal plane, with the plane of each functional pair crossing at approximately right angles. As with the horizontal canals, motion that excites one member of the pair (e.g., the left superior) will inhibit the other member of the pair (the right posterior).

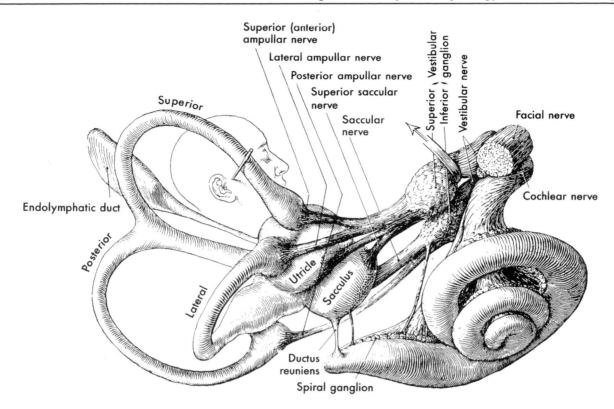

Fig. 5.1 The endolymph-containing membranous labyrinth is bathed in perilymph and is housed within the bony labyrinth. This space is continuous with the endolymph-containing scala media of the cochlea via the ductus reuniens. Used with permission from Bodel M. Three unpublished drawings of the anatomy of the human ear. Philadelphia, PA: W.B. Saunders; 1946.

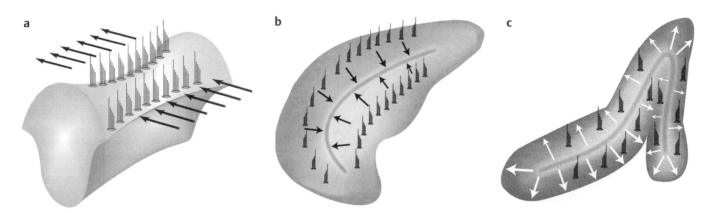

Fig. 5.2 **(a)** The kinocilia and stereocilia of the vestibular hair cells are oriented differently in the cristae than they are in the maculae of the utricle and the saccule. **(b)** In the cristae, the hair cells are polarized all in the same direction, so that a deflection of the cupula produces an excitation or inhibition of all of the hair cells at the same time. **(c)** In the utricle, the hair cells are oriented with the kinocilia toward the striola, whereas in the saccule, the kinocilia are oriented away from the striola. Thus in the maculae, shifts in the otolithic membrane will produce excitation of a portion of the hair cells while simultaneously producing an inhibition of others. Used with permission from Carey JP, Della Santina C. Principles of applied vestibular physiology. In: Cummings CW, ed. Cummings Otolaryngology Head and Neck Surgery. Vol IV. 4th ed. Philadelphia, PA: Elsevier Mosby; 2005:3119, 3121.

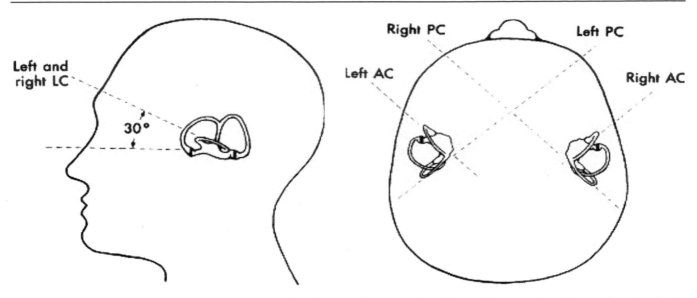

Fig. 5.3 The semicircular canals (SCCs) are arranged in functional pairs, so that the two horizontal canals are a functional pair, whereas the right superior (anterior) canal is paired with the left posterior canal. The two horizontal canals are oriented 30° off the Frankfort horizontal. The RALP and LARP functional pairs are oriented 45° off the mid-sagittal plane. Motion that activates one canal within a functional pair will inhibit its contralateral counterpart. Used with permission from Barber HO, Stockwell CW. Manual of Electronystagmography. St. Louis, MO: Mosby–Year Book; 1976.

The Otolithic Organs

The two otolithic organs are located within the vestibule, the saccule in the medial aspect and the utricle in the posterior superior aspect. Their orientation in space is key to the understanding of their function as sensors of linear motion and head tilt. The maculae of the otolithic organs are analogous functionally to the cristae of the SCCs. The utricular macula is oriented in a nearly horizontal plane, similar to that of the lateral SCC; whereas the saccular macula is oriented in a vertical parasagittal plane. Given these orientations in space, the saccule is designed in such a way that it is responsive to the pull of gravity, craniocaudal motion of the head, and linear acceleration in an anterior-posterior vector. The utricle is oriented nearly horizontally and thus detects head tilt, anterior-posterior acceleration, and lateral motion.

The microstructure of the otolithic organs is somewhat different from that of the cristae ampullares, though their functions are similar. The vestibular hair cells and supporting cells form a sheet of neuroepithelium known as the macula. The cilia of these hair cells are embedded in a trilaminar membrane known as the otolithic membrane. The gel layer is roughly 10 microns in thickness and contains the embedded cilia of the vestibular hair cells. The middle layer of the membrane, also ~ 10 microns thick, is the mesh layer, which is hypothesized to disperse the local shearing forces of the otoconia. The uppermost (otoconial) layer, is ~ 15 microns thick.[2] The otoconia

are calcium salt crystals of varying sizes and shapes that have a density of 2.7 g/mL, twice the specific gravity of endolymph.[2] Near the center of each otolithic membrane is a curvilinear ridge known as the striola. Within the striola, the otoconia are smaller than the surrounding portions of the membrane. Unlike in the cristae, where the kinocilia are polarized all in one direction, the kinocilia of the maculae are oriented around the striola. In the utricle, the kinocilia are oriented toward the striola, whereas in the saccule the kinocilia are oriented away from the striola (see **Fig. 5.2**). Since the striola itself is a curvilinear structure, the hair cells of the maculae are oriented in multiple directions, allowing individual populations of hair cells within each macula to be activated (excited) with a particular motion while others within the same macula are inhibited.

The Internal Auditory Canal (IAC)

The IAC is located within the medial aspect of the petrous portion of the temporal bone, just medial to the vestibule. The IAC, from the porus acusticus medially to the fundus laterally, is oriented in a plane roughly the same as the external auditory canal and contains the seventh and eighth cranial nerve complexes. The facial nerve bundle occupies the anterior superior quadrant of the IAC. In the lateral aspect of the canal near the fundus, the facial nerve is separated from the superior division of the vestibular nerve by the vertical crest (Bill's bar) and the cochlear nerve by the crista transversalis, which also separates the superior and inferior vestibular nerves. Scarpa's ganglia contain cell bodies of the bipolar neurons that make up the vestibular nerves; however, there are no synapses. The anterior inferior cerebellar artery (AICA) arises from the basilar artery next to the junction of the pons and medulla. It runs within the IAC and may be placed between the facial and vestibulocochlear nerve. The labyrinthine artery, which is most commonly a branch of the AICA, is the principal blood supply to the inner ear. A somatic afferent, the nervus intermedius (which contains sensory, special sensory, and parasympathetic fibers) also courses within the IAC adjacent to the facial nerve.

Peripheral Innervation

The superior vestibular nerve provides afferent innervation to the superior SCC, the lateral SCC, and the utricle. The inferior vestibular nerve innervates the posterior SCC and the saccule. The neurons within these nerve bundles are bipolar neurons whose cell bodies lie within Scarpa's ganglia. The nerves project centrally to both the cerebellum and the vestibular nuclei, where they synapse and transmit afferent vestibular inputs and contribute to vestibular reflex pathways.

The vestibular nuclei are located in the pons and the upper portion of the medulla, just lateral to the fourth ventricle. The vestibular nuclear complex is made up of four main nuclei: the superior, lateral, medial (largest), and descending (or inferior) nuclei. Additionally, there are multiple other vestibular nuclei whose roles are more minor and less well understood.

Afferent Projections

The projections from the vestibular nerves to the nuclei are divided into rostral and caudal bundles. The rostral branch projects primarily to the superior and medial vestibular nuclei and the contralateral cerebellum. Caudal fibers project to the medial and descending vestibular nuclei. Additionally there is incoming input from the cerebellar uvula and nodulus, the accessory optic system, and the proprioceptors in the cervical musculature.[3]

There is also spatial orientation of the incoming vestibular input (**Fig. 5.4**). Thus the otolithic organs project primarily to the dorsal portion of the lateral nucleus and the descending (inferior) nucleus. The SCCs project to the superior, medial, and ventral portion of the lateral vestibular nucleus. This is even further divided. The superior SCC projects primarily to the lateral portion of the ipsilateral superior vestibular nucleus, and the horizontal canal projects more

medially within the superior vestibular nucleus. The horizontal SCC is less discriminating and projects to all of the nuclei except the lateral vestibular nucleus. The saccule projects primarily to the ipsilateral lateral nucleus. There is considerable convergence between the SCCs and the otoliths; therefore, one neuron within a nucleus may receive input from several different peripheral end-organs.[3]

An extensive network of second-order commissural projections from the contralateral vestibular nuclei also terminates on the vestibular nuclei. These commissural pathways serve primarily to inhibit second-order vestibular neurons. Thus the stimulation of one second-order vestibular neuron actually serves to indirectly inhibit the second-order neurons on the contralateral side. These commissural pathways originate from all of the vestibular nuclei except the dorsal portion of the lateral vestibular nucleus. Commissural inputs are less intense in the case of saccular input; only 10% of neurons excited by the ipsilateral saccule will be inhibited by commissural input from excitation of the contralateral saccule.

Efferent Projections

Efferent projections from the vestibular nuclei target the occulomotor complex, the spinal cord, the cerebellum, and the cerebral cortex and contribute to the vestibulospinal, vestibulocolic, and vestibulo-ocular reflexes. Their function is to provide input to the muscles involved in postural control and to maintain the head steady in response to changes in the vestibular and visual environments. There is distinct organization of the output of the vestibular nuclei. The main descending outflow tracts from the vestibular nuclei are the medial and lateral vestibulospinal tracts (VST) and the reticulospinal tract. Additionally, a large amount of unnamed output goes to the cerebellum and is important for reflex modulation (**Fig. 5.4**).

The medial and lateral VST are important for the maintenance of head and posture control in response to vestibular and visual input. The medial VST originates in the contralateral medial, superior, and descending vestibular nuclei. The majority of the neurons in this tract originate in the ventral portion of the lateral vestibular nucleus and the medial vestibular nucleus. After crossing the midline, this tract descends in the medial longitudinal fasciculus (MLF) to terminate in the cervical spine, where it provides excitatory inputs to the cervical spinal musculature. This tract mediates postural changes in response to input from the SCCs and plays a role in the cervico-vestibulo-ocular reflexes.

The lateral VST is the main outflow tract involved in the maintenance of antigravity posture in the lower extremities in response to head position changes. It originates primarily from the dorsal por-

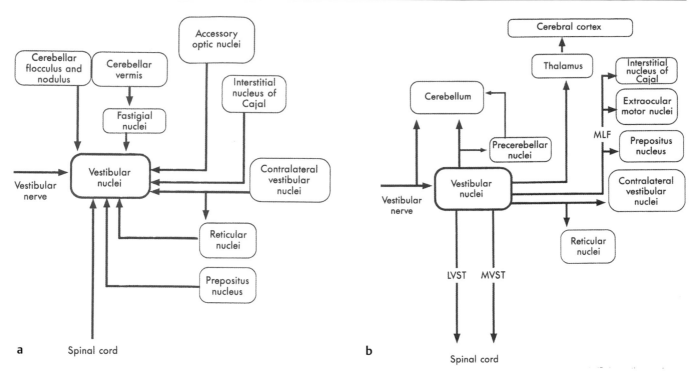

Fig. 5.4 The **(a)** afferent and **(b)** efferent projections of the vestibular nuclei. Used with permission from Lysakowski A. Anatomy of vestibular end organs and neural pathways. In: Cummings CW, ed. Cummings Otolaryngology Head and Neck Surgery. Vol IV. 4th ed. Philadelphia, PA: Elsevier Mosby; 2005:3110.

tion of the lateral vestibular nucleus. The peripheral vestibular input to this portion of the lateral vestibular nucleus is from the otolithic organs and the cerebellum, which explains how the output from the otolithic organs translates into postural control. This tract, unlike the MLF, is an uncrossed descending tract though the spinal cord.

Output from the reticulospinal tract to the cerebellum is important for the vestibular reflexes. The reticulospinal tract contains both crossed and uncrossed fibers. The cerebellum is most important in coordinating the vestibular reflexes, even though it is not part of the actual reflex arc itself. The vestibular output to the nodulus and flocculus reaches the cerebellum mainly through the inferior cerebellar peduncle. The reciprocal input from the cerebellum to the vestibular nuclei is primarily inhibitory in nature.

The vestibulo-ocular reflex (VOR) is important in the maintenance of gaze in response to changes in head position. Both the dorsal and rostral portions of the superior vestibular nuclei are involved in the control of the VOR through projections to the oculomotor nuclei via the MLF. Additionally, there is output from the rostral portion of the medial vestibular nuclei that gives input to the oculomotor nuclei.[3] For details of the VOR, see the section on this reflex in the physiology portion of this chapter.

■ Histology and Cellular Physiology of the Vestibular System

The vestibular hair cells are located within the cristae of the SCCs and the utricular and saccular maculae. There are two types of vestibular hair cells, type I and type II, which are present in a nearly 1:1 ratio within the vestibular end-organs.[4] The hair cells are classified by the type of connection they make with the afferent endplate of the vestibular nerves.

Type I hair cells are surrounded completely by a chalice or calyx type of synaptic ending (**Fig. 5.5**). There are two types of calyx endings, simple and complex. In simple calyx endings, the synaptic endplate surrounds a single type I vestibular hair cell; whereas in complex calyx endings, a synaptic endplate surrounds several nearby type I cells. Recent studies have shown that complex calyx endings are much more common in the central (striolar) region of the macula.[5] Each flask-shaped type I hair cell is associated with a single vestibular nerve endplate. There is no direct efferent innervation of type I cells; rather, the efferent innervation of these hair cells is through indirect contact with the afferent nerve terminals.

Type II hair cells, on the other hand, are more flute- or cylinder-shaped (**Fig. 5.5**). Additionally, these hair cells have connections with several button-type

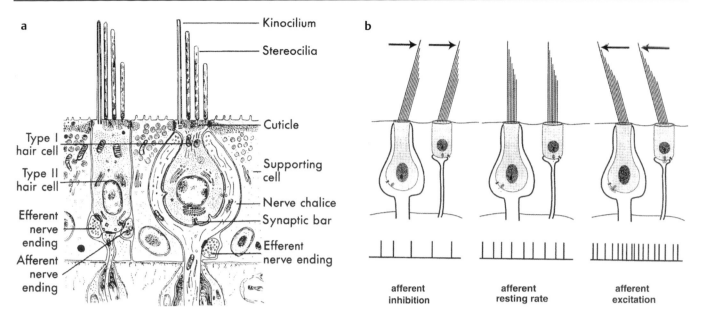

Fig. 5.5 The mammalian vestibular system has two types of vestibular hair cells, type I and type II. **(a)** The type I hair cells are surrounded by a single chalice (calyx) afferent nerve terminal. **(b)** The type II hair cells, however, have button-type synaptic endings with several afferent vestibular nerves. The deflection of the stereocilia toward the kinocilium results in a robust excitation of the hair cell and a resultant increase in the firing rate of the afferent nerves. However, deflection of the stereocilia away from the kinocilium results in inhibition of neurotransmitter release and a slowing of the baseline firing of the afferent nerve.

afferent vestibular nerve endings as well as having direct efferent input from the vestibular nuclei. In the peripheral portion of the macula, the type II cells contact multiple synaptic buttons from multiple nerve cells. In the central striolar portion of the macula, however, there are relatively few synaptic contacts, and each hair cell contacts several synaptic buttons from a small number of vestibular nerve cells.[6,7]

In addition to the vestibular hair cells and the vestibular nerve endings, the maculae and the cristae contain supporting cells. These cells, whose nuclei are located just above the basement membrane, extend from the basement membrane to the apical surface. Each vestibular hair cell is surrounded by several supporting cells. These cells are linked by tight desmosomal junctions that help separate the endolymphatic space from the perilymphatic space. The function of the supporting cells is not well understood, but it is generally felt that they play a role either in the maintenance of the electrolyte composition of the endolymph or in the formation of the cupula and the otolithic membrane.[8] The "dark cells" are separated from the neuroepithelium of the cristae and maculae by a transitional zone.[9] These cells are felt to be important in the production of endolymph due to their structural similarities to the cells of the stria vascularis in the cochlea.

Multiple elongated microvilli, known as stereocilia, occupy the apical ends of both type I and type II vestibular hair cells (**Fig. 5.5**). Although the stereocilia are not true cilia containing dynein arms, each cell contains multiple stereocilia of varying lengths, arranged in a hexagonal pattern around a single longer cilium known as the kinocilium. The kinocilium, in contrast to the stereocilia, is a true cilium with a 9 + 2 arrangement of dynein arms. In the SCCs, the stereocilia and kinocilium of each vestibular hair cell are embedded within the gelatinous matrix of the cupula, which extends to the opposite end of the ampulla. In the otolithic organs, the cilia of the hair cells are embedded in a similar fashion in the gelatinous portion of the otolithic membrane.

Vestibular afferents have a resting firing rate of ~ 80 to 100 Hz.[10] Deflection of the stereocilia toward the kinocilium excites the hair cell. This causes an increase in the release of the neurotransmitter glutamine, and the afferent firing rate increases dramatically. If the stereocilia are deflected away from the kinocilium, then the cell is inhibited, and the firing rate of the vestibular neurons decreases. A basic principle of the vestibular system is that excitatory responses are greater than the inhibitory responses with similar magnitude deflections (**Fig. 5.5**).[11,12]

In each SCC, all the vestibular hair cells are oriented in the same direction along the ridge of the crista. In the lateral (horizontal) canal, these hair cells are oriented so that all the kinocilia are located on the side of the cell nearest the vestibule. In the superior and posterior canals, however, the hair cells are oriented so that the kinocilia are oriented away from the vestibule. Thus, ampullopetal flow of the endolymph (flow toward the ampulla) is excitatory to the horizontal canal, whereas ampullofugal flow (flow away from the ampulla) is excitatory to the superior and posterior canals.[13]

■ Biochemistry of the Endolymph and Perilymph

The ionic makeup of the endolymph and perilymph are very important for the proper function of the vestibular organs. The endolymph has an ionic composition different from any extracellular fluid in the body, resembling intracellular fluid, with high K^+ and low Na^+ concentrations. It has been well established that the cells of the stria vascularis are the source of the endolymph in the scala media of the cochlea. Due to the ultrastructural and immunohistochemical similarities to the cells of the stria vascularis, the "dark cells" of the cristae and maculae have been implicated as the source of the endolymph for the SCCs and the vestibule. Additional research indicates that the cells of the endolymphatic sac contribute to formation and absorption of endolymph. The perilymph is quite different in composition from the endolymph, with high Na^+ and low K^+, much like cerebrospinal fluid and serum. Additionally, perilymph contains β_2-transferrin like CSF. The actual source of perilymph is somewhat more controversial than that of endolymph. Many advocate that CSF is actually an ultrafiltrate of blood serum. There is also some evidence that filtrates of both blood and CSF contribute to the makeup of perilymph.

■ Embryology of the Vestibular System

A comprehensive, detailed description of the embryology of the ear is beyond the scope of this chapter. For more detailed coverage of this subject, please consult more detailed references than the current text.[14,15,16] Inner ear development begins in the third week of gestation and completes its transformation by week 25, with the development of the vestibular end-organs preceding that of the cochlea. Development begins in the third week at the lateral surface of the cephalic embryo between the second and third branchial arches, where the otic placode, an ectodermal derivative, forms. The otic placode invaginates to form the otic pit and eventually the otocyst (otic vesicle) by ~ 30 days' gestation. The otocyst length-

ens and the cranial portion of the vesicle forms the endolymphatic sac, the caudal portion forms the cochlear duct, and the intermediate segment forms the utriculosaccular chamber.[15] The utriculosaccular chamber further subdivides into a utricular chamber, which is the precursor to the utricule and the SCCs, and the saccular chamber, which becomes the saccule and the cochlea.[8,15]

The three SCCs develop as outpouchings from the utricular portion of the utriculosaccular chamber between the sixth and eighth weeks of gestation, beginning as three diverticula that become evident around the fifth week. The superior SCC completes its development by the sixth week of gestation, followed by the posterior canal and finally the lateral canal. It should be noted that the growth rates of the superior and posterior canals are nearly equal, whereas the lateral canal grows at a slower rate. All three canals complete growth by week 18, a full week before any of the canals is encased in bone (weeks 19–23).[17] The later development of the lateral canal explains why it is the most commonly malformed canal.

The utricle, saccule, and cochlea also begin their formation during the sixth week of gestation. As stated earlier, both the cochlea and saccule originate from the saccular portion of the utriculosaccular chamber. During the sixth week, the saccular chamber begins to expand, and the caudal portion of this chamber, which will eventually become the cochlea, begins to coil. The connection between the saccular and the cochlear portion then begins to thin and by the eighth week is visible as the ductus reuniens.[14,15] By the eighth week, the cochlea has completed its first one and a half turns. By the tenth week, the cochlea has completed the total two and a half turns, but it will not reach its adult length until week 20. Though the development of the cochlea is later in gestation than that of the vestibular end-organs, the cochlea is completely encased in bone by week 19.[17]

The sensory epithelium of the otolithic organs and the SCCs develops from a common ectodermal epithelium in the otocyst, first detectable by the third week of gestation. The upper portion develops into the utricle and superior and lateral SCCs, while the lower portion will become the sensory portions of the saccule and posterior canal. By the ninth week, normal histology and afferent neural connections are evident within the sensory organs.[18] The maculae of the otolith organs are the first to develop, between the seventh and twelfth weeks, and they reach adult form between weeks 14 and 16.[8,15] The cristae begin development about one week later (the eighth week) and do not finish their development until about week 23.[8,15] Finally, the organ of Corti does not reach its full development until approximately two weeks later (week 25).[8]

The innervation of the vestibulocochlear apparatus begins in the third week of gestation. Ectoderm of the otocyst gives rise to the common vestibulo-cochlear ganglia. The cells destined to be peripheral cranial nerve fibers migrate distally toward the sensory organs. The nerve fibers of the vestibular nerve divide into superior and inferior portions. These nerve fibers reach the sensory organs by the ninth week and differentiate their connections by the eleventh week. Interestingly, afferent innervation precedes efferent innervation. The portion of the nerve destined to become the cochlear portion reaches the cochlea prior to its final turn, thus accounting for the spiral nature of the nerve endings.[16]

Both the perilymph-filled bony labyrinth and the bony otic capsule are formed from cephalic mesoderm beginning in the seventh week of gestation. The bony labyrinth commences forming in the eighth week as vacuoles within this mesodermal precartilage start to form and coalesce, beginning around the vestibule. This process, which eventually walls off the perilymphatic space, ends by week 24. At the same time, the same precartilage begins ossifying in three layers from 14 ossification centers. This takes place between the eighth and sixteenth weeks. By week 22, the otic capsule has reached its adult size and shape.[17]

■ Physiology

Semicircular Canal Physiology

The SCCs are the vestibular sensory organs responsible for the encoding of rotational movement of the head and body in space. They do this by sensing changes in rotational acceleration of the head. However, due to the internal coding of the canals, the signals they send to the vestibular nuclei more closely approximate rotational head velocity than they do acceleration. The SCCs are exquisitely sensitive to head motion, and it has been reported that they can sense changes in angular acceleration as small as $0.1°/s^2$. To give this some perspective, if you were to spin at this rate, it would take you ~ 90 seconds to complete one full 360° rotation.[19]

The increase in the firing rate of the vestibular hair cells is a complex process that involves opening of multiple ion channels. Stereocilia are linked through tip links connecting each to the next shorter and longer stereocilia. When deflected toward the kinocilium, each stereocilium is pulled toward the next taller stereocilium, and mechanically gated cation channels are opened. This leads to an influx of cations, predominantly in the form of potassium, into the cell, causing a positive deflection of the resting membrane potential and a subsequent opening of the voltage-gated calcium channels at the basolateral aspect of the cells. Subsequently, there is an influx of

calcium and an increase in the release of excitatory neurotransmitter. This release of predominantly glutamine leads to an increase in the firing rate of the afferent vestibular neurons.[20] The increase in the firing rate of the vestibular afferents in response to deflections of the stereocilia in the excitatory direction are more robust than the slowing of the firing in response to an equal deflection in the inhibitory direction (**Fig. 5.5**).

The Horizontal/Lateral Canal

To understand SCC physiology best, it is easiest to break SCCs' function down into individual units and consider their response to physiologic conditions, keeping in mind that few movements are isolated rotations exactly in the plane of a SCC. The SCC is maximally excited or inhibited with rotation in the plane of the canal.

The ampulla of the lateral canal is on the anterior aspect of the canal, and ampullopetal flow of endolymph will result in excitation. As the head turns to the right, the endolymph lags behind the bony canal, creating an effective rotation of the endolymph to the left, which causes a deflection of the cupula toward the vestibule in the right lateral canal. Since the kinocilia of the lateral canals are oriented on the side of the cells closest to the vestibule, this deflection of the cupula causes a deflection of the stereocilia toward the kinocilia. Thus, the cells are activated, there is an increased release of excitatory neurotransmitter, and the afferent firing rate increases. When the head is then turned back to the left, the endolymph lags behind, and the cupula is deflected away from the vestibule, causing inhibition of neuronal firing from the right lateral canal. Since the left lateral canal completes this functional pair, its afferent firing rate will be opposite that of the right lateral canal. Thus, its afferent firing rate will decrease with head turn to the right and will increase with head turn to the left.

The Superior and Posterior Canals and the Hallpike Position

Excitation of the right-anterior-left-posterior (RALP) and left-anterior-right-posterior (LARP) pairs is elicited by ampullofugal flow of endolymph. Also, one must remember that the ampullated ends of the superior and posterior canals are located at the ends of the canals farthest from the crus commune and closest to the vestibule. Thus the ampullated end of the superior canal is located at the anterior-most aspect of the canal, and the ampullated end of the posterior canal is at the inferior-most part of the canal.

The physiology of the superior and posterior canals is best understood by examining the fluid mechanics and activation of each canal during Dix-Hallpike maneuvers. The first step of a right Dix-Hallpike maneuver is to turn the patient's head toward the right side, bringing the LARP functional pair from the 45° off-sagittal plane to a nearly sagittal orientation. The patient is then brought to the supine position with the head hanging slightly lower than the remainder of the body. In right posterior canal BPPV canalithiasis, initially there is a normal shift in the endolymph of the functional pair, thus the patient experiences no vertigo and there is no nystagmus. However, after a short latent period, the otoconia within the right posterior canal will begin to roll under the effects of gravity away from the ampulla. In so doing, the otoconia move the endolymph away from the crista—an ampullofugal flow of the endolymph (exciting stimulus for vertical canals). The cupula is deflected away from the vestibule and toward the kinocilia of the crista of the right posterior canal. Thus, the hair cells in the crista of the right posterior canal are excited and the firing rate of the afferent nerve increases. Since there is no opposing decrease in the firing rate of the left anterior canal, the vestibular nuclei receive conflicting information, the patient experiences intense vertigo, and the examiner detects geotropic nystagmus.

The Otolithic Organs

Unlike the SCCs, the otolithic organs act as linear rather than rotational accelerometers. Recall that the saccule is oriented in the vertical parasagittal plane, whereas the utricle is oriented in approximately the same plane as the horizontal SCC. Due to the specific gravity of the otoconia, the overall specific gravity of the otolithic membranes is approximately twice that of the endolymph, which is especially important in examining the physiology of the saccule.[2] Additionally, one should recall that the makeup of the otolithic membranes makes the otolithic organs sensitive to linear acceleration in the planes parallel to their orientation. In a similar manner, the inelastic properties of the membranes make them insensitive to motion perpendicular to the organ.[2] Type I hair cells are found in the striola, whereas the type II cells are found in the extrastriolar regions. The striolar, type I, regions show tonic-phasic responses to stimuli that increase as the frequency of movement increases. Thus, they are more responsive to the time-rate of deflection. The type II cells in the extrastriolar regions, however, show a tonic response that is more dependent on the amount of kinocilia deflected.

The saccule responds to linear acceleration in the naso-occipital direction as well as in the cranio-caudal direction. Since the otolithic membranes have a higher specific gravity than the endolymph they are bathed in, gravity pulls the membrane toward the

ground. This generates a state of tonic excitation of portions of the saccule, while other regions are tonically inhibited. Thus it is less responsive to gravitational or superior-inferior acceleration than it is to naso-occipital movement.

The utricle is oriented in a nearly horizontal plane, and in its resting state, gravity has very little influence on the firing rate of the utricular hair cells. The utricle senses acceleration in the naso-occipital direction as well as left-to-right motion of the head. Additionally, it senses head tilt, either nose up or nose down, as well as tilt of either ear toward the ground.

In a series of elegant experiments, Jaeger and Haslwanter evaluated the neural responses of the striola to both tilt of the head with left ear down as well as pitch tilt with nose down. They measured the effective deflection of the membrane as well as the time course of the response of the membrane. Finally, they measured the patterns of maximal neural response to tilts in various directions for both otolithic organs.[2] They found that, at all three places tested along the striola, the neural response rates were the same and occurred before the end of the head movement. Additionally, they demonstrated that the decay to baseline firing of each of these places was nearly the same. They also reported that head tilt in different directions led to very different response patterns, but that for a given tilt, the time response patterns of the different positions along the striola remained the same. Finally, they studied the maximum neural responses of both the saccule and the utricle in response to head tilts in many directions. This experiment demonstrated that, overall, the saccular response to tilts was smaller than the utricular response. However, for certain tilts, the response of the saccule was nearly equal to that of the utricle.[2]

■ The Vestibulo-Ocular Reflex (VOR)

The vestibulo-ocular reflex (VOR) stabilizes the eye with respect to the visual world during rapid head motion (**Video 5.1**). This reflex is critical for vision because even a low-velocity slip of a visual image across the retina produces a loss of visual acuity. Since visual information takes over 100 milliseconds to drive eye movement, visual reflexes like the optokinetic reflex (OKR) are adequate to stabilize the eye during low-frequency head movement, but not the high-frequency movements that characterize head motion during normal activity. Such movements require short-latency open-loop reflexes. The VOR, with a minimum latency of less than 10 milliseconds, is well constructed for this role.[21]

The angular VOR (aVOR) is a response to activation of receptors in the SCCs responding to angular acceleration and produces compensatory eye movement equal and opposite to head movements. The linear VOR (lVOR) results from activation of the otolith receptors in response to linear acceleration and produces compensatory eye movements to translational movement.[22] Since a fully compensatory response for translation is highly dependent on the distance to the visual objects that are to be stabilized, the lVOR is heavily influenced by viewing distance, although the response is not driven directly by retinal motion. Both the aVOR and the lVOR are calibrated by feedback from the visual system, which constantly adjusts the gain of the reflexes so that retinal slip is minimized during natural head motion.[23]

Each form of the VOR can be further subdivided into sets of reflexes that act on different extraocular muscles, relying on different sensory inputs, and displaying different response dynamics. Such reflexes, when rotational, always produce a compensatory rotation that is roughly in the plane of the activated canal pair. Also, the vestibular system is organized in a push-pull fashion, with complementary canals providing inputs of opposite sign. Hence, each reflex is subserved by pairs of canals lying in the same plane but with opposite sensitivities (see above). Since there are four vertical canals and two horizontal canals, a simple mental aid is to think of two aVOR reflexes, a horizontal reflex and a vertical reflex. The pathways subserving these reflexes are pictured in **Fig. 5.6**.[24,25,26]

The horizontal VOR is composed of inputs from both lateral SCCs, which have a crossed inhibitory interaction at the level of the medial vestibular nucleus (MVN). Secondary vestibular neurons in the MVN, which are activated by the ipsilateral SCC, excite cells in the contralateral abducens nucleus, which controls cranial nerve VI (CN VI), to produce compensatory eye rotation in the contralateral eye due to activation of the lateral rectus muscle. In addition, interneurons within the contralateral CN VI drive compensatory rotation of the ipsilateral eye by exciting the ipsilateral medial rectus subdivision of the oculomotor nucleus (CN IIImr), producing activation of the ipsilateral medial rectus muscle. In addition, there is a direct ipsilateral excitatory pathway from the MVN to CN IIImr via the ascending tract of Dieters. Furthermore, inhibitory interneurons within the MVN inhibit neurons in the ipsilateral CN VI, producing a disfacilitation of the ipsilateral lateral rectus and the contralateral medial rectus muscles. The resulting rotation of the eye is in the horizontal plane away from the activated lateral canal because the lateral and medial recti have horizontal pulling directions. Finally, there is a projection from the MVN to the prepositus hypoglossi, which projects to the abducens nucleus. This projection is responsible for creating a signal appropriate to drive the discharge of motoneurons, i.e., a signal coding for both eye position and eye velocity.

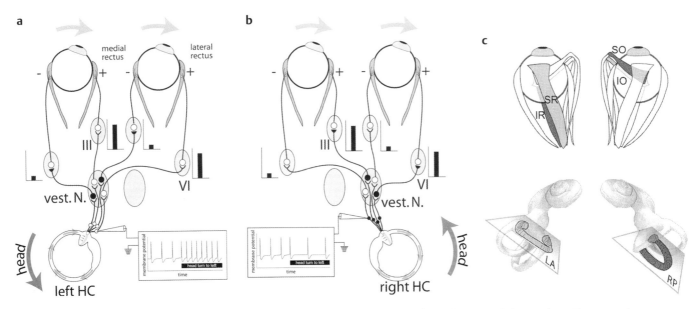

Fig. 5.6 The vestibulo-ocular reflex (VOR) stabilizes visual targets during rapid head motion. **(a)** Angular reflexes produce a compensatory rotation that is roughly in the plane of the activated canal pair. This is done in a push–pull fashion, with contributions from both the excited and inhibited canal. **(b)** Thus, isolated rotation in the plane of the horizontal canals will produce a compensatory activation of the ipsilateral medial rectus and the contralateral lateral rectus, while **(c)** the ipsilateral lateral rectus and contralateral medial rectus are inhibited (relaxed). For details of these neuronal interactions, please see the section "The Vestibulo-ocular Reflex" in this chapter. Used with permission from Carey JP, Della Santina C. Principles of applied vestibular physiology. In: Cummings CW, ed. Cummings Otolaryngology Head and Neck Surgery, Vol IV. 4th ed. Philadelphia, PA: Elsevier Mosby; 2005:3129–3132.

The vertical VOR is subserved by input from the anterior and posterior SCCs (**Fig. 5.6**). Since these are oriented vertically but oblique to the frontal plane, the eye movements that each canal pair produces are both vertical and torsional, matching roughly the plane of the activated canals. The anterior canals produce excitation in secondary vestibular neurons in the superior and ventrolateral medial vestibular nuclei.[27,28] These neurons in turn excite neurons in the contralateral inferior oblique and superior rectus subdivisions of CN III, exciting the ipsilateral superior rectus and the superior oblique muscles. Some anterior canal receiving neurons of the superior vestibular nucleus also inhibit ipsilateral trochlear motoneurons, which in turn disfacilatates the contralateral superior oblique. Other anterior canal receiving neurons of the superior vestibular nucleus inhibit motoneurons in the ipsilateral inferior rectus subdivision of CN III, disfacilitating the ipsilateral inferior rectus. The net result of these changes in muscle activation is elevation of both eyes, with intorsion of the ipsilateral eye and extorsion of the contralateral eye. Therefore, the connections, muscles, and canal planes are all roughly in register. An oculomotor scientist or neurophthalmologist can infer the direction of excitation of the anterior canal by its extraocular muscle connections, while the vestibular scientist or otolaryngologist can likewise reconstruct the connections by recalling the direction of excitation of an individual canal.

Since posterior and anterior canals complement one another, it is not surprising that activation of the posterior canal produces depression of both eyes, with intorsion of the contralateral eye and extorsion of the ipsilateral eye. This is accomplished through excitatory and inhibitory pathways that complement those of the anterior canals. The posterior canals produce excitation in secondary vestibular neurons in the superior and ventrolateral medial vestibular nuclei. Neurons in the ventrolateral medial vestibular nuclei in turn excite neurons in the contralateral inferior rectus subdivision of CN III, exciting the contralateral inferior rectus. Posterior canal receiving neurons of the superior vestibular nucleus excite contralateral trochlear motoneurons, which in turn activate the ipsilateral superior oblique. Some posterior canal receiving neurons of the superior vestibular nucleus inhibit the ipsilateral inferior oblique and superior rectus subdivisions of CN III, disfacilitating the contralateral superior rectus and the ipsilateral inferior oblique muscles. Finally, there is an inhibitory projection from cells receiving input from either vertical canal to the interstitial nucleus of Cajal, which projects to vertical motoneurons. This projection is responsible for creating a signal appropriate to drive the discharge of vertical motoneurons analogous to the activity of neurons in the prepositus hypoglossi in the horizontal system, i.e., a signal

coding for both vertical eye position and vertical eye velocity.

While knowing the central connections of the aVOR pathways is useful to the basic scientist and clinician, a thorough knowledge of the dynamics of the VOR pathways is also useful. As described previously, the semicircular canals generate a signal proportional to eye velocity over a range of frequencies from 0.1 to ~ 1 Hz. The adequate stimulus for activation of hair cells in the semicircular canals is head acceleration. This is phase-shifted 180° relative to eye position, which is the final output of the VOR. The discharge of primary canal afferents is phase-shifted by roughly 90° from acceleration to velocity by the mechanical properties of the cupula. Since the cupula has a fixed time constant, it tends to straighten too rapidly for lower-frequency stimuli, causing the afferent discharge under these conditions to report both head acceleration and velocity. Activation of extraocular muscles and the sluggish mechanical properties of the plant, further shift the phase of the response toward eye position, especially at higher frequencies. Somewhere, however, a further phase-shift of up to 90° must occur to produce the eye-position output of the aVOR. This phase-shift, which is termed neural integration, is produced by the activity of cells in the prepositus hypoglossi for the horizontal VOR and the interstitial nucleus of Cajal for the vertical VOR.[29,30]

Below 0.2 Hz, the response is still phase-advanced with respect to eye position. A further integration is required, where velocity is stored by the brain and played out after the afferent neural discharge has died away. This second integration process is called velocity storage, and it is useful for both phase-shifting the low frequency VOR and integrating output in changing planes of activation over time.

In the vertical system, one final mechanism exists for extending the frequency range of the aVOR. As discussed earlier, the otolithic organs have convergent input to cells in the vestibular nucleus that respond to SCC input. Many of these cells display a response to off vertical axis rotation and contribute to reflexive compensatory eye movements. In the vertical system, this otolith input can provide a dynamic, very-low-frequency boost to the vertical aVOR.[31] Indeed, recent studies suggest that some otolith afferents are activated only during dynamic movement, and are not active during static tilt.[32] Thus, there is a physiologic basis for an unambiguous dynamic otolith response.

Again, the pragmatic value of knowledge of the dynamics of the VOR is that it allows us to understand the abnormalities that result from damage to the vestibular system. Since eye velocity is the dependent variable for many clinical tests of vestibular function, the VOR is the primary neural mechanism that is being probed by such tests. Low-frequency tests of lateral canal function, such as the caloric test, evaluate only a single end-organ across a small portion of its dynamic operating range. Rotational chair tests, which typically focus on lateral canals, reveal different information at different frequencies simply because of the relative contribution of velocity storage and other central processes at each frequency.

Finally, it is important to note that all of these VOR reflexes are modulated by a variety of convergent sensory and motor signals. Individually identified secondary neurons in the aVOR have been shown to discharge for eye position, eye velocity, head velocity, and commanded gaze movements.[33,34] Indeed, even the identified interneuron in the simplest incarnation of the horizontal VOR pauses completely during the rapid saccadic eye movements of head unrestrained gaze shifts.[35] Under these circumstances, the VOR would impede a rapid eye movement that occurs in conjunction with a similarly directed rapid head movement to shift the orientation of the eye toward an interesting object. While the mechanism of this interaction is not fully understood, the result is a complete elimination of the reflex when it is inappropriate in a given context. The significance of these complexities will become increasingly apparent as researchers and clinicians work to develop vestibular neural prostheses and strategies to help patients compensate for vestibular loss.

■ Vestibular Evoked Myogenic Potentials (VEMP)

The vestibular system also affects the tension in other muscle groups. In fact, loud sound stimulus can induce relaxation of flexor muscles. Vestibular evoked myogenic potentials represent this relation and they can be measured in clinic to diagnose vestibular disorders. We typically measure by EMG the relaxation of the ipsilateral sternocleidomastoid muscle (SCM) in response to auditory stimulation (95 dB SPL or tone bursts) to record this reflex.[36] Tonic contraction of the muscle is required to demonstrate the inhibitory response. This response of the SCM is called cervical VEMP (cVEMP) and is selective to the function of the inferior vestibular nerve that innervates the sacculus. The response pathway consists of the saccule, inferior vestibular nerve, lateral vestibular nucleus, lateral vestibulospinal tract, and SCM. Measuring VEMP is very useful to identify disorders solely affecting the inferior vestibular nerve because caloric and rotational testing mainly stimulate the horizontal semicircular canal (superior vestibular nerve).[37]

Patients with profound sensorineural hearing loss can still present cVEMP. However, transmission of the VEMP acoustic stimulus is very sensitive and VEMP are usually absent in the presence of conductive hearing loss. The amplitude of the response, and also the threshold needed to generate it, are measured. Because the absolute amplitudes vary importantly between patients, the more reliable abnormality is detection of a side-to-side difference. Patients with superior semicircular canal dehiscence (SSCD) will present with a lower threshold and increased amplitude, while patients with Meniere's disease can present a higher threshold to cVEMP.[38] In contrast to cVEMP, ocular VEMP (oVEMP) are responses of the extraocular musculature in reaction to sound stimulation of the utricular apparatus and they are recorded from electrodes placed around the eye.

■ Conclusion

This chapter provides a basic overview of the anatomy, histology, and physiology of the peripheral vestibular system and its central connections. The goal is to provide a framework for understanding the clinical examination and disease states described in the other chapters of this text. A complex analysis of central vestibular pathways is outside the scope of this text but relevant connections are presented to understand central contributions to normal end-organ physiology and reflex activity.

Questions

Q1: During the embryogenesis, the organ of Corti reaches its full development at which week?

Q2: Given the orientations of the two otolithic organs in space, which of the utricule and saccule is designed in such a way that it is responsive to the pull of gravity?

Q3: With similar magnitude deflections of the stereocilia in a semicircular canal, which of the excitatory or inhibitory responses is greater?

Q4: Is the ampullopetal flow of the endolymph (flow toward the ampulla) excitatory or inhibitory for the horizontal semicircular canal?

Q5: How will the VEMP threshold and amplitude differ in patients with superior semicircular canal dehiscence (SSCD)?

Answers

A1: Week 25.

A2: Saccule.

A3: Excitatory response is always greater.

A4: Excitatory.

A5: Lower threshold; increased amplitude.

References

1. Money KE, Bonen L, Beatty JD, Kuehn LA, Sokoloff M, Weaver RS. Physical properties of fluids and structures of vestibular apparatus of the pigeon. Am J Physiol 1971;220(1):140–147

2. Jaeger R, Haslwanter T. Otolith responses to dynamical stimuli: results of a numerical investigation. Biol Cybern 2004;90(3):165–175

3. Barmack NH. Central vestibular system: vestibular nuclei and posterior cerebellum. Brain Res Bull 2003;60(5-6):511–541

4. Lindeman HH, Reith A, Winther FO. The distribution of type I and type II cells in the cristae ampullaris of the guinea pig. Acta Otolaryngol 1981;92(3-4):315–321

5. Fernández C, Lysakowski A, Goldberg JM. Hair-cell counts and afferent innervation patterns in the cristae ampullares of the squirrel monkey with a comparison to the chinchilla. J Neurophysiol 1995;73(3):1253–1269

6. Lysakowski A. Synaptic organization of the crista ampullaris in vertebrates. Ann N Y Acad Sci 1996; 781:164–182

7. Lysakowski A, Goldberg JM. A regional ultrastructural analysis of the cellular and synaptic architecture in the chinchilla cristae ampullares. J Comp Neurol 1997;389(3):419–443

8. Lysakowski A. Anatomy of vestibular end organs and neural pathways. In: Cummings CW, ed. Cummings Otolaryngology Head and Neck Surgery. Vol IV. 4th ed. Philadelphia, PA: Elsevier Mosby; 2005:3089–3114

9. Kimura RS. Distribution, structure, and function of dark cells in the vestibular labyrinth. Ann Otol Rhinol Laryngol 1969;78(3):542–561

10. Goldberg JM. Afferent diversity and the organization of central vestibular pathways. Exp Brain Res 2000;130(3):277–297

11. Goldberg JM, Smith CE, Fernández C. Relation between discharge regularity and responses to externally applied galvanic currents in vestibular nerve afferents of the squirrel monkey. J Neurophysiol 1984; 51(6):1236–1256

12. Hudspeth AJ. The cellular basis of hearing: the biophysics of hair cells. Science 1985;230(4727):745–752

13. Wall C, Vrabec JT. Vestibular function and anatomy. In: Bailey BJ, ed. Head & Neck Surgery—Otolaryngology. Vol II. 3rd ed. Philadelphia, PA: Lippincott Williams & Wilkins; 2001:1641–1650

14. Anson BJ, Davies J. Embryology of the ear. In: Paparella MM, Shumrick DA, eds. Otolaryngology. Vol I. 2nd ed. Philadelphia, PA: W. B. Saunders Company; 1980:3–25

15. Wareing MJ, Lalwani AK, Jackler RK. Development of the ear. In: Bailey BJ, ed. Head & Neck Surgery—Otolaryngology. Vol II. 3rd ed. Philadelphia, PA: Lippincott Williams & Wilkins; 1995:22–42

16. Sulik KK. Embryology of the ear. In: Gorlin RJ, Toriello HV, Cohen MM, eds. Hereditary Hearing Loss and Its Syndromes. New York, NY: Oxford University Press; 2001: 1641–1650

17. Jeffery N, Spoor F. Prenatal growth and development of the modern human labyrinth. J Anat 2004; 204(2):71–92

18. Sans A, Dechesne C. Early development of vestibular receptors in human embryos. An electron microscopic study. Acta Otolaryngol Suppl 1985;423:51–58

19. Minor LE, Hullar TA, Zee DS. Anatomy and physiology of the vestibular system. In: Lustig LR, Niparko JK, eds. Clinical Neurotology: Diagnosing and Managing Disorders of Hearing, Balance and the Facial Nerve. London, UK: Martin Dunitz Ltd. (an imprint of Taylor & Francis Group); 2003:37–54

20. Carey JP, Della Santina C. Principles of applied vestibular physiology. In: Cummings CW, ed. Cummings Otolaryngology Head and Neck Surgery. Vol IV. 4th ed. Philadelphia, PA: Elsevier Mosby; 2005:3115–3159

21. Huterer M, Cullen KE. Vestibuloocular reflex dynamics during high-frequency and high-acceleration rotations of the head on body in rhesus monkey. J Neurophysiol 2002;88(1):13–28

22. Paige GD, Seidman SH. Characteristics of the VOR in response to linear acceleration. Ann N Y Acad Sci 1999;871:123–135

23. Broussard DM, Kassardjian CD. Learning in a simple motor system. Learn Mem 2004;11(2):127–136

24. Leigh RJ, Zee DS. The vestibular-optokinetic system. In: Leigh RJ, Zee DS, eds. The Neurology of Eye Movements: Contemporary Neurology Series. 3rd ed. New York, NY: Oxford University Press; 1999:19–89

25. McCrea RA, Strassman A, May E, Highstein SM. Anatomical and physiological characteristics of vestibular neurons mediating the horizontal vestibulo-ocular reflex of the squirrel monkey. J Comp Neurol 1987;264(4):547–570

26. McCrea RA, Strassman A, Highstein SM. Anatomical and physiological characteristics of vestibular neurons mediating the vertical vestibulo-ocular reflexes of the squirrel monkey. J Comp Neurol 1987;264(4):571–594

27. Carpenter MB. Vestibular nuclei: afferent and efferent projections. Prog Brain Res 1988;76:5–15

28. Carpenter MB, Cowie RJ. Connections and oculomotor projections of the superior vestibular nucleus and cell group 'y'. Brain Res 1985;336(2):265–287

29. McCrea RA, Horn AK. Nucleus prepositus. Prog Brain Res 2006;151:205–230

30. Fukushima K. The interstitial nucleus of Cajal in the midbrain reticular formation and vertical eye movement. Neurosci Res 1991;10(3):159–187

31. Brettler SC, Baker JF. Timing of low frequency responses of anterior and posterior canal vestibulo-ocular neurons in alert cats. Exp Brain Res 2003;149(2):167–173

32. Dickman JD, Angelaki DE. Vestibular convergence patterns in vestibular nuclei neurons of alert primates. J Neurophysiol 2002;88(6):3518–3533

33. McCrea RA, Luan H. Signal processing of semicircular canal and otolith signals in the vestibular nuclei during passive and active head movements. Ann N Y Acad Sci 2003;1004:169–182

34. McCrea RA, Gdowski GT. Firing behaviour of squirrel monkey eye movement-related vestibular nucleus neurons during gaze saccades. J Physiol 2003;546(Pt 1): 207–224

35. Fuchs AF, Ling L, Phillips JO. Behavior of the position-vestibular-pause (pvp) interneurons of the vestibulo-ocular reflex during head-free gaze shifts in the monkey [abstract]. J Neurophysiol [serial online]. 2005 Aug 24. Available at: http://jn.physiology.org/cgi/content/abstract/00101.2005v1. Accessed November 4, 2005

36. Welgampola MS, Colebatch JG. Characteristics and clinical applications of vestibular-evoked myogenic potentials. Neurology 2005;64(10):1682–1688

37. Halmagyi GM, Aw ST, Karlberg M, Curthoys IS, Todd MJ. Inferior vestibular neuritis. Ann N Y Acad Sci 2002; 956:306–313

38. Minor LB. Clinical manifestations of superior semicircular canal dehiscence. Laryngoscope 2005; 115(10):1717–1727

6 Laboratory Testing in the Diagnosis and Treatment of Dizziness

Mikhaylo Szczupak and Michael E. Hoffer

■ Introduction

The etiology of dizziness can be determined by history and physical examination alone in the majority of patients, ~ 75% in large series.[1] For cases when the history and physical by themselves do not elucidate a cause, a variety of sophisticated auditory and vestibular tests are available, supplemented by established and emerging imaging techniques to help determine the diagnosis. It is reasonable, then, to ask if there continues to be a role for traditional laboratory testing in the diagnosis of patients presenting with complaints of dizziness.

Recent literature is largely devoid of specific guidelines regarding the use of laboratory tests in the diagnosis and treatment of dizziness. Hoffman et al, in a meta-analysis of over 4,000 patients, demonstrated that less than 1% had abnormal laboratory tests that identified a specific cause for dizziness.[1] Several standard textbooks address laboratory tests for dizziness under the heading for specific diseases or disorders in which the laboratory test would be applicable. Even less attention is directed to the judicious use of tests in the treatment of patients with vertigo. In this chapter, we examine several specific laboratory tests that may be helpful in some cases of dizziness. We provide information about the test and then discuss how we would use the test in the diagnosis and treatment of dizziness.

■ *Treponema pallidum* Serology

Treponema pallidum is the spirochete that causes syphilis. After entering the body, the spirochete can invade any organ system and manifest with a wide array of symptoms. This allows syphilis to closely mimic many other diseases, such as Meniere's disease, autoimmune inner ear disease, and perilymphatic fistula. Audiovestibular symptoms of *Treponema pallidum* infection are known to develop in secondary,

tertiary, and congenital forms of syphilis. In a series of 85 patients diagnosed with otosyphilis, patients presented with symptoms of dizziness ~ 53% of the time.[2] The diagnosis of otosyphilis is often delayed, so this is an important entity to consider in patients with fluctuating or sudden sensorineural hearing loss (SNHL) and/or vestibular symptoms.[3]

Syphilis can be diagnosed accurately with two different types of serologic tests, nontreponemal tests (Venereal Disease Research Laboratory [VDRL] or rapid plasma reagin [RPR]) and treponemal tests (fluorescent treponemal antibody-absorption [FTA-ABS], *Treponema pallidum* passive particle agglutination [TP-PA] assay, or treponemal enzyme immunoassay [EIA]/chemiluminescence immunoassays [CIA]). Nontreponemal tests usually correlate with disease activity and may be used to monitor treatment response. On the other hand, the majority of patients with reactive treponemal tests will remain positive after treatment, so a history must be taken for prior syphilis treatment. The Centers for Disease Control and Prevention (CDC) recommends initial screening by a nontreponemal test, with reactive samples undergoing reflex testing by a treponemal test for confirmation.[4] Syphilis cannot be accurately diagnosed with only one serologic test due to the high rates of false-negatives in persons with primary syphilis and false-positives in persons without syphilis.[4] For economic reasons, the advent of automated EIA/CIA testing in large-volume clinical laboratories has led to reverse sequence testing. This process is defined as initial screening with a treponemal test and reflex testing of reactive samples with a nontreponemal test.[5] Issues arise in determining a diagnosis in patients with discordant results (i.e., reactive treponemal test with nonreactive subsequent nontreponemal test). The CDC continues to recommend the classical serologic testing sequence, but if reverse sequence testing is used, then discordant specimens should be reflexively tested by TP-PA.[6] Discordant samples determined to be reactive by TP-PA testing are considered to indicate past or present syphilis infection, and if serology on TP-PA is nonreactive, then syphilis is unlikely.[6]

Dizziness secondary to syphilis can masquerade as almost any form of dizziness, including patients presenting with episodic vertigo, episodic unsteadiness, and constant unsteadiness while walking. Despite the fact that syphilis can cause any form of dizziness, we obtain syphilis serology only when we cannot make a definitive or even presumptive diagnosis with history, physical exam, or vestibular tests (i.e., when we are completely stumped), or when the individual has a history suggestive of syphilis infection (which can be difficult to obtain). The Tullio phenomenon (dizziness elicited with loud noises or pressure to the ear), which was once thought to be a diagnostic sign of syphilis, can occur with other disorders, such as superior canal dehiscence and Meniere's disease, as well as in posttraumatic dizziness. Patients exhibiting dizziness with noise or pressure should undergo a work-up to rule out the known causes, and then one may think of ordering a syphilis serology more readily in these patients.

■ *Borrelia burgdorferi* Serology

Borrelia burgdorferi is the organism responsible for Lyme disease. The infected *Ixodes* tick transmits the gram-negative spirochete. The disease is named after the community in which it was discovered, Lyme, Connecticut. The CDC guidelines for serologic diagnosis of Lyme disease recommend a two-test approach consisting of EIA/immunofluorescent assay (IFA), with positive and equivocal samples undergoing Western blot (WB).[7] Samples found to be unreactive by EIA/IFA do not need further testing. WB testing parameters vary based on the length of symptoms. Both immunoglobulin (Ig) M and IgG WB must be performed in patients with signs and symptoms for less than or equal to 30 days. Only IgG WB need be performed in patients with signs and symptoms for more than 30 days.

Otolaryngologic manifestations can occur in as many as 75% of cases of Lyme disease.[8] After the facial nerve, the vestibulocochlear nerve is the cranial nerve most commonly affected by this disorder. A variety of balance disorders have been reported in association with Lyme disease, including episodic vertigo, chronic disequilibrium, and episodic disequilibrium with headaches (mimicking migraine disease). Like other spirochete disorders, Lyme disease can mimic a variety of other syndromes. The tick is now indigenous to many parts of the United States and has been identified in Central and South America as well. The onset of symptoms can be remote from the time of the tick bite. When individuals present with dizziness (especially if it is not easy to characterize as a classic disorder), a careful history must be taken for a possible tick bite, including any exposure to areas where ticks tend

to be present. If a positive history of a tick bite or possible travel to endemic regions is obtained, then we obtain serology for *B. burgdorferi*. It does not appear necessary to examine the cerebrospinal fluid (CSF); a simple blood test is often positive in this disorder.

■ Autoimmune Panels

Many investigators have postulated the association of autoimmune disorders with dizziness.[9,10,11,12] The disorders variously termed autoimmune inner ear disease (AIED) or immune-mediated cochleovestibular disorders likely represent a variety of different autoimmune diseases. Cogan's disease is a documented autoimmune disorder that affects the inner ear, and many investigators argue that a certain percentage of Meniere's disease is autoimmune in nature.[12] In general, autoimmune causes of vestibular dysfunction produce symptoms similar to Meniere's disease with episodic vertigo. Auditory symptoms in these patients are usually bilateral, with at least one ear showing a rapid decline in hearing. A variety of laboratory tests have been proposed to evaluate the disorder, including complete blood count with differential white count (CBC), erythrocyte sedimentation rate (ESR), rheumatoid factor, antineutrophil antibodies, anti-double-stranded DNA antibodies, antiphospholipid antibodies, anti-SSA/B antibodies, C3 and C4 complement levels, and Raji cell assay for circulating immune complexes.[12] These tests are standard in the work-up of rheumatologic disorders but are not specific for ear diseases. Sensitivity for each of these tests is, as yet, undetermined for inner ear disease.

Over the years, a variety of more ear-specific tests have been developed, including the lymphocyte migration inhibition assay[13] and the lymphocyte transformation test.[14] Western blot analysis, for the 68-kDa antigen, has largely replaced these tests (OtoBlot). This test and other tests that analyze the levels of heat shock proteins are now commercially available. There is mounting evidence that these tests are valuable for examining individuals with suspected inner ear autoimmune disorders.[15,16] There continues to be a great deal of debate about how and when to use any of these tests in managing patients with balance disorders. Heat shock protein analysis and 68-kDa antigen analysis seem to be the best tests available, with recent data demonstrating a sensitivity of ~ 55% in patients with AIED.[17,18] We perform this analysis when a patient presents with classical AIED symptoms (any balance disorder with progressive bilateral SNHL). We do not routinely perform these tests on other balance disorder patients. OtoBlot tests can be positive in a variety of collagen vascular diseases and in common causes of vertigo, including Meniere's disease.

■ Coagulation Profile and Lipids

Vestibulobasilar occlusive disorders have the potential to produce isolated vestibular disorders, isolated cochlear disorders, or more widespread disorders. Generally, individuals who present with dizziness after a cerebrovascular accident have sudden-onset, profound disequilibrium and gait disturbances (if ambulatory). The etiology of the disorder is often not in doubt and is best analyzed with one of many radiologic tests. Rarely, the occlusive disease occurs in a small vessel and is not apparent on the radiologic exam. In these cases, a complete blood count, coagulation profile, and blood cholesterol and lipid levels may be helpful.[19] We tend not to use these tests but believe they may be valuable in the rare patient presenting with symptoms that appear to be caused by either occlusive disease or transient ischemic attacks in which radiologic or historical evidence is lacking.

■ Thyroid Function Tests

Investigators have debated the role of hypothyroidism in dizziness and disorders that cause dizziness.[20] In patients presenting to the emergency department with sudden-onset dizziness, the incidence of thyroid disorders was found to be 10%, approximately three times greater than the general prevalence.[21] The best single screening test for thyroid hormone levels is to test the level of thyroid-stimulating hormone (TSH). This test is highly accurate, and, if abnormal, a full thyroid panel can be ordered. We feel that thyroid laboratory evaluations are helpful only for patients who have dizziness of unknown etiology and who relate a history of thyroid disorders.

■ Glucose Tolerance Test

Low blood sugar can cause symptoms of lightheadedness and disequilibrium. In many cases, a careful history can elicit a relationship between the episodes to eating, with individuals complaining of symptoms at a given time period after meals or when skipping meals. The treatment of choice for these individuals is dietary management. Before undertaking this process, a confirmatory laboratory test is helpful. A 3- or 5-hour glucose tolerance test is the test of choice. Individuals to be tested come to the laboratory in the morning, having not eaten or taken any liquids for at least 8 hours. A baseline blood sugar is taken, and the patient is instructed to drink a glucose-rich solution. Glucose levels are then taken every hour until completion of the test. Significantly reduced glucose levels at 2 to 3 hours after drinking the solution indicate an abnormal test.

■ Genetic Testing

In recent years, the use of genetic testing in otolaryngology has gained prominence with the discovery of many genes that are known to cause nonsyndromic deafness. In comparison to the genetics of nonsyndromic deafness, the genetics of vestibular disorders are poorly understood. This is likely due to the subjective nature of vestibular symptoms, which are often difficult to objectively measure in the clinical setting.[22]

Autosomal dominant nonsyndromic sensorineural deafness 9 typically presents with early-onset, progressive, high-frequency hearing loss and vertigo, and it has been linked to defects in the *COCH* gene.[22] Usher syndrome is a heterogeneous collection of autosomal recessive disorders that cause the triad of congenital hearing loss, retinitis pigmentosa, and vestibular dysfunction. While there are many different subtypes of Usher syndrome, Usher syndrome type 1 and Usher syndrome type 3 are most commonly linked with vestibular problems. Nine genes have been determined to cause the various Usher syndrome subtypes, with one additional modifier gene.[22] For patients suspected to have one of these conditions, indications for ordering genetic testing are not determined by vestibular symptoms but by the potential for genetic counseling.

■ Conclusion

History and physical examination with the aid of sophisticated auditory testing, vestibular testing, and imaging modalities have largely replaced or made redundant most laboratory tests in the work-up of a patient with balance disorders. Because of the success of other portions of the patient evaluation and because practitioners must become increasingly sensitive to the number of tests that we order, the use of laboratory tests as a routine part of the work-up of a patient with dizziness has become less common. Even in disorders in which the need for laboratory testing is documented (autoimmune disease), there is debate about the best test to order. We do believe that there are a few disorders and circumstances in which laboratory tests are an important part of the diagnosis and treatment. We provide a partial list of these tests in this chapter, but we advise individual practitioners to engage in the same thought process and to make their own decisions about the circumstances in which ordering laboratory tests is appropriate.

References

1. Hoffman RM, Einstadter D, Kroenke K. Evaluating dizziness. Am J Med 1999;107(5):468–478

2. Yimtae K, Srirompotong S, Lertsukprasert K. Otosyphilis: a review of 85 cases. Otolaryngol Head Neck Surg 2007;136(1):67–71

3. Phillips JS, Gaunt A, Phillips DR. Otosyphilis: a neglected diagnosis? Otol Neurotol 2014;35(6):1011–1013

4. Centers for Disease Control and Prevention (CDC). 2015 Sexually Transmitted Diseases Treatment Guidelines. Page last reviewed June 4, 2015. Retrieved from http://www.cdc.gov/std/tg2015/syphilis.htm

5. Centers for Disease Control and Prevention (CDC). Syphilis testing algorithms using treponemal tests for initial screening—four laboratories, New York City, 2005–2006. MMWR Morb Mortal Wkly Rep 2008; 57(32):872–875

6. Centers for Disease Control and Prevention (CDC). Discordant results from reverse sequence syphilis screening—five laboratories, United States, 2006–2010. MMWR Morb Mortal Wkly Rep 2011;60(5):133–137

7. Centers for Disease Control and Prevention (CDC). Recommendations for test performance and interpretation from the Second National Conference on Serologic Diagnosis of Lyme Disease. MMWR Morbid Mortal Wkly Rep 1995;44:590–591

8. Younger DS. Vasculitis of the nervous system. Curr Opin Neurol 2004;17(3):317–336

9. Harris JP, Sharp PA. Inner ear autoantibodies in patients with rapidly progressive sensorineural hearing loss. Laryngoscope 1990;100(5):516–524

10. Rauch SD. Clinical management of immune-mediated inner-ear disease. Ann N Y Acad Sci 1997;830:203–210

11. Rahman MU, Poe DS, Choi HK. Etanercept therapy for immune-mediated cochleovestibular disorders: preliminary results in a pilot study. Otol Neurotol 2001;22(5):619–624

12. Ruckenstein MJ. Autoimmune inner ear disease. Curr Opin Otolaryngol Head Neck Surg 2004;12(5):426–430

13. McCabe BF. Autoimmune inner ear disease: therapy. Am J Otol 1989;10(3):196–197

14. Hughes GB, Moscicki R, Barna BP, San Martin JE. Laboratory diagnosis of immune inner ear disease. Am J Otol 1994;15(2):198–202

15. Billings PB, Keithley EM, Harris JP. Evidence linking the 68 kilodalton antigen identified in progressive sensorineural hearing loss patient sera with heat shock protein 70. Ann Otol Rhinol Laryngol 1995; 104(3):181–188

16. Bloch DB, San Martin JE, Rauch SD, Moscicki RA, Bloch KJ. Serum antibodies to heat shock protein 70 in sensorineural hearing loss. Arch Otolaryngol Head Neck Surg 1995;121(10):1167–1171

17. Bonaguri C, Orsoni JG, Zavota L, et al. Anti-68 kDa antibodies in autoimmune sensorineural hearing loss: are these autoantibodies really a diagnostic tool? Autoimmunity 2007;40(1):73–78

18. Matsuoka AJ, Harris JP. Autoimmune inner ear disease: a retrospective review of forty-seven patients. Audiol Neurootol 2013;18(4):228–239

19. Sauvaget E, Kici S, Petelle B, et al. Vertebrobasilar occlusive disorders presenting as sudden sensorineural hearing loss. Laryngoscope 2004;114(2):327–332

20. Brenner M, Hoistad DL, Hain TC. Prevalence of thyroid dysfunction in patients with Ménière's disease. Arch Otolaryngol Head Neck Surg 2004;130(2):226–228

21. Lok U, Hatipoglu S, Gulacti U, Arpaci A, Aktas N, Borta T. The role of thyroid and parathyroid metabolism disorders in the etiology of sudden onset dizziness. Med Sci Monit 2014;20:2689–2694

22. Eppsteiner RW, Smith RJ. Genetic disorders of the vestibular system. Curr Opin Otolaryngol Head Neck Surg 2011;19(5):397–402

7 Meniere's Disease

Sujana S. Chandrasekhar

■ Introduction

Meniere's disease is a syndrome classically characterized by a quadrad of symptoms occurring episodically: aural fullness, fluctuating sensorineural hearing loss (SNHL), roaring tinnitus, and spinning vertigo, often accompanied by nausea and/or vomiting. This inner ear disorder's pathological correlate is hydrops of the endolymphatic space.[1] It is named for Prosper Meniere, the first individual to describe the symptom complex and who proposed its labyrinthine origin in 1861.[2] The term was applied indiscriminately until the current definition of the disorder was published in 1938 by Hallpike and Cairns,[3] and then in 1995 the American Academy of Otolaryngology–Head and Neck Surgery (AAO-HNS) published clear criteria enabling researchers to communicate coherently.[4] For the purist, the idiopathic constellation of these findings is called *Meniere's syndrome,* while when there is attribution to a specified cause, such as otosyphilis, it is called *Meniere's disease*; however, it is exceedingly rare that a proper etiology is identified, and the terms are generally used interchangeably.

■ Incidence

Vestibular dysfunction in the U.S. population, as estimated from the 2001–2004 National Health and Nutrition Examination Survey (NHANES), affects 35% of U.S. adults 40 years old and older, and 85% of those 80 years old and older.[5] Meniere's disease is a relatively unusual cause of vertigo among all patients with vertigo, as benign paroxysmal positional vertigo (BPPV) and migrainoid vertigo are far more common.[6] The most common vestibular disorder is BPPV, with a cumulative lifetime incidence of 10% by age 89; vestibular migraine is the second most common cause of dizziness, with a lifetime prevalence of 0.98%.

The incidence of Meniere's disease varies from 7.5 to 515 per 100,000 population in published studies from several countries.[7] The most rigorous assessment in the United States, based on the U.S. Health Claims Database, shows 473,000 Meniere's disease diagnoses out of 60 million claims, yielding a prevalence of 190 per 100,000 population.[8] Females are slightly more likely than males to be affected (1.3:1), and although the peak ages affected are between the fourth and sixth decades, Meniere's has been diagnosed in all age groups. Meniere's disease generally presents in only one ear, and in early stages either vestibular or cochlear symptoms may occur in isolation. Only about one-third of cases present with the full quadrad of symptoms.[9]

The published incidence[10] of bilateral involvement varies widely, between 9 and 50%, but is generally accepted to be around 30%. The enormous range appears to reflect a lack of consensus about diagnostic criteria and varying lengths of time of follow-up. A prospective study of 610 patients with disabling unilateral Meniere's disease found only a 5% incidence of contralateral Meniere's disease[11]; however, there was a 16% incidence of isolated hearing loss in the low frequencies in the contralateral ear. Other studies have suggested that there is an increased percentage of bilateral involvement over time.[12,13] There is evidence of immune complexes and circulating complement level abnormalities in Meniere's disease,[14] although the evidence of causal association between allergy and Meniere's disease is inconclusive.[15] The natural course of the disease is variable; up to 60% of patients with severe disease show remission within 2 years of onset and up to 71% within 8 years,[16] but there is a sizeable group of patients with progressive, unremitting disease.[17]

■ Pathophysiology and Possible Causes

The pathologic basis of Meniere's disease is thought to be distortion of the membranous labyrinth, which is characterized by endolymphatic hydrops. In this disorder, endolymph, the potassium-rich fluid in the middle portion of the inner ear, is either overabundantly produced or is inadequately absorbed. Either or both of these conditions results in expansion of the endolymphatic space. It is thought that when Reissner's membrane ruptures due to endolymphatic overpressure, the admixture of endolymph and perilymph results in vertigo, and eventually normal pressures are re-established and the membrane heals. Evidence of both hydrops and healed Reissner's membrane are seen in temporal bone specimens of Meniere's patients. However, although we can produce histopathologic findings of Meniere's disease in animals by disrupting the endolymphatic sac, these same animals do not display the characteristic symptoms of the disorder.[18] There is also lack of specificity in the human temporal bone histopathologic findings, in that endolymphatic hydrops is also seen in patients without the clinical history.[19] Cellular density changes in Reissner's membrane have been described in ears with endolymphatic hydrops with and without Meniere's disease.[20]

Endolymphatic hydrops is most consistently found in the pars inferior of the inner ear, that is, in the cochlea and saccule,[21] as bowing of Reissner's membrane out toward the scala vestibuli and distention of the saccule. When saccular distension is extensive, it can distort the utricle and semicircular canals in the vestibule and the saccular membrane can bulge out to contact the stapes footplate either directly or via fibrous adhesions.[22] The Hennebert sign, described in idiopathic as well as otosyphilitic endolymphatic hydrops, is vertigo produced by pressure insufflation on an intact tympanic membrane, causing stapes footplate movement, and is thought to result from this severe saccular distension.[23] Endolymphatic changes in the pars superior are infrequently seen and include herniation of the utricle into the common crus and displacement of semicircular canal cupulae from their ampullary roof attachment.[24]

Membranous ruptures in the labyrinth have been found in nearly all parts of the inner ear in Meniere's disease.[25] The ruptures appear to be significant in Meniere's pathophysiology in that they allow leakage of the potassium-rich endolymph into the perilymph, bathing the eighth cranial nerve and basal surfaces of the hair cells. This causes direction-changing nystagmus, which is a result of initial excitation from a rise in perilymphatic potassium concentration followed by inhibition due to a blockade of transmitter release. Membrane healing allows restitution of the normal chemical milieu and termination of the vertiginous attack, with hearing improvement. Repeated exposure to potassium's effects is presumably the cause of the chronic inner ear function deterioration that is seen in some cases of Meniere's disease.

Evidence for autoimmune processes causing Meniere's disease exists at the cellular level and, for bilateral disease, in clinical studies. The human endolymphatic sac appears to be the primary immunocompetent structure of the inner ear.[26] It can process antigen, synthesize antibodies, and raise a cellular immune response; its stromal cells contain immunoglobulins A and G and secretory component, and the perisaccular tissues contain macrophages, lymphocytes, and plasma cells. An abnormality of the Thl/Th2 balance in acute low-tone hearing loss, as well as increased natural killer cell activity, has been demonstrated in patients with Meniere's disease.[27] Antibodies against bovine 68-kDa heat shock protein HSP-70, regarded as an indicator of autoimmune ear disease, are elevated in 50% of patients with bilateral Meniere's disease.[28] Additionally, based on the potential role of thrombogenic antiphospholipid antibodies, patients with bilateral Meniere's disease may be more likely to have a systemic autoimmune process than those with unilateral disease.[29]

Other entities[30] implicated in causation include viral infection,[31] both acute and chronic, ischemia of the inner ear and sac,[32] and vascular disease that accounts for the association between Meniere's disease and migraine headaches.[33] This multifactorial list reflects both our lack of complete understanding of the pathophysiology as well as the fact that it is a syndrome, or constellation of symptoms, that we treat, with several potential causes. Clinicians generally lump the disorder into the "hydrops group" or the "migraine group," and management based on the causational belief ensues.

Genetic evaluation is of no value in patients without a suggestive history, as the data from various studies indicate only 5 to 15% heredity.[34] However, a high prevalence of symptoms of Meniere's disease has been described in families with a mutation in the coagulation factor C homology (*COCH*) gene, while no differences were found in the nucleotide sequences of exons 4 and 5 in the *COCH* gene in patients with sporadic Meniere's disease compared with controls.[35] Missense mutations in the *COCH* gene (14ql2-ql3) cause the disorder DFNA9, which is characterized by autosomal dominant SNHL with vestibular symptomatology. Individuals who are homozygous for the mutation appear to have earlier onset of symptoms.[36]

■ Symptoms

The diagnosis of Meniere's syndrome or disease is made clinically, based on the symptoms of aural fullness, fluctuating hearing loss, roaring tinnitus, and episodic vertigo. Classically, the patient experiences all of these symptoms in a single episode. However, in practice, symptoms are rarely "classic," and, especially initially, the patient may present with only cochlear or only vestibular symptoms. Thirty percent of sudden "idiopathic" hearing loss patients, when followed over a year in one study, manifested Meniere's disease.[37] In an acute Meniere's attack, the vertigo lasts several minutes to several hours, with most patients reporting a duration of 2 to 3 hours.[38] After the rotatory vertigo subsides, the patient is unsteady for some period of time (minutes to hours). In general, the length of the postvertiginous disequilibrium is related to the duration of the vertigo; that is, the longer the episode of spinning lasts, the longer the post-episode unsteadiness lasts. The patient is classically symptom-free between episodes. Atypical Meniere's disease includes cochlear hydrops, in which there is aural fullness, tinnitus, and fluctuating SNHL without vertigo, vestibular hydrops in which there is episodic vertigo alone, and attacks that occur without the typical "aura" of ear fullness and tinnitus. The variability of disease presentation contributes to the diagnostic and treatment inconsistencies.

The most debilitating symptom these patients face is episodic rotatory vertigo. When it occurs, it is exacerbated by head movements—the patient generally maintains a static position with the affected ear up to minimize the spinning—and may be accompanied by nausea, vomiting, diarrhea, and sweating. The vertigo causes patients to miss work and personal activities, and its unpredictability is the root of the anxiety seen in Meniere's disease. Two to 6% of patients with Meniere's disease may experience sudden, unexplained falls without vertigo or loss of consciousness,[39] known as *otolithic crises of Tumarkin* (or *drop attacks*, which Tumarkin attributed to acute utriculosaccular dysfunction).[40] Other diagnoses, such as vertebrobasilar insufficiency and migraine, must be ruled out before this diagnosis is made.

Low-frequency SNHL is the typical audiometric finding.[41] The hearing loss in Meniere's disease is typically fluctuating and can be progressive. Although high frequencies are initially preserved, with longer duration of disease, all frequencies may be affected. Hearing loss is effectively managed with hearing aids or, in more severe cases, cochlear implantation. Only 1 to 2% of patients will develop profound hearing loss. Lermoyez described what is frequently encountered in early Meniere's disease, that is, improvement in hearing thresholds in some patients after the vertiginous attack.

Tinnitus is the first presenting symptom in only 5% of patients and is equally divided in early Meniere's disease between mild (38%), moderate (32%), and severe (30%).[42] Intense tinnitus is, however, common in late-stage Meniere's disease. In the author's clinical experience, patients with advanced Meniere's disease are more overwhelmed and disabled by their tinnitus than is published and are willing to sacrifice any remaining hearing if only the tinnitus can be reduced or abolished.

Episodic vertigo is present in 96.2% of patients with Meniere's disease, tinnitus in 91.1%, and ipsilateral hearing loss in 87.7%.[43] Diagnosis and reporting on Meniere's disease was standardized when the AAO-HNS published guidelines for making a diagnosis of "definite" Meniere's disease. The criteria include two or more spontaneous episodes of vertigo, each lasting 20 minutes or longer; hearing loss documented at least once by audiometry; and tinnitus or aural fullness in the affected ear. The disease must be idiopathic, in that other causes have been excluded, typically with brain imaging. Symptoms need not be (and frequently are not) present simultaneously or in the same pattern, especially in the early phases of the disease.

Meniere's disease causes a significant impairment in quality of life that is worse on days of vertiginous attacks.[44] Meniere's patients also have higher incidences of depression and anxiety.[45] A vicious circle of interaction exists between the organic symptoms of Meniere's disease, particularly vertigo and tinnitus, and resultant psychological stress and anxiety.[46,47] Fifty-seven percent of patients have spontaneous cessation of vertigo in 2 years; 71% after 8.3 years.[48] However, there is an average pure-tone hearing loss of 50 dB, a mean speech discrimination score of 53%, and an average caloric response reduction of 50% in patients with long-standing Meniere's disease.[49] Attacks may be few and far between, separated by several months or years, or the patient may experience a months-to-years period of unrelenting, recurring attacks. Patients with Meniere's disease of shorter than 10 years' duration tend to experience less continuous vertigo than those in whom the disease is present for more than 20 years.[50] In those with > 20-year histories, 36% still have attacks one to four times per week, and 75% still consider their attacks to be severe in nature.

Triggers of Meniere's attacks include high salt intake, dehydration, high caffeine intake, and significant emotional stress. Emotional stress increases the risk of experiencing an attack of Meniere's disease during the next hour, and the hazard period is possibly extended up to 3 hours.[51]

Distinction between Meniere's Disease and Vestibular Migraine

Meniere's disease and vestibular migraine share symptoms, and the clinician may confuse one with the other. Additionally, the same patient may have both disorders. Forty-five percent of patients with Meniere's disease have at least one migrainous symptom during their vertiginous attacks as well as an increased lifetime prevalence of migraine.[52] Vestibular migraine is often associated with motion sensitivity, and diagnostic criteria for basilar migraine include vertigo, tinnitus, and hypacusia in the aura symptoms.[53] The categories of migraine accepted by the International Headache Society unfortunately do not reflect the complex presentations of patients suspected of having vestibular migraine, leading clinicians to expand criteria on their own, and that affects comparison of treatment outcomes.[54] However, as vestibular migraine is much more prevalent than Meniere's disease, and given that many of the symptoms overlap, some institutions treat all of Meniere's disease as a cerebrovascular disorder.[55]

■ Diagnosis

The diagnosis of Meniere's disease is based on history and audiometric findings, as detailed in the AAO-HNS Guidelines, which are summarized here:

Certain Meniere's disease:

- Definite Meniere's disease plus histopathological confirmation

Definite Meniere's disease:

- Two or more definitive spontaneous episodes of vertigo, each 20 minutes or longer
- Audiometrically documented hearing loss on at least one occasion
- Tinnitus or aural fullness in the treated ear
- Other causes excluded

Probable Meniere's disease:

- One definitive episode of vertigo
- Audiometrically documented hearing loss on at least one occasion
- Tinnitus or aural fullness in the treated ear
- Other causes excluded

Possible Meniere's disease:

- Episodic vertigo of the Meniere's type without documented hearing loss; or
- Sensorineural hearing loss, fluctuating or fixed, with disequilibrium but without definitive episodes
- Other causes excluded

Despite the guidelines, a survey of neuro-otologists showed that only one-third relied solely on history, physical examination, and audiometry. Two-thirds used adjunctive tests, including electrocochleography, electronystagmography, rotary chair evaluation, vestibular evoked myogenic potentials, head thrust testing, glycerol and furosemide dehydration tests, posturography, auditory brainstem response testing, tympanometry, blood tests, and magnetic resonance imaging (MRI).[56,57]

Electrocochleography (ECoG) is frequently used as a diagnostic tool in Meniere's disease; it is helpful when the results are positive, but a normal ECoG cannot rule out the presence of endolymphatic hydrops.[58] Electrocochleography is based on the presence of a summating potential (SP) and an action potential (AP) generated by the cochlea in response to repeated presentations of sound. In Meniere's disease, due to distension of the basilar membrane into the scala tympani causing increase in the (normal) asymmetry of its vibration, the SP is reported to be larger and more negative than in normal ears. A difference of > 45% SP/AP ratio is abnormal (**Fig. 7.1**).

The sensitivity of a basic ECoG test in evaluating the SP/AP amplitude ratio ranges from 20%[59] to 70%.[60] Modifying the test to measure the SP/AP area ratio is reported to significantly improve detection, to 83%.[61] However, the test is not specific for Meniere's disease, as an abnormal ECoG is characteristic of other disease entities, such as perilymphatic fistula and semicircular canal dehiscence.

Electronystagmography (ENG) or video-ENG (VNG) is a more exact test of vestibular function,[62] and a significantly reduced vestibular response to caloric stimulation is seen in the affected ear in Meniere's disease in 48 to 74% of patients. Additionally, absent caloric response in the affected ear is seen in 6 to 11% of patients.[63] It is very difficult to obtain ENG or VNG evaluation during an acute Meniere's attack, as patients are too ill for testing at that time, and they must be free of central nervous system sedative agents (typically used to "abort" the attacks) for 72 hours prior to the test. Findings are shown in **Fig. 7.2** and include spontaneous nystagmus to the lesioned side and severely reduced caloric response from the affected ear. It is important to remember that a caloric response difference of 20 to 25% between ears is normal, depending upon the individual laboratory's settings. Additionally, testing can be normal between episodes, particularly in early or very sporadic Meniere's disease. ENG has only a 50% total positive rate response in patients with Meniere's disease, indicating limited sensitivity for diagnosis. This modality is of great benefit, however, when deciding on ablation types of therapy for disabling Meniere's disease, as it indicates not only the condition of the affected ear, but the vestibular reserve in the opposite ear, allowing for enhanced patient counseling. Vestibular evoked myogenic potential (VEMP) testing may be of benefit in an early Meniere's diagnosis.[64] VEMPs are auditory evoked potentials that measure small variations in neck muscle (cVEMP) or extraocular muscle (oVEMP) contractions that occur when a sudden burst of sound is introduced to the ear. The linear sensing parts of the saccule cause a brief relaxation of the muscles in the neck that function to keep the

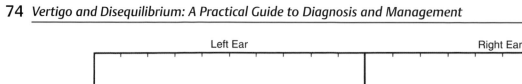

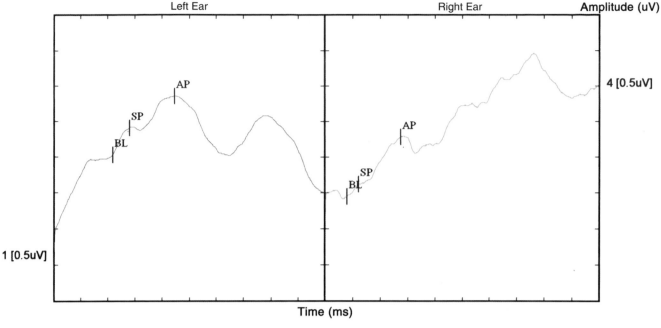

Latencies (ms)							
ECochG							
Waveform	Ear	AP	SP	III	IV	V	BL
1	Left	2.14	1.34	***	***	***	1.05
4	Right	1.31	0.58	***	***	***	0.38

Amplitudes (uV)				
ECochG				
Waveform	BL	AP	SP	SP/AP
1	-2.55	0.83	0.38	46%
4	-2.45	0.83	0.17	21%

Waveforms													
ECochG													
#	Date	Record	Transducer	Intensity	Ear	Rate	Stimulus	Gain	High	Low	Acc	Rej	Epoch
1	5/25/2006	11.1	Insert Phone	95dB nHL	Left	7.7/s	Click-A	100k	5 Hz	1.5 kHz	175	113	5ms
4	5/25/2006	14.2	Insert Phone	95dB nHL	Right	7.7/s	Click-A	100k	5 Hz	1.5 kHz	71	20	5ms

Fig. 7.1 Electrocochleography in left-ear Meniere's disease. Left-ear EcoG SP/AP ratio is 46% (abnormal). SP, summating potential, AP, action potential; BL, baseline.

head erect. The VEMP, therefore, is an inferior vestibular nerve test. Studies have demonstrated that up to 67% of patients with Meniere's attacks had abnormal VEMPs, indicating that the saccule participates in a Meniere's attack; half of the abnormal VEMPs return to normal after 48 hours[65] or after glycerol or furosemide dehydration. In Meniere's disease, an abnormal VEMP test result is seen as a reduction in amplitude of > 40%, or greater than 3:1 ratio (**Fig. 7.3**).

The advantages of using VEMPs for a Meniere's diagnosis are that they can confirm the side of the lesion, they can be used in patients with severe to profound hearing loss, where auditory brainstem response testing cannot, and they can help to distinguish atypical Meniere's disease from superior semi-circular canal dehiscence syndrome or perilymphatic fistula, in which VEMPs are present at abnormally low thresholds (lower than 80 dB) in the affected ear.

The Halmagyi head thrust test[66] is a passive test of unilateral vestibulo-ocular reflex (VOR) gain in which the patient is instructed to view a distant object and to keep his visual focus on that object at all times. The examiner suddenly turns the patient's head to the right or left rapidly through a small arc and then to the opposite side (**Fig. 7.4**). If the VOR gain is normal, or near normal, on the side of the direction of the movement, the eyes will remain on the visual target. However, if the patient exhibits saccadic corrections of the eye, reduced VOR gain on the side of the movement is suggested. Head thrust testing may

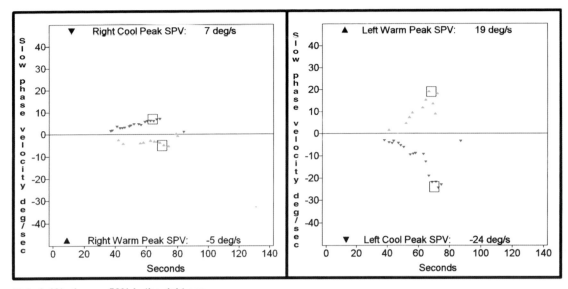

Caloric Weakness: 56% in the right ear

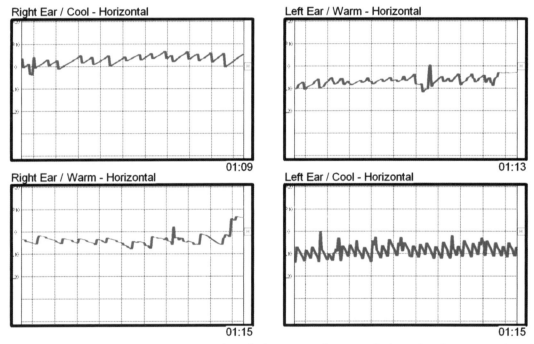

Fig. 7.2 Electronystagmography evaluation in acute right-sided Meniere's disease. Caloric testing shows severely reduced response from the right ear (56% reduced vestibular response).

be of limited benefit if there is less than 50% vestibular weakness.[67]

Osmotic diuretics are able to reduce endolymphatic pressure and volume and hence improve peripheral auditory and vestibular function. After baseline audiometric testing, a dose of glycerol, urea, furosemide, or other osmotic diuretic is administered. Repeat audiometric testing is performed at 3 hours (and sometimes at 1 and 2 hours) after

ingestion. The test is considered positive if (1) there is a 10-dB or greater improvement at two or more frequencies (250 to 2000 Hz), or (2) there is a 12% or greater improvement in speech discrimination scores. Positive dehydration tests are found in 60 to 66% of patients with Meniere's disease.[68,69] The glycerol test is associated with several unpleasant side effects, including headache, nausea, thirst, diarrhea, emesis, diuresis, and dizziness; these are not seen

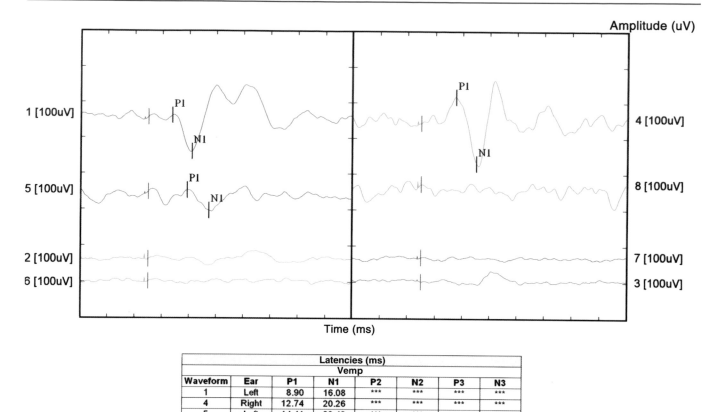

Latencies (ms)							
Vemp							
Waveform	Ear	P1	N1	P2	N2	P3	N3
1	Left	8.90	16.08	***	***	***	***
4	Right	12.74	20.26	***	***	***	***
5	Left	14.41	22.43	***	***	***	***

Waveforms													
Vemp													
#	Date	Record	Transducer	Intensity	Ear	Rate	Stimulus	Gain	High	Low	Acc	Rej	Epoch
1	6/29/2006	5.1	Insert phone	95dB nHL	Left	5.1/s	500 Hz-A	5k	2 Hz	500 Hz	150	0	100ms
2	6/29/2006	5.2	Insert phone	95dB nHL	Left	5.1/s	500 Hz-A	5k	2 Hz	500 Hz	150	0	100ms
3	6/29/2006	6.1	Insert phone	95dB nHL	Right	5.1/s	500 Hz-A	5k	2 Hz	500 Hz	150	0	100ms
4	6/29/2006	6.2	Insert phone	95dB nHL	Right	5.1/s	500 Hz-A	5k	2 Hz	500 Hz	150	0	100ms
5	6/29/2006	7.1	Insert phone	70dB nHL	Left	5.1/s	500 Hz-A	5k	2 Hz	500 Hz	150	0	100ms
6	6/29/2006	7.2	Insert phone	70dB nHL	Left	5.1/s	500 Hz-A	5k	2 Hz	500 Hz	150	0	100ms
7	6/29/2006	8.1	Insert phone	70dB nHL	Right	5.1/s	500 Hz-A	5k	2 Hz	500 Hz	150	0	100ms
8	6/29/2006	8.2	Insert phone	70dB nHL	Right	5.1/s	500 Hz-A	5k	2 Hz	500 Hz	150	0	100ms

Fig. 7.3 Vestibular evoked myogenic potential (VEMP) testing. This patient had atypical left-ear symptoms; VEMP testing is more consistent with superior semicircular canal dehiscence syndrome or perilymphatic fistula due to the early latency of PI (8 milliseconds versus normal of 15 milliseconds) and the existence of an amplitude on the left at 70 dB (wave 5). Vestibular evoked myogenic potential amplitudes generally disappear at 80 dB.

with furosemide.[70] Because dehydration tests are relatively specific for endolymphatic hydrops, they may be useful in confirming the presence of disease in patients with atypical presentations. However, because the tests are relatively insensitive, they are not useful to rule out endolymphatic hydrops or as screening tests for the disease. Tests are more likely negative very early and very late in the course of disease, although the stage of the disease is not predictable from the results of the dehydration testing.[71]

Rotary chair testing is of benefit in acute Meniere's disease as well as in determining the level of residual deficit in poorly compensated but inactive disease.

Findings include reduced response to the velocity step of rotation on the affected side and offset to that side during sinusoidal rotation. Some literature suggests that computerized dynamic posturography (CDP) evaluation can be of benefit in classifying Meniere's disease patients as acute (recent post-attack), subacute (late post-attack), or inactive.[72] The value of CDP, however, lies primarily in objective assessment of quality-of-life issues in the disease, such as balance dysfunction, which is seen in chronic or poorly compensated Meniere's.

Auditory brainstem response (ABR) testing is primarily employed to rule out retrocochlear pathology

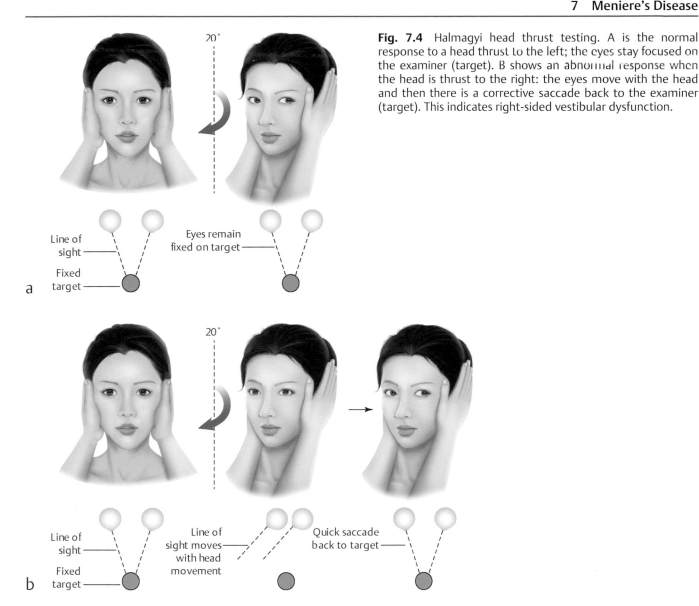

Fig. 7.4 Halmagyi head thrust testing. A is the normal response to a head thrust to the left; the eyes stay focused on the examiner (target). B shows an abnormal response when the head is thrust to the right: the eyes move with the head and then there is a corrective saccade back to the examiner (target). This indicates right-sided vestibular dysfunction.

in these patients; however, attempts have also been made to use ABR as an objective method to indicate endolymphatic hydrops.[73] The traveling-wave velocity test, which uses derived ABRs, has been shown to be altered, reflecting endolymphatic hydrops in 27% of the asymptomatic (contralateral) ears of unilateral Meniere's disease patients.[74] Cochlear hydrops analysis masking procedures (CHAMPs) is an ABR test masked at different frequencies with high-pass noise masking. In Meniere's patients CHAMPs show that the masking noise is insufficient, such that an undermasked wave V is still present similar to that with clicks alone. This is not true in non-Meniere's ears.[75] The CHAMPs test may prove to be of use in objectively distinguishing active Meniere's disease and in tracking changes in severity of disease.[76]

Tympanometric evaluation of Meniere's patients reveals reduced resonant frequency in the affected ear, with consistently increased width of conductance tympanograms at 2 kHz in these patients. In one study, while more than 95% of normal subjects had a negative test, 56.5% of affected ears and 45.8% of nonaffected ears of Meniere's patients had a positive test.[77] As detailed previously in this chapter, metabolic screening, including carbohydrate and lipid metabolism and thyroid function tests, has not proved useful in the diagnosis of Meniere's disease, and the use of laboratory tests is generally limited to the treponemal antigen test for syphilis and suitable tests for patients in whom autoimmune disease is highly suspected.

Magnetic resonance imaging (MRI) is generally employed to rule out retrocochlear pathology as a cause for the symptoms; however, some studies have found smaller and shorter endolymph drainage systems or inflammatory changes in the endolymphatic sac in Meniere's disease patients.[78,79] High-resolution MRI can be used to image the endolymphatic duct and sac. One study correlated visible abnormalities and the lack of a visible endolymphatic duct and sac with the clinical course of Meniere's disease.[80] Intratympanic injection of gadolinium and 3D FLAIR MRI may be more conclusive for Meniere's; in patients with clinically and ECoG-confirmed definitive Meniere's disease,[81] the degree of impairment of perilymph enhancement directly correlated with degree of otovestibular dysfunction, and in all normals there was no impairment of perilymph enhancement.[82,83,84] However, the diagnosis of Meniere's disease still cannot be made by MRI.[85] Twenty-three patients with Meniere's disease and 50 controls were evaluated by high-resolution computed tomography (HRCT) and MRI.[86] The percentage of nonvisualized vestibular aqueduct on HRCT was significantly lower in the control group (3.4%) than in either the involved (27.8%) or uninvolved (22.2%) ears of the study group. There was no difference between diseased and nondiseased ears in the Meniere's group. MRI showed the endolymphatic duct and sac system in 64.1% of controls and only 39.1% of subjects ($p = 0.05$). Computed tomography (CT) is not overly useful in confirming the diagnosis of Meniere's disease, with the possible exception being that the vestibular aqueduct may be narrow in some cases, as shown in **Fig. 7.5**. MR images in Meniere's disease are seen in **Fig. 7.6**.

■ Treatment

To standardize result reporting for Meniere's disease and therapy, the then-American Academy of Ophthalmology and Otolaryngology (AAOO) devised a system in 1972 that was later revised by the AAO-HNS in 1985 and again in 1995.[4] Because of the capriciousness of behavior and treatment response identified in the initial AAOO system, adherence to the 1995 guidelines, which demand 18- to 24-month follow-up and strict mathematical comparison of pre- and posttreatment vertigo (**Table 7.1**), would be very useful to enhance our understanding of this disorder. Unfortunately, only 50% of papers in peer-reviewed, English-language publications between January 1989 and December 1999 used the guidelines.[87]

The same study of neuro-otologists quoted above regarding diagnosis revealed the following about treatment. Conservative medical management is preferred; when this fails, the preferred initial invasive intervention is endolymphatic sac surgery in 50%, intratympanic gentamicin in 39%, local overpressure using the Meniett device in 9%, and vestibular nerve section in 2%. Over the last decade and a half, intratympanic steroid injection for Meniere's disease has increased in popularity.[88] Overall, clinicians continue to turn toward less invasive means to treat medically recalcitrant Meniere's disease. The treatment of the disease continues to be one of palliation and support.

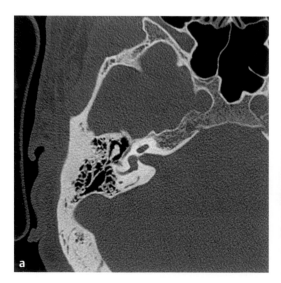 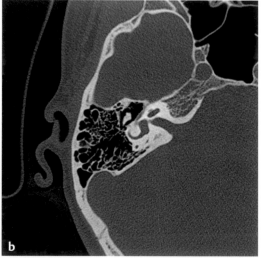

Fig. 7.5 High-resolution computed tomography imaging of **(a)** a normal vestibular aqueduct in a non-Meniere's patient compared with **(b)** a narrow vestibular aqueduct in a patient with Meniere's disease. Courtesy of Linda Heier, MD.

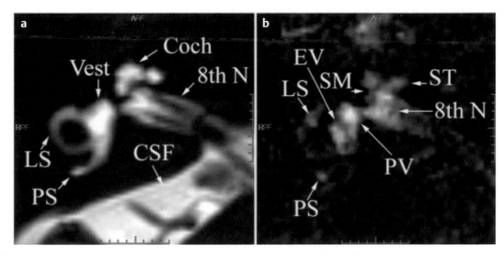

Fig. 7.6 MRI of a 72-year-old patient with Meniere's disease on the right side at 4 h postintravenous injection of Gd-DTPA-BMA at a single dosage. **(a)** Anatomy is demonstrated by T2-weighted MRI. **(b)** Uptake of Gd-DTPA-BMA in the inner ear is shown using a heavy T2-weighted FLAIR sequence. Obvious enlargement of the scala media (SM) at the basal turn is a sign of endolymphatic hydrops and was observed in the cochlea. Coch, cochlea; CSF, cerebrospinal fluid; 8th N, cochleo-vestibular nerve; EV, endolymph in the vestibulum; LS, lateral semicircular canal; PS, posterior semicircular canal; PV, perilymph in the vestibulum; ST, sinus tympani; Vest, vestibulum.

Medical Treatment

There is no cure per se for Meniere's disease; however, aggressive medical management results in dramatic or complete reduction in symptoms in 80 to 90% of patients.[89,90] Management differs during acute attacks and in the intervening periods between episodes and is based primarily on collective anecdotal experience, as there is a paucity of evidence-based management guidelines in the literature.[91] The overriding philosophy of all Meniere's disease treatments is to be as noninvasive and nondestructive as possible for as long as possible and to remain cognizant of the relatively high likelihood of eventual bilateral disease. Treatments are grouped into categories: conservative (medical) or either nondestructive or destructive interventional. Physicians can be divided into a "hydrops group" and a "migraine group" and, within their groups, follow a relatively universal protocol through the categories.

Hydrops Group Protocol

As a baseline for therapy, all patients are given a low-salt diet (~ 1500 to 2000 mg/day of sodium). Most patients are also given oral diuretics, preferably of the potassium-sparing variety, and are counseled about potassium replacement, either dietary or medicinal. Although many believe that salt restriction and diuretics are the mainstay of therapy,[92] with control of vertigo in 58% and stabilization of hearing in 69%,[93] other studies show no diuretic effect.[94] A Cochrane review showed no articles supporting diuretic use that met currently accepted review standards.[95] Nonetheless, diuretics are employed almost universally. The diuretics are continued until all aural symptoms have disappeared, with the exception of tinnitus, which may always remain present. In general, patients are asked to withdraw diuretic therapy gradually while monitoring symptoms and

Table 7.1 AAO-HNS guidelines on reporting vertigo in Meniere's disease

Numerical Value*	Class
0	A (complete control of definitive spells)
1–40	B
41–80	C
81–120	D
> 120	E
Secondary treatment initiated because of disability from vertigo	F

*Numerical value = $(X/Y) \times 100$, where X = average number of definitive spells per month for the 6-month period 18 to 24 months after therapy, and Y = average number of definitive spells per month for the 6-month period before therapy.

are counseled to maintain a low-salt diet. In this author's experience, patients may respond to either hydrochlorothiazide or acetazolamide at different points in their disease. Often, recurrent symptoms in the face of ongoing diuretic use will respond to a change in the type of diuretic.

Migraine Group Protocol

Sodium restriction is not directly advocated in migraine treatment; however, reduction of monosodium glutamate (MSG) intake as part of sodium restriction may be helpful, as glutamate is a known migraine trigger,[96] and a low-sodium diet is useful for control of hypertension, which is a vascular risk factor.[97]

Avoidance of migraine food triggers, such as monosodium glutamate, chocolate, red wine, fermented dairy products including yogurt, and aged or pickled foods, is advocated by the migraine group. As well, in the hydrops group, patients are counseled against caffeine, nicotine, and alcohol intake. Adequate hydration is encouraged. There is no scientific evidence to support this; however, there is a great deal of anecdotal experience in its favor. Vitamins are also encouraged anecdotally, primarily lipoflavinoids with extra B and C, niacin (B_3), and magnesium.

Agents like amitriptyline, β-blockers, calcium channel blockers, acetazolamide, and topiramate are commonly used for migraine prophylaxis as well as for vestibular symptoms in migraineurs, and are used at some "migraine group" centers for Meniere's disease. Again, controlled studies on the utility of these agents in Meniere's disease are lacking.

Papaverine is employed for its vasodilatory capability, despite evidence that it does not directly affect cochlear blood flow.[98] If diuretics alone fail, some physicians add a calcium channel blocker (first choice is nimodipine, 30 mg twice a day, and second choice is amlodipine, 5 mg per day) with good success.

There is evidence for a role of environmental and food allergies in Meniere's disease, in both unilateral and bilateral cases. 734 patients with Meniere's disease and 172 non-Meniere's otology patients were administered the same survey.[99] Of the Meniere's patients, 59.2% reported possible airborne allergies, 40.3% had or suspected food allergies, and 37% had confirmatory skin or in vitro tests for allergy. In the control group, 42.7% reported having or suspecting airborne allergies, and 25% had or suspected food allergies. The differences were statistically significant. A study[100] of 113 Meniere's disease patients treated with allergy desensitization and diet showed a significant improvement from pretreatment to posttreatment in both allergy and Meniere's symptoms compared with Meniere's disease patients not treated for allergies. Of the treated patients, 47.9%

achieved AAO-HNS class A or B vertigo control, and 61.4% had stable or improved hearing.

Histamine receptors have been found within the endolymphatic sac, and betahistine (a structural analog of histamine) is a mainstay of Meniere's therapy in several countries. Normal dosages are 12 to 16 mg up to three times per day.[101] A study of very-high-dose betahistine between 288 and 480 mg/day showed fewer patients reporting vertiginous attacks with higher dosages of medication.[102] Side effects of high-dose betahistine include gastrointestinal complaints, fatigue, and altered taste, and these may be significant. Additionally, there is a possibility of migraine as a confounder in the association of allergy and Meniere's disease.[15] Despite the lack of definitive studies, it behooves the treating physician to be cognizant of a possible allergy contribution in treating Meniere's disease.

During acute episodes of vertigo, vestibular sedatives, such as prochlorperazine, dimenhydrate, meclizine, promethazine, and diazepam, are prescribed. Rarely are these medications required on an ongoing basis, except in a few individuals with chronic unremitting vestibulopathy near the end stage of the disease. Additionally, ondansetron, a commonly used antiemetic for chemotherapy that is available as an orally disintegrating tablet, can greatly reduce the severe nausea and vomiting that can occur in acute Meniere's attacks.

Steroid Therapy

Systemic corticosteroids are frequently used when the patient is in the throes of an acute episode or when the time between episodes is short. As an example, in patients experiencing attacks every 2 to 3 days, systemic steroids are used to break the cycle. The dosage ranges from 0.5 to 1 mg/kg body weight for a short period of 5 to 10 days, depending on the severity of the attack, the patient's medical condition, gender, stress level, and his or her prior response to steroids.[103] Despite over 60 years of steroid use for inner ear disorders, a thorough review of the literature points out that there is limited understanding of their mechanism of action in reversing hearing loss or vestibular dysfunction.[104] However, the review is able to assert the following: (1) the statement that "steroids have no positive impact on hearing and vestibular dysfunction" is a misconception; (2) hearing loss that is steroid responsive is not necessarily immune-mediated, despite the steriod-responsiveness seen in autoimmune inner ear disorders[105]; (3) there are inner ear tissue-specific and challenge-specific transcriptional effects of glucocorticoids; and (4) the dose regimen for systemic steroid therapy should not be fixed; rather, it should be adjusted for age, sex, season, time of day, and lifestyle.

Intratympanic steroids for Meniere's disease are discussed in detail in the next section, because they can be categorized as interventional, nondestructive treatment.

Several herbal and other alternative remedies are in use for Meniere's disease[106]; the most common ones are discussed here. *Ginkgo biloba* is touted for vertigo and tinnitus relief, but adequate studies are not available. The dosage considered appropriate is 240 mg/day.[107] Patients should be cautioned about its effects as a blood thinner. Lysine is a commonly occurring amino acid that is popular in France for vertigo treatment.[108] Vertigo-heel is a homeopathic combination of cocculus, conium, ambra, and mineral oil. One study reported 57% subjective improvement with three tablets three times daily for 2 weeks.[109] Alternative medicine websites, such as www.cancertutor.com, also list "known" causes of Meniere's disease to be avoided "at all costs." These include aspartame, monosodium glutamate, hydrolyzed vegetable protein, and cysteine. Evidence supporting these claims is not available.

Interventional, Nondestructive Treatment

Intratympanic (IT) application of steroids for inner ear perfusion results in significantly higher drug levels in inner ear fluids than are achieved with systemic application.[110,111] The initial studies on IT steroid perfusion were done in patients with sudden sensorineural hearing loss or autoimmune ear disease. A Cochrane Review of IT steroids for Meniere's disease[88] was able to include only a single 2-year prospective, placebo-controlled, double-blind, randomized trial[112] of IT dexamethasone (4 mg/mL) given daily for 5 consecutive days that utilized the 1995 AAO-HNS criteria. In the treatment group, complete vertigo control (class A) was achieved in 82% and substantial control (class B) in 18%. Thirty-six percent of the control group needed other treatment for continuing vertigo and were therefore failures (class F); 57% of the remainder achieved class A, 29% class C, and 14% class F. In addition to vertigo control, the treatment group had 48% improvement in tinnitus and aural fullness and 35% in hearing loss, compared with only 20 and 10% in the control group. A study[113] of 22 patients given IT methylprednisolone and/or dexamethasone for acute Meniere's disease showed 54.5% short-term vertigo control; after 12 months, that percentage decreased to 18.2%. Another study[114] of 50 patients with either classic Meniere's disease or cochlear hydrops given from one to three IT dexamethasone (16 mg/mL) injection(s) demonstrated 40% significant acute hearing improvement and 56% no change in hearing acuity. Five of eight with improvement who were followed over 3 to 6 months

had lasting improvement over their baseline; the other three deteriorated back to the pretreatment hearing level. Inner ear steroid perfusion is generally employed in acute, severe cases of vertigo and hearing loss as a means of rapid salvage.[115]

The basic technique for intratympanic infusion[11] is to have the patient lie back at 45 to 60 degrees with the affected ear up. The canal is inspected under the microscope, and 0.5 ml of the solution to be injected is drawn up into a 1 ml syringe that is loaded with a 22-gauge spinal needle. A small amount of phenol applied with a right-angle double-pronged applicator to just blanch the anterosuperior quadrant of the tympanic membrane is very effective in providing anesthesia during the procedure. Two small myringotomies are made in the anterosuperior quadrant of the tympanic membrane with the tip of the needle, one just below the other. The medication is infused into the middle ear space via the inferior perforation. The infusion is stopped when air bubbles and then liquid start to escape from the superior hole. The patient then lies in that position for 20 minutes, without swallowing, so as to not lose much of the solution into the nasopharynx via the Eustachian tube. This technique is employed for both dexamethasone and gentamicin perfusion.

Local overpressure treatment delivered to the ear via a pressure-equalizing tube was approved for use in the United States in 2000 as the Meniett device. A systematic review[116] of 18 papers and a meta-analysis of 12 suggested that the Meniett device is effective for both vertigo and hearing loss in Meniere's disease, while remaining nondestructive. A randomized, placebo-controlled study[117] of 40 patients (20 treated and 20 controls) followed for 8 weeks revealed significant improvement in the patient's functional level and vertigo as evaluated by the visual analog scale, reduction in frequency of vertiginous attacks, and no difference in perception of hearing, tinnitus, and aural pressure. Eighteen other patients were followed for a mean of 18 months with the overpressure device,[118] and 12 (67%) showed significant improvement of one or more Meniere's symptoms. Sixty-seven percent had significant improvements when rated on the six-point functional scale. There were no changes in caloric function, and the six patients without improvement had previously had either surgery or IT gentamicin treatment. Overpressure therapy in guinea pigs with experimental hydrops[119] appears to suppress development of hydrops and improve cochlear function without destroying the inner ear. This treatment would be recommended for individuals for whom first-line medical management has failed, and prior to recommending destructive intervention.

The data just mentioned are confounded by the fact that simple insertion of ventilation tubes across the tympanic membrane has at least some efficacy in

Meniere's treatment. One study[120] of seven patients followed for 2 and 4 years after tube insertion showed that five of seven had substantial vertigo control and one had limited vertigo control at 24 months; four of seven and three of seven, respectively, had those outcomes at 48 months.

Endolymphatic sac decompression (ELSD) and shunting (ELSS) are hearing-preserving surgical interventions for Meniere's disease that is refractory to medical management. The premise is that the increased pressure in endolymphatic hydrops is alleviated by decompressing the mastoid bone off the sac and/or by opening the sac and shunting the fluid off, either (previously) into the subarachnoid space or (currently) into the mastoid bone.[121] An infamous "sham" study, published in 1981,[122] quoting an 81% vertigo control rate attributed to placebo, caused significant reduction of enthusiasm for endolymphatic surgery; a reassessment of the data[123] in 2000 showed a significant improvement in vertigo control for endolymphatic sac surgery over placebo. This surgical intervention remains the most popular one in use today.[56] A systematic review and meta-analysis of endolymphatic sac surgery[124] included 36 papers and concluded that ELSD and ELSS are effective at controlling vertigo in both short- and long-term in at least three-fourths of Meniere's patients who had previously failed medical management. Of interest, hearing outcomes seemed to be better without Silastic shunting once the sac was opened. In contrast, a Cochrane review update on surgery for Meniere's disease[125] was able to include only two trials, one comparing endolymphatic sac surgery with ventilation tubes and one with simple mastoidectomy, and found no beneficial effect. Quality-of-life assessments show 87% improvement[126] and significant improvement in physical health, as well as physical and social functioning,[127] after ELSD. Studies of surgical efficacy of both ELSD and ELSS vary from < 60% resolution of vertigo to 94% and 95% improvement, and 37 to 78% resolution of vertigo.[128,129] Long-term outcomes of ELSD and ELSS are very good; after a mean follow-up of 55 months, 81% of patients treated with ELSD[130] showed significant improvement in functionality, from median level 4 to 2, and long-term vertigo control was 72% in class A or B. Fifty-one percent of patients were in hearing stage I or II, with 18% showing hearing improvement and 64% remaining stable. A variation on sac surgery that appears to be beneficial involves topical steroid application to the opened sac at the time of ELSS. A series of 12 patients treated with ELSS and steroid application followed for 6 to 14 months showed complete vertigo control, improved hearing, and reduction in tinnitus in all but one.[131]

Interventional, Destructive Treatment

Aminoglycoside therapy for refractory Meniere's disease was first proposed by Schuknecht in 1956.[132] Successful bilateral ablation, unfortunately, results in gait disturbance and oscillopsia. Subsequent reports of use of streptomycin for chemical labyrinthectomy admonished that dosage was not yet able to be properly controlled.[133] At present, IT application of gentamicin is an accepted and frequently utilized therapy in Meniere's disease. Gentamicin is primarily vestibulotoxic, and the target appears to be the dark cells near the crista ampullaris,[134] although all portions of the inner ear may be affected.[135] Animal studies[136] have indicated improved inner ear absorption kinetics when the gentamicin is delivered in a sustained-release fashion; this is confirmed with human studies using a round window microcatheter.[137] Fourteen studies were included in a review of IT gentamicin for Meniere's disease.[138] Data were pooled. Class A vertigo control was achieved in 457 (71.4%) of 559 patients, class B in 16.1%, class C in 4.3%, class D in 2.4%, class E in 2.9%, and class F in 2.9%. Overall, IT gentamicin was successful in treating Meniere's disease in 87.5%. Quality of life was remarkably improved after IT gentamicin treatment, and hearing loss was not significant except in the 11 patients (1.8%) who experienced total deafness. Functional evaluation of post-treatment angular vestibulo-ocular reflex (aVOR) comparing gentamicin instillation in 17 patients and surgical unilateral vestibular destruction in 13 patients,[139] revealed that IT gentamicin resulted in decreased gains attributable to each semicircular canal on the treated side and minimal effect on the contralateral canals. There was no difference between patients who received a single IT injection and those who received two or three injections. Gain decreases were not as severe as those observed after surgical destruction, suggesting that IT gentamicin causes only a partial vestibular lesion. However, patients must be warned that usually 2 to 3 days after the first and second injection, they will experience a severe vertiginous episode as some of the vestibular cells die, analogous to what happens in a vestibular nerve section.

A meta-analysis[140] of 15 trials of IT gentamicin with 627 patients showed that vertigo control was effective and cochleotoxicity was unlikely, and was unrelated to treatment regimens of titration versus fixed application. The recommendation of the authors was titration with low-dose medication. Conversely, another meta-analysis[141] published that same year concluded that the titration method of gentamicin delivery demonstrated significantly better complete (81.7%) and effective (96.3%) vertigo control than other methods. The low-dose method of delivery demonstrated significantly worse complete vertigo control (66.7%) and trends toward worse effective vertigo control (86.8%) compared with other methods. The weekly method of delivery trended toward less overall hearing loss (13.1%), and the multiple daily method demonstrated significantly more overall hearing loss (34.7%). No significant difference in profound hearing loss was found between groups, nor did degree of vestibular ablation correlate with the resulting vertigo control or hearing loss status.

A study[142] compared IT dexamethasone, IT gentamicin, and ELSD for intractable vertigo in Meniere's disease. The regimen studied was used in 24, 16, and 25 patients, respectively, and each achieved satisfactory control of vertigo in 72%, 75%, and 52% of patients, respectively. Two patients in the gentamicin group had total hearing loss; hearing was stable or improved in 62% of the dexamethasone group. The study authors' treatment protocol is medical management for 6 months, followed by IT dexamethasone. After 3 more months, symptomatic patients with no hearing undergo IT gentamicin and those with hearing undergo ELSD. If that also fails, the patients become candidates for labyrinthectomy or vestibular nerve section.

This is a common treatment paradigm for Meniere's disease. A survey of otologists and neuro-otologists published in 2001 reflected the previous decade's experience in vertigo.[143] The number of vestibular neurectomies, endolymphatic sac surgeries, and labyrinthectomies had all decreased, while office-administered IT gentamicin therapy increased rapidly throughout the entire 10-year period, and by 1999 it had become the most frequently used invasive treatment for Meniere's disease. Surgeons now seem to reserve inpatient procedures for cases where IT gentamicin fails to control vertigo.

Cochleosacculotomy is a transcanal surgical option for elderly patients with refractory Meniere's disease and poor hearing.[144] With the increased use of IT medications, this procedure has waned in popularity.

Selective vestibular nerve section (VNS) is an excellent surgical option but involves a craniectomy for access. It is employed when most other means of treatment have been exhausted but hearing is such that it can be preserved. When hearing is poor, transmastoid labyrinthectomy (TL) is an excellent surgical intervention for recalcitrant disease.

In one study comparing VNS, ELSS, and TL, most patients had Meniere's disease for longer than 1 year and more than 20% for longer than 5 years.[145] In that study, 38% of patients undergoing VNS were disabled preoperatively, compared with 22% and 23%, respectively, of those undergoing ELSS or TL. Class A vertigo control was seen in 70.6% and to class B in another 11.8% after VNS; for ELSS, the percentages were 47.3% and 25.5%, respectively, and for TL, 95.2%

and 4.8%. Functionality was equivalent between VNS and ELSS patients at 2 years and was much better for the TL patients. At 18 to 24 months, 22% of VNS and ELSS patients had pure tone average (PTA) worsen by > 15 dB, and 28% had speech discrimination scores (SDS) worsen by > 15%. The conclusions of the study were that ELSS remains a valid option, that VNS vertigo control rates are comparable with those of gentamicin instillation, and that labyrinthectomy has outstanding vertigo control rates as well as patient perception of benefit.

A review[146] of 210 patients who had undergone VNS and had 2 years of follow-up revealed the following (**Video 7.1**). Patients suffered from vertigo for a mean of 32.2 months before surgery. Disease became bilateral in 5.7% of patients during the follow-up period. Vertigo control was 90.1% class A and 4.3% class B. Hearing preservation was excellent, and complication rates were low (2.5%). Another study[147] comparing 25 patients undergoing gentamicin injection and 39 patients undergoing VNS revealed no significant hearing loss in the VNS group, compared with an average elevation of pure-tone thresholds of 13 dB and reduction in SDS of 13% ($p = 0.006$). Vertigo control was class A or B in 92% of VNS patients compared with 66% of injection patients. The conclusion was that gentamicin causes a higher level of hearing loss related to treatment, and VNS has higher vertigo control rates.

The question has been raised whether combining ELSS with VNS will improve hearing outcomes compared with VNS alone. Fifteen patients in the combination group and eight in the VNS-only group were followed for more than 16 months.[148] Hearing was worse in 11 patients and 5 patients, respectively. There was no benefit for either hearing or tinnitus when ELSS was combined with VNS.

■ Atypical Meniere's Disease

Bilateral Meniere's disease occurs in 30 to 50% of cases and is a possibility that must always be kept in mind when treating these patients. Particular attention must be paid in bilateral cases to evaluation of possible autoimmunity, possible allergic Meniere's disease, and possible otosyphilis. It is because of the risk of eventual bilaterality that physicians are very methodical, conservative, and stepwise in their treatment regimens. In the small subgroup of patients who have bilateral, severe, progressive disease resulting in disabling vertigo and severe to profound hearing loss, aggressive chemical labyrinthectomy with gentamicin to alleviate vertigo and use of a cochlear implant for hearing restoration is valid treatment.[149]

Migraine disorder can mimic the symptoms of Meniere's disease. In fact, Prosper Meniere's himself noted the association of headache and vertigo in his original paper on the subject.[150] The entity currently is variously described as vestibular migraine, migraine-related vestibulopathy, or migrainous vertigo. The murky waters of making this diagnosis are made even more so by a lack of clear criteria for vestibular migraine, unlike the AAO-HNS criteria for Meniere's disease. The utility of VEMP in distinguishing between Meniere's disease and migraines is under investigation.

General criteria for diagnosing migraine headaches[151] are five headaches lasting 4 to 72 hours, with each headache having two of the following characteristics: unilaterality, pulsatility, inhibition or prohibition of daily activities, and exacerbation by physical activity. Additionally, the headaches must be accompanied by phonophobia, photophobia, nausea, and/or vomiting. Basilar migraine and benign paroxysmal vertigo of childhood (a type of migraine disorder[152]) are specifically associated with a sensation of dizziness or vertigo. Proposed criteria for diagnosis of definite and probable migrainous vertigo are as follows.[153] Definite migrainous vertigo has a history of episodic moderate vertigo, migraine, and at least one characteristic migraine symptom during two vertiginous attacks. Probable migrainous vertigo has a history of episodic moderate vertigo with at least one of the following: migraine, migrainous symptoms during vertigo, migraine-specific vertigo triggers (such as foods, olfactory/ visual stimuli, hormonal changes, and/or sleep disturbances), or response to antimigraine therapy.

The problem becomes even more difficult to dissect out when one considers that the lifetime prevalence of migraine in adults is 16%,[154] compared with 0.2% for Meniere's disease. The prevalence of migraine was found to be only 22% in patients with classic Meniere's disease but 81% in patients with (atypical) vestibular Meniere's disease[155]; more recently, 56% prevalence of migraines was found among patients with Meniere's disease, as defined by the 1995 guidelines.[156] As a rule of thumb, hearing loss is an occasional, mild, and nonprogressive feature of migrainous vertigo, while it is a regular accompaniment of Meniere's disease.[157] However, in the Meniere's patient with a history of migraine, one must consider antimigraine medication as part of the treatment regimen.

Pediatric Meniere's disease is a rare entity, comprising, at most, 3% of vertigo in childhood.[158] Diagnosis is based on criteria already discussed; it may take years for the full symptomatology to develop. Treatment is medically conservative, but these cases may require chemical labyrinthectomy or VNS at a higher rate than adult-onset Meniere's disease.[159,160] Most pediatric vertigo is a migraine variant.[161]

■ Conclusion

Meniere's disease diagnosis is based on clinical history, physical examination, and audiometry. Additional testing is reserved for unusual presentations or for preoperative testing and counseling. As with any other unilateral pathology of the ear, retrocochlear work-up is mandatory. Special attention to allergy evaluation and possible migraine is warranted. Adherence to the 1995 AAO-HNS guidelines for diagnosis will enable the clinician to maximize treatment outcomes. Results of any treatment regimen must be determined after 18 to 24 months in light of the fluctuating nature of the disease.

Treatment is primarily aggressive medical management, which should achieve symptom control in up to 90% of patients. Cases refractory to traditional medical management are pursued with interventional treatment in a stepwise fashion, from intratympanic application of steroids and endolymphatic sac surgery to destructive procedures, such as gentamicin chemical labyrinthectomy, vestibular nerve section, and transmastoid labyrinthectomy. Auditory and psychological support is essential. The future of research in this field lies in understanding the mechanisms of inner ear injury in Meniere's disease and fine-tuning treatment regimens that curtail vertigo and tinnitus while preserving hearing.

References

1. Schuknecht HF. The pathophysiology of Meniere's disease. Am J Otol 1984;5(6):526–527

2. Baloh RW. Prosper Ménière and his disease. Arch Neurol 2001;58(7):1151–1156

3. Hallpike CS, Cairns H. Observations on the pathology of Meniere's syndrome. Proc R Soc Med 1938;31(11):1317–1336

4. Monsell EM, Balkany TA, Gates GA, et al. Committee on hearing and equilibrium guidelines for the diagnosis and evaluation of therapy in Meniere's disease. Otolaryngol Head Neck Surg 1995;113(3):181–185

5. Agrawal Y, Carey JP, Della Santina CC, Schubert MC, Minor LB. Disorders of balance and vestibular function in US adults: data from the National Health and Nutrition Examination Survey, 2001-2004. Arch Intern Med 2009;169(10):938-44.

6. Harcourt J, Barraclough K, Bronstein AM. Meniere's disease: clinical review. BMJ 2014;349:1–5

7. Havia M, Kentala E, Pyykkö I. Prevalence of Ménière's disease in general population of Southern Finland. Otolaryngol Head Neck Surg 2005;133(5):762–768

8. Harris JP, Alexander TH. Current-day prevalence of Ménière's syndrome. Audiol Neurootol 2010;15(5):318–322

9. Kentala E. Characteristics of six otologic diseases involving vertigo. Am J Otol 1996;17(6):883–892

10. Perez R, Chen JM, Nedzelski JM. The status of the contralateral ear in established unilateral Ménière's disease. Laryngoscope 2004;114(8):1373–1376

11. Thomas K, Harrison MS. Long-term follow up of 610 cases of Ménière's disease. Proc R Soc Med 1971;64(8):853–857

12. Paparella MM, Griebie MS. Bilaterality of Meniere's disease. Acta Otolaryngol 1984;97(3-4):233–237

13. Enander A, Stahle J. Hearing in Ménière's disease. A study of pure-tone audiograms in 334 patients. Acta Otolaryngol 1967;64(5):543–556

14. Xenellis J, Morrison AW, McClowskey D, Festenstein H. HLA antigens in the pathogenesis of Meniere's disease. J Laryngol Otol 1986;100(1):21–24

15. Weinreich HM, Agrawal Y. The link between allergy and Ménière's disease. Curr Opin Otolaryngol Head Neck Surg 2014;22(3):227–230

16. Silverstein H, Smouha E, Jones R. Natural history vs. surgery for Ménière's disease. Otolaryngol Head Neck Surg 1989;100(1):6–16

17. Torok N. Old and new in Ménière disease. Laryngoscope 1977;87(11):1870–1877

18. Fukuda S, Keithley EM, Harris JP. The development of endolymphatic hydrops following CMV inoculation of the endolymphatic sac. Laryngoscope 1988;98(4):439–443

19. Rauch SD, Merchant SN, Thedinger BA. Meniere's syndrome and endolymphatic hydrops. Double-blind temporal bone study. Ann Otol Rhinol Laryngol 1989;98(11):873–883

20. Cureoglu S, Schachern PA, Paul S, Paparella MM, Singh RK. Cellular changes of Reissner's membrane in Meniere's disease: human temporal bone study. Otolaryngol Head Neck Surg 2004;130(1):113–119

21. Schuknecht HF. Endolymphatic hydrops: can it be controlled? Ann Otol Rhinol Laryngol 1986;95(1 Pt 1):36–39

22. Horner KC. Review: morphological changes associated with endolymphatic hydrops. Scanning Microsc 1993;7(1):223–238

23. Nadol JB Jr. Positive Hennebert's sign in Meniere's disease. Arch Otolaryngol 1977;103(9):524–530

24. Rizvi SS. Investigations into the cause of canal paresis in Ménière's disease. Laryngoscope 1986;96(11):1258–1271

25. Schuknecht HF. Meniere's disease: a correlation of symptomatology and pathology. Laryngoscope 1963;73:651–665

26. Tomiyama S, Yagi T, Sakagami M, Fukazawa K. Immunological pathogenesis of endolymphatic hydrops and its relation to Ménière's disease. Scanning Microsc 1993;7(3):907–919, discussion 919–920

27. Fuse T, Hayashi T, Oota N, et al. Immunological responses in acute low-tone sensorineural hearing loss and Ménière's disease. Acta Otolaryngol 2003;123(1):26–31

28. Rauch SD, San Martin JE, Moscicki RA, Bloch KJ. Serum antibodies against heat shock protein 70 in Ménière's disease. Am J Otol 1995;16(5):648–652

29. Ruckenstein MJ, Prasthoffer A, Bigelow DC, Von Feldt JM, Kolasinski SL. Immunologic and serologic testing in patients with Ménière's disease. Otol Neurotol 2002;23(4):517–520, discussion 520–521

30. Paparella MM, Djalilian HR. Etiology, pathophysiology of symptoms, and pathogenesis of Meniere's disease. Otolaryngol Clin North Am 2002;35(3):529–545, vi

31. Selmani Z, Marttila T, Pyykkö I. Incidence of virus infection as a cause of Meniere's disease or endolymphatic hydrops assessed by electrocochleography. Eur Arch Otorhinolaryngol 2005;262(4):331–334

32. Friberg U, Rask-Andersen H. Vascular occlusion in the endolymphatic sac in Meniere's disease. Ann Otol Rhinol Laryngol 2002;111(3 Pt 1, 3 Pt l):237–245

33. Boyev KP. Meniere's disease or migraine? The clinical significance of fluctuating hearing loss with vertigo. Arch Otolaryngol Head Neck Surg 2005;131(5):457–459

34. Kotimaki J. Meniere's disease in Finland. An epidemiological and clinical study on occurrence, clinical picture and policy. Acta Univ. Oul. D 747. Oulu, Finland: Oulu University Press; 2003. Available at http://herkules.oulu.fi/issn03553221

35. Sanchez E, López-Escámez JA, López-Nevot MA, López-Nevot A, Cortes R, Martin J. Absence of COCH mutations in patients with Meniere disease. Eur J Hum Genet 2004;12(1):75–78

36. Fransen E, Verstreken M, Verhagen WI, et al. High prevalence of symptoms of Ménière's disease in three families with a mutation in the COCH gene. Hum Mol Genet 1999;8(8):1425–1429

37. Penido NO, Cruz OL, Zanoni A, Inoue DP. Classification and hearing evolution of patients with sudden sensorineural hearing loss. Braz J Med Biol Res 2009;42(8):712–716

38. Barber HO. Meniere's disease: symptomatology. In: Oosterveld WJ, ed. Meniere's Disease: A Comprehensive Appraisal. New York, NY: John Wiley; 1983:25–34

39. Pillsbury HC III, Postma DS. Lermoyez' syndrome and the otolithic crisis of Tumarkin. Otolaryngol Clin North Am 1983;16(1):197–203

40. Tumarkin A. The otolithic catastrophe: a new syndrome. BMJ 1936;2(3942):175–177

41. Belinchon A, Perez-Garrigues H, Tenias JM, Lopez A. Hearing assessment in Menière's disease. Laryngoscope 2011;121(3):622–626

42. Havia M, Kentala E, Pyykkö I. Hearing loss and tinnitus in Meniere's disease. Auris Nasus Larynx 2002;29(2):115–119

43. Paparella MM, Mancini F. Vestibular Meniere's disease. Otolaryngol Head Neck Surg 1985;93(2):148–151

44. Anderson JP, Harris JP. Impact of Ménière's disease on quality of life. Otol Neurotol 2001;22(6):888–894

45. Söderman AC, Bagger-Sjöbäck D, Bergenius J, Langius A. Factors influencing quality of life in patients with Ménière's disease, identified by a multidimensional approach. Otol Neurotol 2002;23(6):941–948

46. Celestino D, Rosini E, Carucci ML, Marconi PL, Vercillo E. Ménière's disease and anxiety disorders. Acta Otorhinolaryngol Ital 2003;23(6):421–427

47. Orji F. The influence of psychological factors in Menière's disease. Ann Med Health Sci Res 2014;4(1):3–7

48. Silverstein H, Smouha E, Jones R. Natural history vs. surgery for Ménière's disease. Otolaryngol Head Neck Surg 1989;100(1):6–16

49. Friberg U, Stahle J, Svedberg A. The natural course of Meniere's disease. Acta Otolaryngol Suppl 1984; 406:72–77

50. Havia M, Kentala E. Progression of symptoms of dizziness in Ménière's disease. Arch Otolaryngol Head Neck Surg 2004;130(4):431–435

51. Söderman AC, Möller J, Bagger-Sjöbäck D, Bergenius J, Hallqvist J. Stress as a trigger of attacks in Ménière's disease. A case-crossover study. Laryngoscope 2004;114(10):1843–1848

52. Radtke A, Lempert T, Gresty MA, Brookes GB, Bronstein AM, Neuhauser H. Migraine and Ménière's disease: is there a link? Neurology 2002;59(11):1700–1704

53. Furman JM, Marcus DA. Migraine and motion sensitivity. Continuum (Minneap Minn) 2012;18(5 Neuro-otology):1102–1117

54. Sargent EW. The challenge of vestibular migraine. Curr Opin Otolaryngol Head Neck Surg 2013;21(5):473–479

55. Foster CA. Optimal management of Ménière's disease. Ther Clin Risk Manag 2015;11:301–307

56. Kim HH, Wiet RJ, Battista RA. Trends in the diagnosis and the management of Meniere's disease: results of a survey. Otolaryngol Head Neck Surg 2005;132(5):722–726

57. Pierce NE, Antonelli PJ. Endolymphatic hydrops perspectives 2012. Curr Opin Otolaryngol Head Neck Surg 2012;20(5):416–419

58. Kim HH, Kumar A, Battista RA, Wiet RJ. Electrocochleography in patients with Meniere's disease. Am J Otolaryngol 2005;26(2):128–131

59. Margolis RH, Rieks D, Fournier EM, Levine SE. Tympanic electrocochleography for diagnosis of Ménière's disease. Arch Otolaryngol Head Neck Surg 1995;121(1):44–55

60. Ferraro JA, Tibbils RP. SP/AP area ratio in the diagnosis of Ménière's disease. Am J Audiol 1999;8(1):21–28

61. Devaiah AK, Dawson KL, Ferraro JA, Ator GA. Utility of area curve ratio electrocochleography in early Meniere disease. Arch Otolaryngol Head Neck Surg 2003;129(5):547–551

62. Haid CT, Watermeier D, Wolf SR, Berg M. Clinical survey of Meniere's disease: 574 cases. Acta Otolaryngol Suppl 1995;520(Pt 2):251–255

63. Minor LB, Schessel DA, Carey JP. Ménière's disease. Curr Opin Neurol 2004;17(1):9–16

64. Magliulo G, Cianfrone G, Gagliardi M, Cuiuli G, D'Amico R. Vestibular evoked myogenic potentials and distortion-product otoacoustic emissions combined with glycerol testing in endolymphatic hydrops: their value in early diagnosis. Ann Otol Rhinol Laryngol 2004;113(12):1000–1005

65. Kuo SW, Yang TH, Young YH. Changes in vestibular evoked myogenic potentials after Meniere attacks. Ann Otol Rhinol Laryngol 2005;114(9):717–721

66. Halmagyi GM, Curthoys IS. A clinical sign of canal paresis. Arch Neurol 1988;45(7):737–739

67. Park HJ, Migliaccio AA, Della Santina CC, Minor LB, Carey JP. Search-coil head-thrust and caloric tests in Ménière's disease. Acta Otolaryngol 2005;125(8):852–857

68. Klockhoff I, Lindblom U. Glycerol test in Ménière's disease. Acta Otolaryngol 1966;224:224, 449

69. Snyder JM. Predictability of the glycerin test in the diagnosis of Ménière's disease. Clin Otolaryngol Allied Sci 1982;7(6):389–397

70. Futaki T, Kitahara M, Morimoto M. A comparison of the furosemide and glycerol tests for Meniere's disease. With special reference to the bilateral lesion. Acta Otolaryngol 1977;83(3–4):272–278

71. Paparella MM. Methods of diagnosis and treatment of Meniére's disease. Acta Otolaryngol Suppl 1991;485:108–119

72. Soto A, Labella T, Santos S, et al. The usefulness of computerized dynamic posturography for the study of equilibrium in patients with Meniere's disease: correlation with clinical and audiologic data. Hear Res 2004;196(1–2):26–32

73. Thornton AR, Farrell G. Apparent travelling wave velocity changes in cases of endolymphatic hydrops. Scand Audiol 1991;20(1):13–18

74. Friedrichs I, Thornton AR. Endolymphatic hydrops in asymptomatic ears in unilateral Ménière's disease. Laryngoscope 2001;111(5):857–860

75. Don M, Kwong B, Tanaka C. A diagnostic test for Ménière's disease and cochlear hydrops: impaired high-pass noise masking of auditory brainstem responses. Otol Neurotol 2005;26(4):711–722

76. Le CH, Truong AQ, Diaz RC. Novel techniques for the diagnosis of Ménière's disease. Curr Opin Otolaryngol Head Neck Surg 2013;21(5):492–496

77. Franco-Vidal V, Legarlantezec C, Blanchet H, Convert C, Torti F, Darrouzet V. Multifrequency admittancemetry in Ménière's disease: a preliminary study for a new diagnostic test. Otol Neurotol 2005;26(4):723–727

78. Albers FWJ, Van Weissenbruch R, Casselman JW. 3DFT-magnetic resonance imaging of the inner ear in Ménière's disease. Acta Otolaryngol 1994;114(6):595–600

79. Fitzgerald DC, Mark AS. Endolymphatic duct/sac enhancement on gadolinium magnetic resonance imaging of the inner ear: preliminary observations and case reports. Am J Otol 1996;17(4):603–606

80. Tanioka H, Kaga H, Zusho H, Araki T, Sasaki Y. MR of the endolymphatic duct and sac: findings in Meniere disease. AJNR Am J Neuroradiol 1997;18(1):45–51

81. Naganawa S, Nakashima T. Visualization of endolymphatic hydrops with MR imaging in patients with Ménière's disease and related pathologies: current status of its methods and clinical significance. Jpn J Radiol 2014;32(4):191–204

82. Fukuoka H, Takumi Y Tsukada K, et al. Comparison of the diagnostic value of 3T MRI after intratympanic injection of GBCA, electrocochleograpy, and the glycerol test in patients with Meniere's disease. Acta Otolaryngol 2012;132:141-145

83. Fiorino F, Pizzini FB, Beltramello A, Mattellini B, Barbieri F. Reliability of magnetic resonance imaging performed after intratympanic administration of gadolinium in the identification of endolymphatic hydrops in patients with Ménière's disease. Otol Neurotol 2011;32(3):472–477

84. Gürkov R, Flatz W, Louza J, Strupp M, Ertl-Wagner B, Krause E. In vivo visualized endolymphatic hydrops and inner ear functions in patients with electrocochleographically confirmed Ménière's disease. Otol Neurotol 2012;33(6):1040–1045

85. Lorenzi MC, Bento RF, Daniel MM, Leite CC. Magnetic resonance imaging of the temporal bone in patients with Ménière's disease. Acta Otolaryngol 2000;120(5):615–619

86. Xenellis J, Vlahos L, Papadopoulos A, Nomicos P, Papafragos K, Adamopoulos G. Role of the new imaging modalities in the investigation of Meniere's disease. Otolaryngol Head Neck Surg 2000;123(1 Pt 1):114–119

87. Thorp MA, Shehab ZP, Bance ML, Rutka JA; AAO-HNS Committee on Hearing and Equilibrium. The AAO-HNS Committee on Hearing and Equilibrium guidelines for the diagnosis and evaluation of therapy in Meniere's disease: have they been applied in the published literature of the last decade? Clin Otolaryngol Allied Sci 2003;28(3):173–176

88. Phillips JS, Westerberg B. Intratympanic steroids for Ménière's disease or syndrome. Cochrane Database Syst Rev 2011;(7):CD008514

89. Harris J, ed. Meniere's Disease. The Hague, The Netherlands: Kugler Publishers; 1999

90. Glasscock ME III, Gulya AJ, Pensak ML, Black JN Jr. Medical and surgical management of Meniere's disease. Am J Otol 1984;5(6):536–542

91. Thorp MA, Shehab ZP, Bance ML, Rutka JA. Does evidence-based medicine exist in the treatment of Ménière's disease? A critical review of the last decade of publications. Clin Otolaryngol Allied Sci 2000;25(6):456–460

92. Jackson CG, Glasscock ME III, Davis WE, Hughes GB, Sismanis A. Medical management of Ménière's disease. Ann Otol Rhinol Laryngol 1981;90(2 Pt 1):142–147

93. Klockhoff I, Lindblom U. Ménière's disease and hydrochlorothiazide (Dichlotride)—a critical analysis of symptoms and therapeutic effects. Acta Otolaryngol 1967;63(4):347–365

94. van Deelen GW, Huizing EH. Use of a diuretic (Dyazide) in the treatment of Ménière's disease. A double-blind cross-over placebo-controlled study. ORL J Otorhinolaryngol Relat Spec 1986;48(5):287–292

95. Thirlwall AS, Kundu S. Diuretics for Ménière's disease or syndrome. Cochrane Database Syst Rev 2006;3(3):CD003599

96. Chan K, MaassenVanDenBrink A. Glutamate receptor antagonists in the management of migraine. Drugs 2014;74(11):1165–1176

97. Ha SK. Dietary salt intake and hypertension. Electrolyte Blood Press 2014;12(1):7–18

98. Ohlsén KA, Didier A, Baldwin D, Miller JM, Nuttall AL, Hultcrantz E. Cochlear blood flow in response to dilating agents. Hear Res 1992;58(1):19–25

99. Derebery MJ, Berliner KI. Prevalence of allergy in Meniere's disease. Otolaryngol Head Neck Surg 2000;123(1 Pt 1):69–75

100. Derebery MJ. Allergic management of Meniere's disease: an outcome study. Otolaryngol Head Neck Surg 2000;122(2):174–182

101. Lacour M, van de Heyning PH, Novotny M, Tighilet B. Betahistine in the treatment of Ménière's disease. Neuropsychiatr Dis Treat 2007;3(4):429–440

102. Lezius F, Adrion C, Mansmann U, Jahn K, Strupp M. High-dosage betahistine dihydrochloride between 288 and 480 mg/day in patients with severe Ménière's disease: a case series. Eur Arch Otorhinolaryngol 2011;268(8):1237–1240

103. Beeson PB. Age and sex associations of 40 autoimmune diseases. Am J Med 1994;96(5):457–462

104. Trune DR, Canlon B. Corticosteroid therapy for hearing and balance disorders. Anat Rec (Hoboken) 2012;295(11):1928–1943

105. Haynes BF, Pikus A, Kaiser-Kupfer M, Fauci AS. Successful treatment of sudden hearing loss in Cogan's syndrome with corticosteroids. Arthritis Rheum 1981;24(3):501–503

106. Hain TC, Uddin M. Pharmacological treatment of vertigo. CNS Drugs 2003;17(2):85–100

107. Seidman MD, Keate B. Re: myths in neurotology, revisited: smoke and mirrors in tinnitus therapy. [letter to the editor] Otol Neurotol 2002;23(6):1013–1015, author reply 1015–1016

108. Rascol O, Hain TC, Brefel C, Benazet M, Clanet M, Montastruc JL. Antivertigo medications and drug-induced vertigo. A pharmacological review. Drugs 1995; 50(5):777–791

109. Claussen CF, Bergmann J, Bertora G, Claussen E. [Clinical experimental test and equilibrimetric measurements of the therapeutic action of a homeopathic drug consisting of ambra, cocculus, conium and mineral oil in the diagnosis of vertigo and nausea]. Arzneimittelforschung 1984;34(12):1791–1798

110. Banerjee A, Parnes LS. Intratympanic corticosteroids for sudden idiopathic sensorineural hearing loss. Otol Neurotol 2005;26(5):878–881

111. Chandrasekhar SS. Intratympanic dexamethasone for sudden sensorineural hearing loss: clinical and laboratory evaluation. Otol Neurotol 2001;22(1):18–23

112. Garduño-Anaya MA, Couthino De Toledo H, Hinojosa-González R, Pane-Pianese C, Ríos-Castañeda LC. Dexamethasone inner ear perfusion by intratympanic injection in unilateral Ménière's disease: a two-year prospective, placebo-controlled, double-blind, randomized trial. Otolaryngol Head Neck Surg 2005; 133(2):285–294

113. Dodson KM, Woodson E, Sismanis A. Intratympanic steroid perfusion for the treatment of Ménière's disease: a retrospective study. Ear Nose Throat J 2004; 83(6):394–398

114. Hillman TM, Arriaga MA, Chen DA. Intratympanic steroids: do they acutely improve hearing in cases of cochlear hydrops? Laryngoscope 2003; 113(11):1903–1907

115. Sennaroğlu L, Dini FM, Sennaroğlu G, Gursel B, Ozkan S. Transtympanic dexamethasone application in Ménière's disease: an alternative treatment for intractable vertigo. J Laryngol Otol 1999;113(3):217–221

116. Ahsan SF, Standring R, Wang Y. Systematic review and meta-analysis of Meniett therapy for Meniere's disease. Laryngoscope 2015;125(1):203–208

117. Thomsen J, Sass K, Odkvist L, Arlinger S. Local overpressure treatment reduces vestibular symptoms in patients with Meniere's disease: a clinical, randomized, multicenter, double-blind, placebo-controlled study. Otol Neurotol 2005;26(1):68–73

118. Rajan GP, Din S, Atlas MD. Long-term effects of the Meniett device in Ménière's disease: the Western Australian experience. J Laryngol Otol 2005;119(5):391–395

119. Chi F-L, Liang Q, Wang Z-M. Effects of hyperbaric therapy on function and morphology of guinea pig cochlea with endolymphatic hydrops. Otol Neurotol 2004;25(4):553–558

120. Sugawara K, Kitamura K, Ishida T, Sejima T. Insertion of tympanic ventilation tubes as a treating modality for patients with Meniere's disease: a short- and long-term follow-up study in seven cases. Auris Nasus Larynx 2003;30(1):25–28

121. Brackmann DE, Nissen RL. Ménière's disease: results of treatment with the endolymphatic subarachnoid shunt compared with the endolymphatic mastoid shunt. Am J Otol 1987;8(4):275–282

122. Thomsen J, Bretlau P, Tos M, Johnsen NJ. Placebo effect in surgery for Ménière's disease. A double-blind, placebo-controlled study on endolymphatic sac shunt surgery. Arch Otolaryngol 1981;107(5):271–277

123. Welling DB, Nagaraja HN. Endolymphatic mastoid shunt: a reevaluation of efficacy. Otolaryngol Head Neck Surg 2000;122(3):340–345

124. Sood AJ, Lambert PR, Nguyen SA, Meyer TA. Endolymphatic sac surgery for Ménière's disease: a systematic review and meta-analysis. Otol Neurotol 2014;35(6):1033–1045

125. Pullens B, Verschuur HP, van Benthem PP. Surgery for Ménière's disease. Cochrane Database Syst Rev 2013;2:CD005395

126. Kato BM, LaRouere MJ, Bojrab DI, Michaelides EM. Evaluating quality of life after endolymphatic sac surgery: The Ménière's Disease Outcomes Questionnaire. Otol Neurotol 2004;25(3):339–344

127. Durland WF Jr, Pyle GM, Connor NP. Endolymphatic sac decompression as a treatment for Meniere's disease. Laryngoscope 2005;115(8):1454–1457

128. Glasscock ME III, Jackson CG, Poe DS, Johnson GD. What I think of sac surgery in 1989. Am J Otol 1989;10(3):230–233

129. Kitahara M, Kitajima K, Yazawa Y, Uchida K. Endolymphatic sac surgery for Meniere's disease: eighteen years' experience with the Kitahara sac operation. Am J Otol 1987;8(4):283–286

130. Ostrowski VB, Kartush JM. Endolymphatic sac-vein decompression for intractable Meniere's disease: long term treatment results. Otolaryngol Head Neck Surg 2003;128(4):550–559

131. Kitahara T, Takeda N, Mishiro Y, et al. Effects of exposing the opened endolymphatic sac to large doses of steroids to treat intractable Meniere's disease. Ann Otol Rhinol Laryngol 2001;110(2):109–112

132. Schuknecht HF. Ablation therapy for the relief of Meniere's disease. Trans Am Laryngol Rhinol Oto 1 Soc 1956;(60th Meeting):589–600

133. Silverstein H. Streptomycin treatment for Meniere's disease. Ann Otol Rhinol Laryngol Suppl 1984; 112:44–48

134. Cureoglu S, Schachern PA, Paparella MM. Effect of parenteral aminoglycoside administration on dark cells in the crista ampullaris. Arch Otolaryngol Head Neck Surg 2003;129(6):626–628

135. Imamura S, Adams JC. Distribution of gentamicin in the guinea pig inner ear after local or systemic application. J Assoc Res Otolaryngol 2003;4(2):176–195

136. Balough BJ, Hoffer ME, Wester D, O'Leary MJ, Brooker CR, Goto M. Kinetics of gentamicin uptake in the inner ear of Chinchilla langier after middle-ear administration in a sustained-release vehicle. Otolaryngol Head Neck Surg 1998;119(5):427–431

137. Hoffer ME, Kopke RD, Weisskopf P, et al. Use of the round window microcatheter in the treatment of Meniere's disease. Laryngoscope 2001;111(11 Pt 1): 2046–2049

138. Huon L-K, Fang T-Y, Wang P-C. Outcomes of intratympanic gentamicin injection to treat Ménière's disease. Otol Neurotol 2012;33(5):706–714

139. Carey JP, Minor LB, Peng GC, Della Santina CC, Cremer PD, Haslwanter T. Changes in the three-dimensional angular vestibulo-ocular reflex following intratympanic gentamicin for Ménière's disease. J Assoc Res Otolaryngol 2002;3(4):430–443

140. Cohen-Kerem R, Kisilevsky V, Einarson TR, Kozer E, Koren G, Rutka JA. Intratympanic gentamicin for Ménière's disease: a meta-analysis. Laryngoscope 2004;114(12):2085–2091

141. Chia SH, Gamst AC, Anderson JP, Harris JP. Intratympanic gentamicin therapy for Ménière's disease: a meta-analysis. Otol Neurotol 2004;25(4):544–552

142. Sennaroglu L, Sennaroglu G, Gursel B, Dini FM. Intratympanic dexamethasone, intratympanic gentamicin, and endolymphatic sac surgery for intractable vertigo in Meniere's disease. Otolaryngol Head Neck Surg 2001;125(5):537–543

143. Silverstein H, Lewis WB, Jackson LE, Rosenberg SI, Thompson JH, Hoffmann KK. Changing trends in the surgical treatment of Ménière's disease: results of a 10-year survey. Ear Nose Throat J 2003;82(3):185–187, 191–194

144. Rosenberg SI. Vestibular surgery for Ménière's disease in the elderly: a review of techniques and indications. Ear Nose Throat J 1999;78(6):443–446

145. Kaylie DM, Jackson CG, Gardner EK. Surgical management of Meniere's disease in the era of gentamicin. Otolaryngol Head Neck Surg 2005;132(3):443–450

146. Goksu N, Yilmaz M, Bayramoglu I, Bayazit YA. Combined retrosigmoid retrolabyrinthine vestibular nerve section: results of our experience over 10 years. Otol Neurotol 2005;26(3):481–483

147. Hillman TA, Chen DA, Arriaga MA. Vestibular nerve section versus intratympanic gentamicin for Meniere's disease. Laryngoscope 2004;114(2):216–222

148. Moody-Antonio S, House JW. Hearing outcome after concurrent endolymphatic shunt and vestibular nerve section. Otol Neurotol 2003;24(3):453–459

149. Morgan M, Flood L, Hawthorne M, Raje S. Chemical labyrinthectomy and cochlear implantation for Menière's disease—an effective treatment or a last resort? J Laryngol Otol 1999;113(7):666–669

150. Meniere P. Pathologie auriculaire: memoires sur une lesion de l' oreille interne donnant lieu a des symptoms de congestion cerebrale apoplectiforme. Gaz Med Fr 1861;16:597–601

151. Headache Classification Subcommittee of the International Headache Society. The international classification of headache disorders. Cephalalgia 2004;24(Suppl 1):9–160

152. Koenigsberger MR, Chandrasekhar SS. [An infant with dizziness]. Rev Neurol 1995;23(Suppl 3):S410–S417

153. Neuhauser H, Leopold M, von Brevern M, Arnold G, Lempert T. The interrelations of migraine, vertigo, and migrainous vertigo. Neurology 2001;56(4):436–441

154. Rasmussen BK, Jensen R, Schroll M, Olesen J. Epidemiology of headache in a general population—a prevalence study. J Clin Epidemiol 1991;44(11):1147–1157

155. Rassekh CH, Harker LA. The prevalence of migraine in Ménière's disease. Laryngoscope 1992;102(2):135–138

156. Radtke A, Lempert T, Gresty MA, Brookes GB, Bronstein AM, Neuhauser H. Migraine and Ménière's disease: is there a link? Neurology 2002;59(11):1700–1704

157. Neuhauser H, Lempert T. Vertigo and dizziness related to migraine: a diagnostic challenge. Cephalalgia 2004;24(2):83–91

158. Meyerhoff WL, Paparella MM, Shea D. Ménière's disease in children. Laryngoscope 1978;88(9 Pt 1):1504–1511

159. See GB, Mahmud MR, Zurin AA, Putra SH, Saim LB. Vestibular nerve section in a child with intractable Ménière's disease. Int J Pediatr Otorhinolaryngol 2002;64(1):61–64

161. Moody-Antonio S, House JW. Hearing outcome after concurrent endolymphatic shunt and vestibular nerve section. Otol Neurotol 2003;24:453–459

160. Akagi H, Yuen K, Maeda Y, et al. Ménière's disease in childhood. Int J Pediatr Otorhinolaryngol 2001;61(3):259–264

8 Benign Paroxysmal Positional Vertigo

Judith White

◼ Introduction

Benign paroxysmal positional vertigo (BPPV) is a commonly recognized vestibular disorder. Earlier estimates of the incidence of BPPV range from 10.7[1] to 64[2] per 100,000, with increases of 38% with each decade of life, but later data suggest that the disorder may be more common. In a 2000 study, Oghalai et al noted that 9% of randomly selected geriatric patients in an urban clinic who had undergone positional testing had positive results and undiagnosed BPPV.[3]

In 1952, Dix and Hallpike described the characteristic ipsidirectional torsional nystagmus provoked by the head maneuver they developed to identify BPPV.[4] During this maneuver, the patient's head is turned 45° to one side while he or she is seated. The patient is then moved quickly to a supine position with the neck slightly extended and the head remaining turned. When the lower ear is affected, nystagmus is seen. The patient is then brought back up to a sitting position, and the nystagmus is noted to reverse direction. The maneuver is then performed on the other side. The characteristic nystagmus occurs after a delay of several seconds, declines after 10 to 30 seconds, and diminishes with repeated positional testing in the same sitting.[4,5] Although the maneuver needs no special equipment, visualization of the nystagmus can be aided by the use of infrared video or optical Frenzel lenses, which eliminate visual fixation.

Approximately 94% of BPPV cases involve the posterior semicircular canal.[6] Lateral (horizontal) semicircular canal (LSC) involvement is the next most common. Lateral semicircular canal benign paroxysmal positional vertigo (LSC-BPPV) was first described by Cipparrone et al[7] and McClure[8] in 1985, and is characterized by nystagmus provoked by supine bilateral head turns and beating toward the lower ear. There are now known to be two distinct subtypes of LSC-BPPV based on the direction of horizontal nystagmus during supine head turns: geotropic and apogeotropic. Geotropic LSC-BPPV beats toward the lower ear on supine positional testing and is characterized by short latency and prolonged duration of horizontal nystagmus with poor fatigability. Apogeotropic LSC-BPPV, thought to be more rare, was not reported until later by Pagnini et al[9] and Baloh et al (**Video 8.1**).[10] Apogeotropic LSC-BPPV is characterized by similar short-latency and prolonged-duration horizontal nystagmus, but the direction beats away from the lower ear on supine positional testing (**Video 8.2**). Geotropic LSC-BPPV is thought to be caused by otoconial debris moving under the influence of gravity within the long arm of the LSC stimulating utriculopetal endolymph flow in the supine position with the affected ear down (**Fig. 8.1**). Different factors are likely responsible for apogeotropic LSC-BPPV, including otoconial debris that adheres to the cupula of the LSC, causing the cupula to become gravity sensitive (cupulolithiasis), and otoconia trapped in the proximal segment of the LSC near the cupula (**Fig. 8.2**).[7,8,9,10,11,12]

Posterior semicircular canal (PSC) BPPV is likely caused by otoconia that detach from the utricle and fall into the PSC (canaliths). Schuknecht[13] was the first to suggest that these basophilic deposits on the cupula of the PSC are the cause of BPPV. However, further work and intraoperative observations suggest that they are likely to be free-floating in the PSC, where they act as a plunger, rendering the canal gravitationally sensitive (**Video 8.3** and **Video 8.4**).[14,15]

Benign paroxysmal positional vertigo is usually idiopathic but can occur after head trauma or in association with other ear disorders, such as vestibular neuritis or labyrinthitis.[16,17,18,19] Certain positions are likely to provoke vertigo, including lying back in bed, arising quickly, looking up, or reclining for dental or hairdressing procedures.

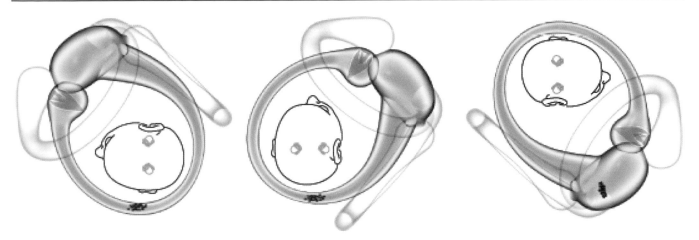

Fig. 8.1   Geotropic lateral semicircular canal benign paroxysmal positional vertigo affecting the left ear. Used with permission from White J. Benign paroxysmal positional vertigo: how to diagnose and quickly treat it. Cleve Clin J Med 2004;71(9):722–728.

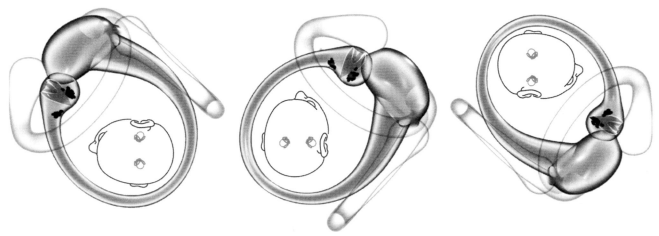

Fig. 8.2   Apogeotropic lateral semicircular canal benign paroxysmal positional vertigo affecting the left ear. Used with permission from White J. Benign paroxysmal positional vertigo: how to diagnose and quickly treat it. Cleve Clin J Med 2004;71(9):722–728.

■ Treatment

Treatment Maneuvers

Initially, BPPV treatments were exercise based and emphasized compensation and habituation.[20,21] Vestibular suppressant medication is not as effective as exercise treatments.[22,23] Specific canalith repositioning maneuvers based on an improved understanding of the pathophysiology of BPPV have been developed in the past 15 years and are now the standard of treatment. These maneuvers include the Semont,[24] the Epley,[25] and the particle repositioning maneuvers[15] for PSC-BPPV, the last of which is a modified

Epley maneuver without mastoid vibration. A commonly used term for the modified Epley maneuver is *canalith repositioning maneuver* (**Fig. 8.3**) (**Video 8.5**).

Identification of the involved canal is necessary before appropriate maneuvers can be chosen. Although Dix-Hallpike positioning is highly sensitive to PSC-BPPV, it lacks sensitivity in LSC-BPPV (**Video 8.6**). For this reason, positional/positioning testing should include Dix-Hallpike positioning to head-hanging right and left positions and supine positional testing in the head-centered supine, right ear down, and left ear down positions. Dix-Hallpike was entirely negative in two published patients whose horizontal nystagmus with lateral supine head turns reached 12 deg/s and 16 deg/s.[26] In most of the other patients with LSC-BPPV,

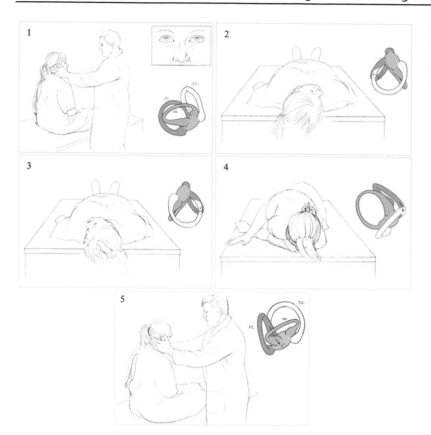

Fig. 8.3 Canalith repositioning maneuver for right posterior semicircular canal benign paroxysmal positional vertigo. Used with permission from White J. Benign paroxysmal positional vertigo: how to diagnose and quickly treat it. Cleve Clin J Med 2004;71(9):722–728.

the Dix-Hallpike positioning nystagmus had a lesser velocity than that seen on supine positional testing. My preference is to perform the head-centered supine and supine left and right ear down positions before returning the patient to sit, and next performing the Dix-Hallpike maneuvers, to increase sensitivity and diagnostic accuracy for LSC-BPPV.

The identification of the involved ear in LSC-BPPV can be especially difficult because the canals are coplanar, and nystagmus is seen in both lateral supine positions. Order effect and head tilt may affect the direction of nystagmus.[27] In geotropic LSC-BPPV, the nystagmus is worse with the affected ear down. Treatment for geotropic horizontal semicircular canal-benign paroxysmal positional vertigo (HSC-BPPV) consists of 360° roll maneuvers toward the unaffected ear, beginning with the patient in the supine position with the head flexed 0° to 30° and laterally rotated toward the affected ear, and proceeding in 90° increments every 30 to 60 seconds toward the unaffected ear.[28] The Gufoni maneuver is also highly effective and is performed with the patient beginning in the sitting position and lying quickly to the unaffected side and then rotating the head 45° downward, maintaining the position for 2 to 3 minutes as described in Appiani et al.[12]

Treatment for apogeotropic LSC-BPPV consists of a variety of maneuvers because none is univer-

sally effective. Identification of the affected ear can be more challenging in apogeotropic LSC-BPPV. Nystagmus is usually worse with the affected ear up, and nystagmus is occasionally seen in the sitting or supine position that usually beats toward the involved side.[29] The Lempert 360° roll maneuver toward the unaffected ear may be used first. The modified Gufoni maneuver can be performed with the patient beginning in the sitting position and lying quickly to the affected side and then rotating the head 45° upward, maintaining the position for 2 to 3 minutes, as described by Appiani et al.[12] The Vannucchi-Asprella maneuvers are performed with the patient rapidly moving from the sitting to the supine position then turning the head rapidly to the unaffected side and returning to sitting, where the head is then returned to midline. This maneuver is repeated five to eight times in rapid succession.[30]

Anterior semicircular canal BPPV is a controversial entity. Some investigators suggest the paroxysmal nystagmus has a pure or torsional downbeat component, in contrast to the nystagmus with PSC-BPPV, which has a vertical upbeat component. Because the same maneuvers used to treat PSC-BPPV appear effective for possible anterior canal involvement (although they may be performed on the contralateral side in some reports), the question may have more theoretical than clinical relevance.

Treatment Efficacy

A patient's response to treatment is assessed using self-reported vertigo frequency and severity and with objective assessment using repeated Dix-Hallpike testing. Several authors have noted a poor correlation between self-report and Dix-Hallpike testing results. For example, Pollack et al,[31] Dornhoffer and Colvin,[32] and Ruckenstein[33] found that 22 to 38% of patients continue to report symptoms despite negative Dix-Hallpike testing, whereas Sargent et al[34] noted reports of subjective improvement despite persistent positive Dix-Hallpike results in his study sample. Lynn et al[35] suggested that objective Dix-Hallpike testing should be considered the gold standard of outcome measures in BPPV. Controlled trials performed without Dix-Hallpike testing at outcome[36] are generally excluded from evidence-based reviews.

The impact of canalith repositioning on the quality of life in patients with BPPV has been demonstrated using the Medical Outcomes Study 36-item Short Form (SF-36)[37] and the Dizziness Handicap Inventory Short Form (DHI-S).[38] In one study, patients with active BPPV scored worse than population norms on both measures, which improved 1 month after canalith repositioning maneuvers were performed (DHI-S mean decrease 8.1, $p < 0.001$, $n = 40$).[39] In addition, SF-36 subscales normalized ($p < 0.05$).[40]

Benign paroxysmal positional vertigo is believed to be self-limiting, although Baloh and Honrubia reported symptoms that persisted for more than 1 year in one-third of their 240 patients with BPPV.[41] The inclusion of a randomized control group allows the spontaneous rate of remission to be compared with the effect of canalith repositioning.

Recurrence is common after successful canalith repositioning for BPPV. Treatment is commonly effective in eliminating the current episode but does not prevent additional episodes. Although the average recurrence rate is ~ 15% per year,[25,42,43] reported rates have ranged from 5% per year[44] to 45% at 30 weeks.[45]

Conversion between canals can occasionally occur, usually between posterior and horizontal canals when the patient is retested with Dix-Hallpike positioning after canalith repositioning has been performed (**Fig. 8.4**). It is heralded by the development of brisk horizontal nystagmus and responds well to a 360° supine roll maneuver toward the good side.

Patients were usually advised to keep their head elevated for 24 to 48 hours after the positioning procedure and to avoid lying on the affected side for 5 days, all of which theoretically allows the free-floating canalith debris to settle back into the utricle rather than return to the semicircular canal. Several studies have suggested that these instructions do not increase treatment efficacy.[46,47,48] Massoud and Ireland[47] studied outcomes for the particle repositioning maneuver ($n = 46$) in patients who were randomized

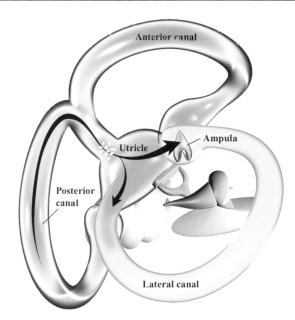

Fig. 8.4 Conversion of posterior semicircular canalithiasis to lateral canalithiasis. Courtesy of The Cleveland Clinic Foundation.

to postprocedure restrictions or control, with follow-up at 1 week. Ninety-six percent of the 23 patients in the control group resolved their BPPV, compared with 88% of the patients who received postprocedure restrictions. The difference did not reach statistical significance, possibly due to the small sample size. Numerous centers continue to observe postprocedure restrictions based on anecdotal experience.

Complications associated with canalith repositioning include conversion of the canalith to a different canal, resulting in alteration of the nystagmus type and/or direction.[49,50] This complication can be treated effectively, however, with additional maneuvers at the same sitting. Other complications include an isolated report of fainting, sweating, pallor, and hypotension during maneuvers accompanied by severe vertigo,[50] possibly reflecting vasovagal response.

In a recently published evidence-based review,[51] the uncontrolled case report efficacy for a single treatment session for PSC-BPPV is 78% (range 53 to 99%, including 22 studies) (**Table 8.1**). The treatment efficacy increases with repeated sessions and usually reaches at least 90%. Nine placebo-controlled trials consisting of 505 patients were evaluated with meta-analysis (**Table 8.2; Fig. 8.5**).

Heterogeneity testing did not show a significant difference between the studies included in the analysis ($c^2 = 11.74$; df = 8; $p < 0.16$) (**Table 8.3**). The mean follow-up was 16 days. The risk of persistent BPPV without treatment was 69%. The risk of persistent BPPV after a single canalith repositioning treatment was 28%. This difference was statistically significant

Table 8.1 Case series and reports: Uncontrolled, single-treatment session unless noted, with Dix-Hallpike at follow-up

Publication	Number of patients	Procedure	Percentage cured	Time
Beynon et al[45]	51	Particle	82%	1–2 weeks
Dal et al[58]	64	Canalith	77%	2–5 days
Dornhoffer & Colvin[32]	52	Canalith	99%	6–8 weeks
Epley[25]	30	Epley	80%	1–2 weeks
Fife[59]	46	Canalith	93% *	1 week
Furman & Cass[42]	151	Canalith	87%	unclear
Hain et al[60]	94	Canalith	61% †	1 week
Herdman et al[61]	30	Epley	57% ‡	1–2 weeks
	30	Semont	70% ‡	1–2 weeks
Honrubia et al[6]	250	Epley	88% §	1 month
Korres et al[62]	110	Canalith	86%	2 weeks
Levrat et al[63]	278	Semont	63%	1 week
Macias et al[64]	259	Canalith	75%	likely 1 week
Massoud & Ireland[47]	50	Semont	94%	1 week
	26	Epley	91%	1 week
Nuti et al[48]	56	Semont	89%	1 week
Parnes & Price-Jones[15]	50	Particle	69%	1 month
Pollak et al[31]	58	Particle	74%	1 month
Ruckenstein[33]	86	Epley	78%	2 week
Sargent et al[34]	168	Canalith	90%	6 weeks
Serafini et al[65]	160	Semont	53%	2 days
Smouha[66]	27	Epley	63%	2 weeks
Tirelli et al[67]	118	Canalith	81%	8 weeks
Wolf et al[68]	102	Epley	78%	1–2 weeks

Used with permission from White J, Sawides P, Cherian N, Oas J. Canalith repositioning for benign paroxysmal positional vertigo. Otol Neurotol 2005;26:704–710.

Note: Mean, 22 reports; 78%. "Epley," "Particle," and "Canalith" reflect designations used by authors to describe the Epley maneuver or some modification of it. "Semont" refers to the Semont liberatory maneuver.

* 1 to 3 sessions, single-treatment session, data not available.

† 50% of patients had Dix-Hallpike at follow-up.

‡ 63% of patients had Dix-Hallpike at follow-up.

§ 1 or 2 sessions, single-treatment session, data not available.

Table 8.2   Controlled randomized trials with Dix-Hallpike at follow-up

Publication	Study Design	Treatment	Number Entered/Analyzed	Outcome	Follow-Up
Angeli et al[69]	Prospective randomized	Canalith versus control	47/47	Dix-Hallpike	1 month
Asawavichianginda et al[70]	Prospective randomized	Canalith versus control	85/70	Dix-Hallpike symptoms	1 month (1 week, 2 weeks, 3 months, 6 months)
Froehling et al[71]	Prospective well-randomized double blind	Canalith versus sham	50/50	Dix-Hallpike symptoms	10 days
Li[72]	Prospective randomized	Epley* versus control	60/60	Dix-Hallpike symptoms	1 week
Lynn et al[35]	Prospective well-randomized double blind	Canalith versus sham	36/33	Dix-Hallpike symptoms diary	1 month
Simhadri et al[73]	Prospective well-randomized single blind (patient)	Canalith versus sham	40/40	Dix-Hallpike symptoms	1 month (1 week, 3 months, 6 months)
Soto Varela et al[74]	Prospective randomized	Semont, Epley, Brandt-Daroff †	106/106	Dix-Hallpike symptoms	1 week (1 month, 3 months)
Wolf et al[75]	Prospective randomized	Epley control	41/41	Dix-Hallpike symptoms	1 week (1 month, 3 months)
Yimtae et al[50]	Prospective randomized single blinded (blind assessment)	Canalith versus control	58/56	Dix-Hallpike symptoms	1 week (2 weeks, 3 weeks, 1 month)

Used with permission from White J, Sawides P, Cherian N, Oas J. Canalith repositioning for benign paroxysmal positional vertigo. Otol Neurotol 2005;26:704–710.
* Results from the Epley maneuver with and without oscillation are combined.
† Brandt-Daroff group outcome (7/29 negative Dix-Hallpike at follow-up) was similar to control group data obtained from the other eight trials and was included.

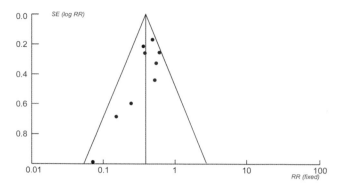

Fig. 8.5 Funnel plot of the included trials. The overall effect estimate (RR) is indicated by the vertical dotted line. Effect estimate (RR) is measured on the x-axis, SE (logRR) is measured on the y-axis, and 95% CI lines are indicated by the gray dotted lines. Studies included in this analysis are evenly distributed within the inverse funnel shape around the total line (as indicated by the 95% CI lines), and therefore there is no indication of publication bias. Used with permission from White J, Savvides P, Cherian N, Oas J. Canalith repositioning for benign paroxysmal positional vertigo. Otol Neurotol 2005;26:704–710.

($Z = 9.09$; $p < 0.00001$). The relative risk (risk of BPPV in the treatment group compared with the control group) was 39% (95% CI, 0.32 to 0.48), representing a relative risk reduction of 61% (1 minus relative risk). The absolute risk reduction was 41% (used to estimate the treatment effect considering the actual frequency of the disorder in both groups). The number needed to treat (NNT) was 2 (whole number rounded from 2.38).

This number indicates that two patients would need to be treated to achieve a favorable outcome compared with no treatment. An NNT within the range of 2 to 3 indicates that a treatment is very effective.[52]

Additional analysis of the three controlled trials that included blinded placebo-controlled outcome was performed (**Table 8.4; Fig. 8.6**). One hundred forty-one patients were included. The mean follow-up was 13 days. Heterogeneity analysis indicated that heterogeneity between studies was not significant ($c^2 = 3.88$; df = 2; $p < 0.14$). The risk of persistent BPPV without treatment was 67%, whereas the risk of persistent BPPV after a single canalith repositioning treatment was 31%. The effect of treatment was significant ($Z = 2.52$; $p < 0.0001$). The relative risk was 47% (95% CI, 0.32 to 0.68). The relative risk reduction was 53%, the absolute risk reduction was 36%, and the NNT was 3 (rounded to whole number from 2.78). These data suggest that the results from the blinded and unblinded controlled clinical trials were comparable.

Funnel plot analysis for publication bias demonstrated no evidence of publication bias (see **Fig. 8.4**). Standard errors [log(effect estimate)] are evenly distributed within the area defined by the 95% CI lines (**Fig. 8.7**).

The results of this meta-analysis of nine controlled studies consisting of 505 patients suggest that canalith repositioning is a safe and effective treatment for PSC-BPPV. A single treatment session successfully resolves positional nystagmus 72% of the time; symptoms spontaneously resolve at 3 weeks in one-third of patients.

Table 8.3 Relative risk, heterogeneity, and overall effect in nine controlled trials of canalith repositioning for BPPV—positive Dix-Hallpike is outcome

Study	Treatment n/N	Control n/N	Weight %	RR, fixed (95% CI)
Wolf et al[68]	8/31	5/10	4.63	0.52 (0.22, 1.22)
Lynn et al[35]	2/18	11/15	7.35	0.15 (0.04, 0.58)
Asawavichianginda et al[70]	3/34	13/36	7.73	0.24 (0.08, 0.78)
Sridhar et al[73]	1/20	14/20	8.57	0.07 (0.01, 0.49)
Froehling et al[71]	8/24	16/26	9.40	0.54 (0.28, 1.03)
Yimtae et al[50]	12/29	20/29	12.25	0.60 (0.36, 0.99)
Angeli et al[69]	10/28	18/19	13.13	0.38 (0.23, 0.63)
Li[72]	18/37	23/23	17.37	0.49 (0.35, 0.68)
Soto Varella et al[74]	21/77	22/29	19.57	0.36 (0.24, 0.55)
Totals	83/298	142/207	100	0.39 (0.32, 0.48)

Used with permission from White J, Sawides P, Cherian N, Oas J. Canalith repositioning for benign paroxysmal positional vertigo. Otol Neurotol 2005;26:704–710.
Note: Test for heterogeneity: $c^2 = 11.74$, df = 8 ($p = 0.16$). Test for overall effect: $Z = 9.09$ ($p < 0.00001$). BPPV, benign paroxysmal positional vertigo; RR, relative risk; CI, confidence interval.

Table 8.4 Relative risk, heterogeneity, and overall effect in three controlled trials of canalith repositioning for BPPV with blinded follow-up—positive Dix-Hallpike is outcome

Study	Treatment n/N	Control n/N	Weight %	RR, fixed (95% CI)
Lynn et al[35]	2/18	11/15	25.34	0.15 (0.04, 0.58)
Froehling et al[71]	8/24	16/26	32.43	0.54 (0.28, 1.03)
Yimtae et al[50]	12/29	20/29	42.23	0.60 (0.36, 0.99)
Totals	22/71	47/70	100	0.47 (0.32, 0.68)

Used with permission from White J, Savvides P, Cherian N, Oas J. Canalith repositioning for benign paroxysmal positional vertigo. Otol Neurotol 2005;26:704–710.

Note: Test for heterogeneity: c^2 = 3.88, df = 2 (p = 0.14). Test for overall effect: Z = 3.92 (p < 0.0001). BPPV, benign paroxysmal positional vertigo; RR, relative risk; CI, confidence interval.

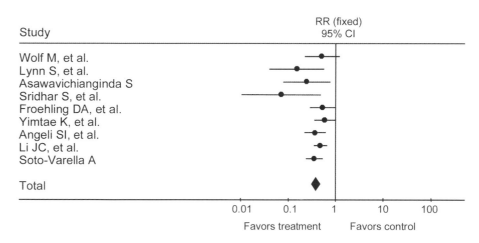

Fig. 8.6 Forest plot, controlled randomized trials of canalith repositioning for BPPV. The confidence interval for each study is represented by a horizontal line, and the point estimate is represented by a square. The size of the square corresponds with the weight of the study in the meta-analysis. The confidence interval for the overall effect estimate is represented by the diamond shape. Data are displayed on a logarithmic scale. Used with permission from White J, Savvides P, Cherian N, Oas J. Canalith repositioning for benign paroxysmal positional vertigo. Otol Neurotol 2005;26:704–710.

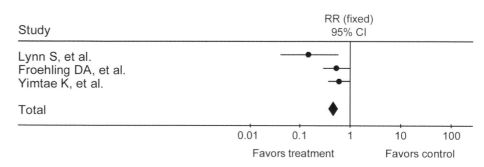

Fig. 8.7 Forest plot, controlled randomized blinded trials of canalith repositioning for BPPV. The confidence interval for each study is represented by a horizontal line, and the point estimate is represented by a square. The size of the square corresponds with the weight of the study in the meta-analysis. The confidence interval for the overall effect estimate is represented by the diamond shape. Data are displayed on a logarithmic scale. Used with permission from White J, Savvides P, Cherian N, Oas J. Canalith repositioning for benign paroxysmal positional vertigo. Otol Neurotol 2005;26:704–710.

The efficacy of canalith repositioning for LSC-BPPV depends on the type of nystagmus observed. For geotropic LSC-BPPV, treatments reportedly alleviate symptoms in 75 to 100% of patients.[12,26,29,30] Apogeotropic LSC-BPPV is more difficult to treat. The same maneuvers used to treat the geotropic variant are commonly used to treat the apogeotropic variant: e.g., the 360° roll maneuver; however, this maneuver is effective only when the otoconial debris can be mobilized. Reports suggest that apogeotropic nystagmus can be converted to geotropic nystagmus if the otoconial debris can be mobilized from near the cupula into the posterior portion of the LSC during repositioning maneuvers.[29,30] This conversion predicts excellent treatment response. Casani used the Gufoni procedure in nine apogeotropic LSC-BPPV patients with a 44% success rate.[12] Asprella et al described related techniques of rapid supine head turns in the Vannucchi-Asprella technique with somewhat better results[30] and White et al[26] reported a 50% success rate. Cupulolithiasis of the HSC explains many of the features of apogeotropic LSC-BPPV, including its persistence and resistance to treatments shown to be successful with canalithiasis, such as roll maneuvers.

On the other hand, it is also possible that some apogeotropic LSC-BPPV cases represent a subtype of vestibular neuritis. The superior vestibular nerve innervates the LSC crista, superior canal crista, macula utriculi, and dorsum of the macula sacculi. Nadol[53] has shown degeneration of the LSC crista in association with superior division vestibular neuritis. Neuritis could also affect the utricular nerve, thus removing otolith inhibition from the LSC efferents at the level of the vestibular nuclei. Animal experiments have demonstrated that apogeotropic horizontal nystagmus develops in cats after unilateral utricular nerve inactivation.[54] Gacek[55] theorizes that a loss of inhibitory otolith input is responsible for some cases of PSC-BPPV, a model that can also be considered in apogeotropic LSC-BPPV. Otolith-canal mismatch or neural degeneration may also explain the persistence of apogeotropic LSC-BPPV despite aggressive therapy aimed at particle repositioning or liberation.

Surgical Treatment

Plugging of the involved semicircular canal may be a consideration in cases of BPPV with unquestionable localization to the semicircular canal involved and persistent symptoms and has been used successfully in cases of resistant PSC-BPPV.[56] Difficulties in definitively identifying the affected side make the procedure less appealing in LSC-BPPV than in PSC-BPPV. Horii et al[57] recently reported on a case of LSC-BPPV that did not improve when treated with plugging of the lateral semicircular canal and required additional treatment on the unoperated side (**Video 8.7**).

References

1. Mizukoshi K, Watanabe Y, Shojaku H, et al. Epidemiological study on benign paroxysmal positional vertigo. Acta Otolaryngol 1988;(Suppl 447):67–72

2. Froehling D, Silverstein MD, Mohr DN, Beatty CW, Offord KP, Ballard DJ. Benign positional vertigo: incidence and prognosis in a population-based study in Olmsted County Minnesota. Mayo Clin Proc 1991;66:596–601

3. Oghalai JS, Manolidis S, Barth JL, Stewart MG, Jenkins HA. Unrecognized benign paroxysmal positional vertigo in elderly patients. Otolaryngol Head Neck Surg 2000;122(5):630–634

4. Dix MR, Hallpike CS. The pathology, symptomatology and diagnosis of certain common disorders of the vestibular system. Proc R Soc Med 1952;45(6):341–354

5. Baloh RW, Sakala SM, Honrubia V. Benign paroxysmal positional nystagmus. Am J Otolaryngol 1979;1(1):1–6

6. Honrubia V, Baloh RW, Harris MR, Jacobson KM. Paroxysmal positional vertigo syndrome. Am J Otol 1999;20(4):465–470

7. Cipparrone L, Corridi G, Pagnini P. Cupulolitiasi. In: Nistagmografia e patologia vestibolare periferica. Milano, Italie: VGiornata Italiana di Nistagmografia Clinica; 1985:6–53

8. McClure JA. Horizontal canal BPV. J Otolaryngol 1985;14(1):30–35

9. Pagnini P, Vannucchi P, Nuti D. Le nystagmus apogeotropique dans le vertige paroxystique positionelle benin du canal semicirculaire horizontal. La revue d'Otoneurologie Francaise 1994;12:304–307

10. Baloh RW, Yue Q, Jacobson KM, Honrubia V. Persistent direction-changing positional nystagmus: another variant of benign positional nystagmus? Neurology 1995;45(7):1297–1301

11. Fife TD. Recognition and management of horizontal canal benign positional vertigo. Am J Otol 1998; 19(3):345–351

12. Ciniglio Appiani G, Catania G, Gagliardi M, Cuiuli G. Repositioning maneuver for the treatment of the apogeotropic variant of horizontal canal benign paroxysmal positional vertigo. Otol Neurotol 2005;26(2):257–260

13. Schuknecht HF. Cupulolithiasis. Arch Otolaryngol 1969;90(6):765–778

14. Hall SF, Ruby RR, McClure JA. The mechanics of benign paroxysmal vertigo. J Otolaryngol 1979;8(2):151–158

15. Parnes LS, Price-Jones RG. Particle repositioning maneuver for benign paroxysmal positional vertigo. Ann Otol Rhinol Laryngol 1993;102(5):325–331

16. Schuknecht HF. Mechanism of inner ear injury from blows to the head. Ann Otol Rhinol Laryngol 1969;78(2):253–262

17. Barber HO. Positional nystagmus, especially after head injury. Laryngoscope 1964;74:891–944

18. Barber HO. Head injury audiological and vestibular findings. Ann Otol Rhinol Laryngol 1969;78(2):239–252

19. Spector M. Positional vertigo after stapedectomy. Ann Otol Rhinol Laryngol 1961;70:2511–2514

20. Cawthorne T. The physiologic basis for head exercises. J Chart Soc Physiother 1944;30:106–107

21. Brandt T, Daroff RB. Physical therapy for benign paroxysmal positional vertigo. Arch Otolaryngol 1980;106(8):484–485

22. McClure JA, Willet JM. Lorazepam and diazepam in the treatment of BPPV. J Otolaryngol 1980;9:472–477

23. Fujino A, Tokumasu K, Yosio S, Naganuma H, Yoneda S, Nakamura K. Vestibular training for benign paroxysmal positional vertigo. Its efficacy in comparison with antivertigo drugs. Arch Otolaryngol Head Neck Surg 1994;120(5):497–504

24. Semont A, Freyss G, Vitte E. Curing the BPPV with a liberatory maneuver. Adv Otorhinolaryngol 1988;42:290–293

25. Epley JM. The canalith repositioning procedure: for treatment of benign paroxysmal positional vertigo. Otolaryngol Head Neck Surg 1992;107(3):399–404

26. White JA, Coale KD, Catalano PJ, Oas JG. Diagnosis and management of lateral semicircular canal benign paroxysmal positional vertigo. Otolaryngol Head Neck Surg 2005;133(2):278–284

27. Bisdorff AR, Debatisse D. Localizing signs in positional vertigo due to lateral canal cupulolithiasis. Neurology 2001;57(6):1085–1088

28. Lempert T, Tiel-Wilck K. A positional maneuver for treatment of horizontal-canal benign positional vertigo. Laryngoscope 1996;106(4):476–478

29. Asprella Libonati G. Diagnostic and treatment strategy of lateral semicircular canal canalolithiasis. Acta Otorhinolaryngol Ital 2005;25(5):277–283

30. Asprella Libonati G, Gagliardi G, Cifarelli D, Larotonda G. "Step by step" treatment of lateral semicircular canal canalolithiasis under videonystagmoscopic examination. Acta Otorhinolaryngol Ital 2003;23(1):10–15

31. Pollak L, Davies RA, Luxon LL. Effectiveness of the particle repositioning maneuver in benign paroxysmal positional vertigo with and without additional vestibular pathology. Otol Neurotol 2002;23(1):79–83

32. Dornhoffer JL, Colvin GB. Benign paroxysmal positional vertigo and canalith repositioning: clinical correlations. Am J Otol 2000;21(2):230–233

33. Ruckenstein MJ. Therapeutic efficacy of the Epley canalith repositioning maneuver. Laryngoscope 2001;111(6):940–945

34. Sargent EW, Bankaitis AE, Hollenbeak CS, Currens JW. Mastoid oscillation in canalith repositioning for paroxysmal positional vertigo. Otol Neurotol 2001;22(2):205–209

35. Lynn S, Pool A, Rose D, Brey R, Suman V. Randomized trial of the canalith repositioning procedure. Otolaryngol Head Neck Surg 1995;113(6):712–720

36. Blakley BW. A randomized, controlled assessment of the canalith repositioning maneuver. Otolaryngol Head Neck Surg 1994;110(4):391–396

37. Ware JE Jr, Sherbourne CD. The MOS 36-item Short-Form Health Survey (SF-36). I. Conceptual framework and item selection. Med Care 1992;30(6):473–483

38. Jacobson GP, Newman CW. The development of the Dizziness Handicap Inventory. Arch Otolaryngol Head Neck Surg 1990;116(4):424–427

39. Lopez-Escamez JA, Gamiz MJ, Fernandez-Perez A, Gomez-Fiñana M, Sanchez-Canet I. Impact of treatment on health-related quality of life in patients with posterior canal benign paroxysmal positional vertigo. Otol Neurotol 2003;24(4):637–641

40. Gámiz MJ, Lopez-Escamez JA. Health-related quality of life in patients over sixty years old with benign paroxysmal positional vertigo. Gerontology 2004;50(2):82–86

41. Baloh RW, Honrubia V. Clinical Neurophysiology of the Vestibular System. 2nd ed. Phildelphia, PA: FA Davis Co; 1990

42. Furman JM, Cass SP. Benign paroxysmal positional vertigo. N Engl J Med 1999;341(21):1590–1596

43. Nunez RA, Cass SP, Furman JM. Short- and long-term outcomes of canalith repositioning for benign paroxysmal positional vertigo. Otolaryngol Head Neck Surg 2000;122(5):647–652

44. Sakaida M, Takeuchi K, Ishinaga H, Adachi M, Majima Y. Long-term outcome of benign paroxysmal positional vertigo. Neurology 2003;60(9):1532–1534

45. Beynon GJ, Baguley DM, da Cruz MJ. Recurrence of symptoms following treatment of posterior semicircular canal benign positional paroxysmal vertigo with a particle repositioning manoeuvre. J Otolaryngol 2000;29(1):2–6

46. Marciano E, Marcelli V. Postural restrictions in labyrintholithiasis. Eur Arch Otorhinolaryngol 2002;259(5):262–265

47. Massoud EA, Ireland DJ. Post-treatment instructions in the nonsurgical management of benign paroxysmal positional vertigo. J Otolaryngol 1996;25(2):121–125

48. Nuti D, Nati C, Passali D. Treatment of benign paroxysmal positional vertigo: no need for postmaneuver restrictions. Otolaryngol Head Neck Surg 2000;122(3):440–444

49. Herdman SJ, Tusa RJ. Complications of the canalith repositioning procedure. Arch Otolaryngol Head Neck Surg 1996;122(3):281–286

50. Yimtae K, Srirompotong S, Srirompotong S, Sae-Seaw P. A randomized trial of the canalith repositioning procedure. Laryngoscope 2003;113(5):828–832

51. White J, Savvides P, Cherian N, Oas J. Canalith repositioning for benign paroxysmal positional vertigo. Otol Neurotol 2005;26(4):704–710

52. Smeeth L, Haines A, Ebrahim S. Numbers needed to treat derived from meta-analyses—sometimes informative, usually misleading. BMJ 1999;318(7197):1548–1551

53. Nadol JB Jr. Vestibular neuritis. Otolaryngol Head Neck Surg 1995;112(1):162–172

54. Fluur E. Positional and positioning nystagmus as a result of utriculocupular integration. Acta Otolaryngol 1974;78(1-2):19–27

55. Gacek RR. Pathology of benign paroxysmal positional vertigo revisited. Ann Otol Rhinol Laryngol 2003;112(7):574–582

56. Parnes LS. Update on posterior canal occlusion for benign paroxysmal positional vertigo. Otolaryngol Clin North Am 1996;29(2):333–342

57. Horii A, Imai T, Mishiro Y, et al. Horizontal canal type BPPV: bilaterally affected case treated with canal plugging and Lempert's maneuver. ORL J Otorhinolaryngol Relat Spec 2003;65(6):366–369

58. Dal T, Ozlüoğlu LN, Ergin NT. The canalith repositioning maneuver in patients with benign positional vertigo. Eur Arch Otorhinolaryngol 2000;257(3):133–136

59. Fife TD. Bedside cure for benign positional vertigo. BNI Q 1994;10:2–8

60. Hain TC, Helminski JO, Reis IL, Uddin MK. Vibration does not improve results of the canalith repositioning procedure. Arch Otolaryngol Head Neck Surg 2000;126(5):617–622

61. Herdman SJ, Tusa RJ, Zee DS, Proctor LR, Mattox DE. Single treatment approaches to benign paroxysmal positional vertigo. Arch Otolaryngol Head Neck Surg 1993;119(4):450–454

62. Korres S, Balatsouras DG, Kaberos A, Economou C, Kandiloros D, Ferekidis E. Occurrence of semicircular canal involvement in benign paroxysmal positional vertigo. Otol Neurotol 2002;23(6):926–932

63. Levrat E, van Melle G, Monnier P, Maire R. Efficacy of the Semont maneuver in benign paroxysmal positional vertigo. Arch Otolaryngol Head Neck Surg 2003;129(6):629–633

64. Macias JD, Massingale S, Gerkin RD. Efficacy of vestibular rehabilitation therapy in reducing falls. Otolaryngol Head Neck Surg 2005;133(3):323–325

65. Serafini G, Palmieri AM, Simoncelli C. Benign paroxysmal positional vertigo of posterior semicircular canal: results in 160 cases treated with Semont's maneuver. Ann Otol Rhinol Laryngol 1996;105(10):770–775

66. Smouha EE. Time course of recovery after Epley maneuvers for benign paroxysmal positional vertigo. Laryngoscope 1997;107(2):187–191

67. Tirelli G, D'Orlando E, Zarcone O, Giacomarra V, Russolo M. Modified particle repositioning procedure. Laryngoscope 2000;110(3 Pt 1):462–468

68. Wolf JS, Boyev KP, Manokey BJ, Mattox DE. Success of the modified Epley maneuver in treating benign paroxysmal positional vertigo. Laryngoscope 1999;109(6):900–903

69. Angeli SI, Hawley R, Gomez O. Systematic approach to benign paroxysmal positional vertigo in the elderly. Otolaryngol Head Neck Surg 2003;128(5):719–725

70. Asawavichianginda S, Isipradit P, Snidvongs K, Supiyaphun P. Canalith repositioning for benign paroxysmal positional vertigo: a randomized, controlled trial. Ear Nose Throat J 2000;79(9):732–734, 736–737

71. Froehling DA, Bowen JM, Mohr DN, et al. The canalith repositioning procedure for the treatment of benign paroxysmal positional vertigo: a randomized controlled trial. Mayo Clin Proc 2000;75(7):695–700

72. Li JC. Mastoid oscillation: a critical factor for success in canalith repositioning procedure. Otolaryngol Head Neck Surg 1995;112(6):670–675

73. Simhadri S, Panda N, Raghunathan M. Efficacy of particle repositioning maneuver in BPPV: a prospective study. Am J Otolaryngol 2003;24(6):355–360

74. Soto Varela A, Bartual Magro J, Santos Pérez S, et al. Benign paroxysmal vertigo: a comparative prospective study of the efficacy of Brandt and Daroff exercises, Semont and Epley maneuver. Rev Laryngol Otol Rhinol (Bord) 2001;122(3):179–183

75. Wolf M, Hertanu T, Novikov I, Kronenberg J. Epley's manoeuvre for benign paroxysmal positional vertigo: a prospective study. Clin Otolaryngol Allied Sci 1999;24(1):43–46

9 The Pathology and Treatment of Benign Paroxysmal Positional Vertigo

Richard R. Gacek

Introduction

Benign paroxysmal positional vertigo (BPPV), described by Barany in 1921,[1] is the most common balance complaint encountered in practice. It is unique in that it is the only clinical form of disequilibrium that is triggered by a change in head position. True, the vertigo experience is brief (less than 1 minute), but it can be so severe during driving, bending, etc., as to be a cause of serious injury. Occasionally, patients may have such a severe episode of vertigo, nausea, and emesis that they require hospitalization.

Since a tilted head position is provocative, BPPV was first assumed to be an otolith disorder. Dix and Hallpike supported this interpretation with histopathologic evidence of utricular end-organ degeneration in the temporal bone of a patient suffering from BPPV.[2] Furthermore, Citron and Hallpike demonstrated that a change in head position provoked the rotatory nystagmus seen in BPPV.[3] Although the use of Frenzel glasses during the Hallpike test is desirable to prevent the patient's fixation on the surround (thus diminishing the eye response), the test may be used without enhancement to detect symptomatic BPPV.[2] The subjective response without nystagmus may be used to identify patients who have a less severe response to provocation with the head in the down and to the side position.[4]

The typical ocular response is the onset of a rotatory and vertical nystagmus after a short (1 to 2 second) latency that has a duration of 10 to 20 seconds.[2] Nystagmus re-appears briefly on the return to the sitting position. Repeat of the test will produce a reduced response and symptoms. This important feature of fatigability is indicative of a peripheral cause, rather than central cause, of the BPPV.

However, focus on the role of otolith organ function in BPPV was changed by the experimental demonstrations that the nystagmus response was elicited by semicircular canal activation and not by otolith stimulation.[5] These findings were supported by temporal bone histopathologic evidence presented by Lindsay and Hemenway showing complete degeneration of the superior vestibular division leaving the inferior division and its sense organs intact in a patient with BPPV after an acute episode of vestibular neuronitis. Both physiologic[6] and anatomic[7] laboratory observations confirmed that the posterior canal sense organ activates the vestibulo-ocular pathway to the contralateral inferior rectus and ipsilateral superior oblique extraocular muscles. These findings supported the contention that posterior canal activation was responsible for the rotatory and vertical nystagmus response characteristic of BPPV.

Pathology

One of the concepts based on morphologic evidence gained from human temporal bones that provided a logical explanation for symptoms was that presented by Schuknecht and Ruby.[8] They found basophilic deposits embedded in the cupula of the posterior canal sense organ of a few patients who had experienced BPPV during life. Since this material stained blue with the hematoxylin and eosin stain that also stained the otoconia of the otolith organs, it was assumed the deposits were derived from otoconia. As otoconia have a high specific gravity (2.7), it was logical to conclude that the cupular mass converted the sense organ into one that was sensitive to gravity. Thus the concept of cupulolithiasis was formulated.

About the same time, selective denervation of the posterior canal sense organ (singular neurectomy) of the lower ear in the provocative position completely and permanently relieved the syndrome.[9,10] This result settled the question of whether it was the up- or downmost ear in the provocative position that is responsible for the clinical findings in BPPV. Later, Parnes and McClure added the observation that the free-floating particles could be seen in the limb of the posterior canal in patients undergoing occlusion of the canal for BPPV.[11] The terms *cupulolithiasis* and *canalolithiasis* were coined to refer to the fixed and free-floating types of deposits in the posterior semicircular canal.

Naturally, a series of head maneuvers were developed to reposition free-floating deposits from the posterior canal aupulla and/or membranous canal through the common crus and into the utricle, where they could no longer activate the canal receptor.[12,13] Although the short-term relief of BPPV by these particle repositioning maneuvers was promising,[14] subsequent reports with longer (> 6 months) follow-up and comparison with no treatment revealed equivalent rates of relief.[15,16]

Additional morphologic observations cast doubt on the validity of the lithiasis concept. Cupular deposits have been found in several temporal bones without a history of positional vertigo. Temporal bone studies describing the incidence of cupular deposits in normal pediatric[17] and adult temporal bones[18,19] indicated that the frequency and size of deposits increases with age. Cupular deposits therefore may be a morphologic change associated with the aging labyrinth. In one report, Parnes observed particles floating in the posterior canal limb in only one-third of 22 patients undergoing canal occlusion for BPPV that did not improve with repositioning maneuvers.[20]

Therefore, inactivation of the posterior canal seems to be a permanent solution to chronic (> 1 year) BPPV demonstrated by a rotatory and vertical nystagmus provoked by head down and to the side position. Positional vertigo and nystagmus following provocation may indicate similar activation of either the lateral or anterior semicircular canals. These are identified by the appropriately directed nystagmus after provocation (horizontal or vertical downbeat). The results of one form of de-activation of the posterior canal (singular neurectomy) to relieve BPPV are presented here and compared with posterior canal occlusion. We also suggest a neurologic basis for this neuropathy that may explain some inadequacies in the purely mechanistic concept of BPPV.

■ Singular Neurectomy (SN)

The author performed 286 singular neurectomies over the period 1972 to 2012. The procedures were performed in 275 patients; 11 of the patients underwent sequentially a contralateral SN for bilateral BPPV. All of the patients experienced chronic (> 1 year) BPPV of the posterior canal demonstrated by a rotatory/vertical nystagmus when placed in the Hallpike provocative position and observed without Frenzel glasses or eye muscle recording. They all had contrast CT or MRI of the brain and no other neurologic deficits. Most had completed a trial of physical therapy. All had hearing tests that were normal for their age.

In the group of 275 patients, there were 196 females and 79 males. The median age of the group was 59 years, with a range of 21 to 93 years. The etiologies of their BPPV fell into three groups: idiopathic (209), trauma (43), and following other surgery under general anesthesia (23).

- The idiopathic group experienced a sudden onset of prolonged vertigo (hours to days) without hearing loss. BPPV followed recovery from the acute vestibular insult (vestibular neuronitis).
- The trauma group suffered a concussive injury to the head with or without loss of consciousness.
- The other surgery group noted onset of BPPV after abdominal, orthopedic, gynecologic, or sinus surgery, all under general anesthesia.

Technique of Singular Neurectomy

The SN procedure may be performed under local anesthesia with sedation or under general anesthesia via intubation. The exposure is through a speculum inserted into the ear canal, with or without support by a speculum holder. After elevation of a tympanomeatal flap, the structures in the posterior half of the middle ear are exposed. Curettage of the posterior and superior bony ear canal may be required for a full view of the round window niche (RWN) and the incudostapedial joint (**Fig. 9.1** and **Fig. 9.2**).

Often there is a mucous membrane fold that may partially or completely obscure the RWN. After removal of this fold with picks or hooks, the rim of the RWN must be removed with a small (1 mm) diamond bur until a full view of the round window membrane (RWM) is obtained. This can be confirmed by downward displacement of the incudostapedial joint.

The drilling on the floor of the RWN is performed with a 1-mm diamond bur. The depression created is inferior to the posterosuperior portion of the RWM. At the depth of 1 to 3 mm, the singular nerve will be encountered in one of three locations (**Fig. 9.1**). The most common is where the white myelinated nerve is partially exposed. Less often, the full width of the nerve may be fully exposed. Rarely, the nerve is not seen because it lies superiorly (under the RWM). This position can be confirmed by the patient's response (if under local anesthesia) to probing with a pick or small hook. The patient will feel vertigo or pain with this stimulation. The proximal end of the singular canal is then lightly drilled with a 0.5-mm diamond bur to cause osteogenesis in the canal lumen. The tympanomeatal flap is returned to anatomic position. The patient usually stays in hospital overnight, but some patients may be discharged the same day.

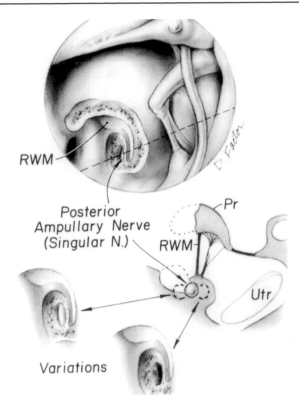

Fig. 9.1 Drawing of the surgical exposure in a left middle ear showing the anatomic relationship of the singular nerve to the round window membrane (RWM). The variation in location of the nerve is illustrated in the lower scheme taken at the level indicated by the *dashed line*. Pr, promontory; Utr, ultricular nerve. Used with permission from Gacek RR. Pathophysiology and management of cupulolithiasis. Am J Otolaryngol 1985;6:66–74.

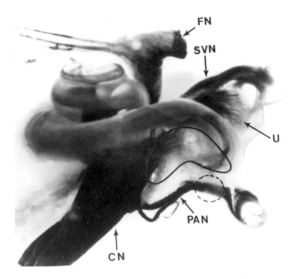

Fig. 9.2 Relationship of the posterior ampullary (singular) nerve (PAN) to the round window membrane (RWM) (*solid line*) is shown in this dissection of the inner ear and its innervation. *Dashed line* marks the location for transection of the singular neurectomy. CN, cochlear nerve; FN, facial nerve; SVN, superior vestibular division; U, utricular nerve. Used with permission from Gacek RR. Transection of the posterior ampullary nerve for relief of benign paroxysmal vertigo. Ann Otol Rhinol Laryngol 1974;88:596.

Confirmation of posterior canal ablation is seen with a spontaneous downbeat vertical nystagmus immediately after surgery.

Results

Singular neurectomy completely relieved vertigo in 276 procedures (96.5%), and partially or failed to relieve vertigo in 3.4% of the 286 procedures. Importantly, a permanent sensorineural hearing loss (SNHL) occurred in 11 of the 286 singular neurectomies. The hearing loss was significant and ranged from severe to mild or moderate.

Possibly because the technique of SN was found to be too difficult and SN was associated with an unacceptably high risk of SNHL, other methods of deactivating the function of the posterior canal were explored. Parnes and McClure[11] described the procedure of fenestrating the limb of the posterior canal in the mastoid compartment and then occluding the lumen of the canal, thus immobilizing the endo-lymph-containing membranous canal and preventing movement of the loose otoconia. This procedure had been used successfully in physiologic animal studies and was found to be accomplished without causing hearing loss.

The procedure as described is performed under general anesthesia through an intact canal wall mastoidectomy and requires hospitalization for several days for the patient to recover. Temporary SNHL may follow, but it recovers with time. The provoked nystagmus response is not eliminated after the surgery but requires several days to 1 week to be absent following provocation. Permanent SNHL may occur in ~ 3% of patients after posterior canal occlusion.[21]

The time course for relief of BPPV and the temporary hearing loss associated with this procedure imply a surgical labyrinthitis is responsible for the reduction in vestibular sensitivity, with the gradient of pathology extending from the posterior canal sense organ to the remainder of the labyrinth. One may assume, then, that the beneficial effects on BPPV are engendered by a degenerative effect, with maximum effect on the posterior canal sense organ. A similar clinical experience is the post-stapedectomy relief of vertigo in patients with otosclerosis. Postoperative vestibular function in these patients has been shown to be decreased.[22]

Several features of BPPV are not accounted for by a purely mechanical alteration in labyrinth physiology. These are: (1) the latency, limited duration, and fatigability of the rotatory nystagmus despite sustained provocation; (2) the absence of nystagmus in the presence of subjective symptoms with provocation in some patients; and (3) the absence of basophilic deposits in the cupula and membranous posterior canal in many donor temporal bones with a history of BPPV.[23]

It has been suggested[3,24] that a neural component may account for BPPV, thus explaining these features. We have carefully measured the neural components to the vestibular sense organs in the temporal bone from five patients with a history of BPPV during life.[23] These temporal bones revealed a 50% loss of superior division vestibular neurons in all five. Caloric responses were normal in four of the temporal bones. There was also a 50% loss of inferior vestibular division neurons in three of the temporal bones, with the other two containing a 30% loss of inferior division neurons. There was degeneration of saccular ganglion cells in the latter two temporal bones (**Fig. 9.3** and **Fig. 9.4**).

This series of temporal bones suggests that degeneration of the saccular ganglion may play a key role in BPPV. The interaction between otolith and canal receptors is important to the pathophysiology of BPPV. Considerable evidence supports an interactive relationship between otolith and canal sense organs.[25,26,27] In patients as well as laboratory animals, excitation of otolith organs exerts an inhibitory effect on the canal response (nystagmus) to rotational or caloric stimulation.[28,29] Loss of an otolith's inhibitory effect, therefore, could permit a stronger canal response (vertigo and nystagmus) when the crista is stimulated.

The loss of saccular input could be inflammatory or mechanical. The largest categories of patients in this series were those whose symptoms of BPPV appeared following vestibular neuronitis. There is ample evidence that this vestibulopathy is caused by neurotropic viruses (e.g., herpes). The second largest group of patients requiring SN was the group suffering head trauma, where the loss of otoconia would render the saccule inactive. The inactivation of virus to its latent state in vestibular neuronitis and the replenishment of otoconia to the saccular macule would be responsible for resolution of positional vertigo. Such a neural interaction is likely to take place in the vestibular nuclei, specifically the medial nucleus where excitatory vestibulo-ocular neurons are located.[30] The medial nucleus receives input from both canal and otolith first-order neurons.[31] It also contains large populations of vestibulo-ocular (VO) and commissural neurons.[7] Although all first-order vestibular input utilizes glutamate neurotransmission and is excitatory, vestibular nerve stimulation inhibits some neurons in the vestibular nuclei.[32] The inhibitory postsynaptic potentials due to activation of inhibitory neurons are disynaptic, likely commissural neurons in the medial nucleus. Therefore, the proposed neural reflex for the otolith effect on the VO pathway generated by canal input is excitation of commissural neurons, which then inhibit VO neurons in the medial vestibular nucleus (**Fig. 9.5**).

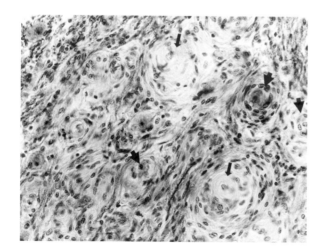

Fig. 9.3 High-power photomicrograph of the saccular ganglion in a 75-year-old woman with a 10-year history of posterior canal BPPV. There are several ganglion cells underlying degeneration (*arrows*) by hyperplasia of satellite cells. Used with permission from Gacek RR. A perspective on recurrent vertigo. ORL 2013;75:91–107.

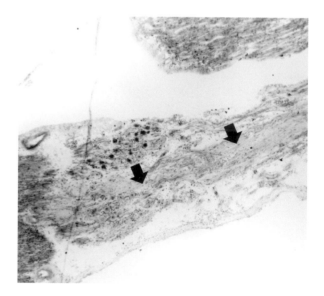

Fig. 9.4 This temporal bone from a 65-year-old man with a 6-month history of posterior canal BPPV shows focal degeneration of saccular ganglion cells and dendrites (*arrows*). Used with permission from Gacek RR. A perspective on recurrent vertigo. ORL 2013;75:91–107.

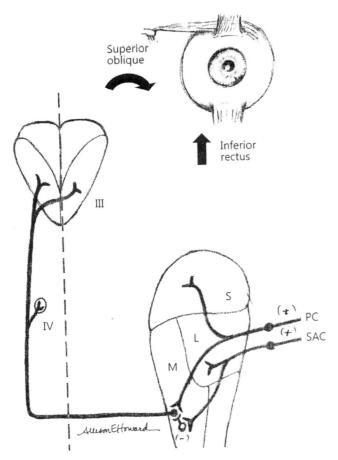

Fig. 9.5 The proposed neural pathways in posterior canal BPPV are shown in this diagram. S, L, M, superior, lateral, and medial vestibular nuclei; PC, posterior ampullary (singular) nerve; SAC, saccular nerve; III, oculomotor nucleus; IV, trochlear nucleus. Used with permission from Gacek RR. A perspective on recurrent vertigo. ORL 2013;75:91–107.

■ Surgical Technique

BPPV—Posterior Canal Plugging

Perform this only after particle repositioning maneuvers by trained therapists or MDs fail to control symptoms. Less than 1% of patients require surgical intervention. The surgical success rate for this procedure is over 90%. The surgery itself is relatively straight forward. The patient is prepped and draped as for standard mastoid surgery. A standard postauricular incision is made, followed by a cortical mastoidectomy—identifying the lateral semicircular canal (LSC), incus, tegmen, and, typically, the sigmoid sinus. Once this is accomplished, the posterior semicircular canal is identified. It lies directly posterior and perpendicular to the LCS.

Prior to drilling more bone to locate the PSC, a saline-soaked gelfoam pledget can be placed in the antrum to reduce the amount of blood and bone dust entering the middle ear space. A diamond burr is used to skeletonize and blue-line the PSC, so that a 1 × 3 mm oval window of bone over the midportion of the PSC is opened to expose, but not violate, the membranous labryrinth.

The next step is to plug the PSC. To accomplish this, connective tissue and/or bone dust is typically used to compress the canal and then sealed with bone wax/dust/fascia. If the membrane is violated, the canal is still packed the same way. In order to prevent hearing loss and significant post-op dizziness, suctioning over the canal defect is to be avoided. The incision is then closed.

Note that using this surgical procedure on elderly patients may result in significant vestibulitis or even a hypoactive vestibular system.

■ Medical Treatment of BPPV

Since there is some question about the effectiveness of physical therapy as a nonsurgical treatment of BPPV, medical treatment is desired. There is some evidence that suggests that BPPV may be the clinical expression of a viral neuropathy. In addition to the two temporal bones with vestibular ganglion cell degeneration in the series reported in 2004, there is the clinical experience that BPPV often follows an episode of vestibular neuronitis and that it often is present on the same side as MD or vestibular neuronitis.

Using the neural pathway depicted in **Fig. 9.5**, a simple explanation would be viral downregulation of the saccular ganglion, removing its normal inhibitory effect on the input of neurons supplying the posterior canal sense organs. Using antiviral medication (Acyclovir), we have been able to control BPPV in 60% of patients presenting acutely.[33] It is presumed that in those patients who experience relief of BPPV on antiviral medication, the saccular ganglion cells have recovered their function after the virus is put back into latency. The patients who do not respond to the antiviral have a sufficiently large loss of saccular ganglion cells to allow the BPPV to persist. A similar relationship exists between the utricular macula and the lateral and superior semicircular canal sense organs. Those forms of BPPV, indicated by the direction of nystagmus on provocation, are much less frequent in occurrence than that based in the posterior canal.

The anatomic alignment of hair cells, with polarization of hair cells in part of the otolith sense organ affecting a canal sense organ, is illustrated by the human labyrinth shown in **Fig. 9.6** and **Fig. 9.7**.

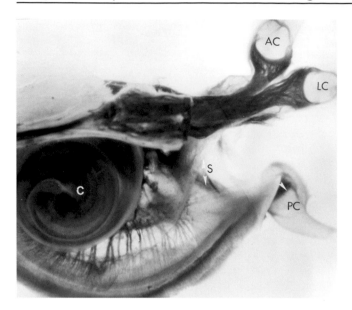

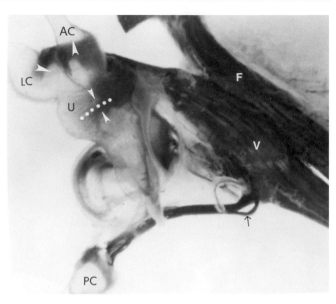

Fig. 9.6 Dissection of the human labyrinth and nerve supply viewed from the middle ear. *Arrowheads* indicate the polarization of hair cells in the posterior canal crista (PC) and the saccular macula (S). AC, anterior canal crista; C, cochlea; LC, lateral crista. Used with permission from Gacek RR. Fusion as an evolutionary principle of the vertebrate labyrinth. Ann Otol Rhinol Laryngol 2009;118:845–851.

Fig. 9.7 View of the labyrinth from above demonstrates the polarization of hair cells in the utricular acula (U), the anterior canal (AC), and the lateral canal (LC) cristae. F, facial nerve in the internal auditory canal; PC, posterior canal crista; V, vestibular nerve trunk. Used with permission from Gacek RR. Fusion as an evolutionary principle of the vertebrate labyrinth. Ann Otol Rhinol Laryngol 2009;118:845–851.

Arrows representing the inferior half of the saccular macula and the posterior canal crista demonstrate this alignment. The polarization of hair cells in the two halves of the utricular macula is similar to that in the anterior and lateral canal cristae. Thus, the physiologic basis for provoked positional vertigo has a firm anatomic basis.

■ Conclusion

Benign paroxysmal positional vertigo is a common clinical vestibular disorder that is usually controlled by nonsurgical treatment. However, in a small number of patients who experience BPPV for longer than 1 year, surgical relief is highly effective.

References

1. Barany R. Diagnose von Krankheitserscheinungen im Bereiche des Otolithenapparates. Acta Otolaryngol 1921;2:434–437

2. Dix MR, Hallpike CS. The pathology, symptomatology and diagnosis of certain common disorders of the vestibular system. Ann Otol Rhinol Laryngol 1952;61:987–1016

3. Citron L, Hallpike CS. Observations upon the mechanism of positional nystagmus of the so-called benign paroxysmal type. J Laryngol Otol 1956;70(5):253–259

4. Tirelli G, D'Orlando E, Giacomarra V, Russolo M. Benign positional vertigo without detectable nystagmus. Laryngoscope 2001;111(6):1053–1056

5. Hemenway WG, Lindsay JR. Postural vertigo due to unilateral sudden partial loss of vestibular function. Ann Otol Rhinol Laryngol 1956;65(3):692–706

6. Cohen B, Suzuki JI. Eye movements induced by ampullary nerve stimulation. Am J Physiol 1963;204:347–351

7. Gacek RR. Anatomical demonstration of the vestibulo-ocular projections in the cat. Acta Otolaryngol Suppl 1971;293:1–63

8. Schuknecht HF, Ruby RR. Cupulolithiasis. Adv Otorhinolaryngol 1973;20:434–443

9. Gacek RR. Transection of the posterior ampullary nerve for the relief of benign paroxysmal positional vertigo. Ann Otol Rhinol Laryngol 1974;83(5):596–605

10. Gacek RR. Technique and results of singular neurectomy for the management of benign paroxysmal positional vertigo. Acta Otolaryngol 1995;115(2):154–157

11. Parnes LS, McClure JA. Posterior semicircular canal occlusion for intractable benign paroxysmal positional vertigo. Ann Otol Rhinol Laryngol 1990;99(5 Pt 1): 330–334

12. Semont A, Freyss G, Vitte E. Curing the BPPV with a liberatory maneuver. Adv Otorhinolaryngol 1988; 42:290–293

13. Epley JM. The canalith repositioning procedure: for treatment of benign paroxysmal positional vertigo. Otolaryngol Head Neck Surg 1992;107(3):399–404

14. Herdman SJ, Tusa RJ, Zee DS, Proctor LR, Mattox DE. Single treatment approaches to benign paroxysmal positional vertigo. Arch Otolaryngol Head Neck Surg 1993;119(4):450–454

15. Asawavichianginda S, Isipradit P, Snidvongs K, Supiyaphun P. Canalith repositioning for benign paroxysmal positional vertigo: a randomized, controlled trial. Ear Nose Throat J 2000;79(9):732–734, 736–737

16. Blakley BW. A randomized, controlled assessment of the canalith repositioning maneuver. Otolaryngol Head Neck Surg 1994;110(4):391–396

17. Bachor E, Wright CG, Karmody CS. The incidence and distribution of cupular deposits in the pediatric vestibular labyrinth. Laryngoscope 2002;112(1):147–151

18. Moriarty B, Rutka J, Hawke M. The incidence and distribution of cupular deposits in the labyrinth. Laryngoscope 1992;102(1):56–59

19. Naganuma H, Kohut RI, Ryu JH, et al. Basophilic deposits on the cupula: preliminary findings describing the problems involved in studies regarding the incidence of basophilic deposits on the cupula. Acta Otolaryngol Suppl 1996;524(Suppl 524):9–15

20. Parnes LS. Update on posterior canal occlusion for benign paroxysmal positional vertigo. Otolaryngol Clin North Am 1996;29(2):333–342

21. Gacek R, McKenna M. Surgical treatment for benign paroxysmal positional vertigo. In: Nadol JB, McKenna MJ, eds. Surgery of the Ear and Temporal Bone. Philadelphia, PA: Lippincott Williams & Wilkins; 2005: 391–402

22. Cody DTR, Baker HL Jr. Otosclerosis: vestibular symptoms and sensorineural hearing loss. Ann Otol Rhinol Laryngol 1978;87(6 Pt 1):778–796

23. Gacek RR. Pathology of benign paroxysmal positional vertigo revisited. Ann Otol Rhinol Laryngol 2003;112(7):574–582

24. Brandt T. Vertigo: Its Multisensory Syndromes. Berlin, Germany: Springer-Verlag; 1991:139–151

25. Fluur E, Mellström A. Saccular stimulation and oculomotor reactions. Laryngoscope 1970;80(11):1713–1721

26. Fluur E, Mellström A. The otolith organs and their influence on oculomotor movements. Exp Neurol 1971;30(1):139–147

27. Fluur E, Siegborn J. The otolith organs and the nystagmus problem. Acta Otolaryngol 1973;76(6):438–442

28. Benson AJ. Interactions between semicircular canals and gravireceptors. In: Busby DE, ed. Recent Advances in Aerospace Medicine. Dordrecht, The Netherlands: D. Reidel; 1970:249–261

29. Raphan T, Cohen B, Henn V. Effects of gravity on rotatory nystagmus in monkeys. Ann N Y Acad Sci 1981; 374:44–55

30. Highstein SM. The organization of the vestibulo-oculomotor and trochlear reflex pathways in the rabbit. Exp Brain Res 1973;17(3):285–300

31. Gacek RR. The course and central termination of first order neurons supplying vestibular endorgans in the cat. Acta Otolaryngol Suppl 1969;254:1–66

32. Wilson VJ, Mellville Jones G. Labyrinthine Input to the Brain. New York, NY: Plenum Press; 1979:127–167

33. Gacek RR. A perspective on recurrent vertigo. ORL J Otorhinolaryngol Relat Spec 2013;75(2):91–107

10 Labyrinthitis

Sean O. McMenomey and Samuel P. Gubbels

■ Introduction

Inflammation of the delicate structures of the inner ear is referred to as labyrinthitis. Suppurative labyrinthitis describes a fulminant, pyogenic infection of the inner ear producing severe symptoms, which can be life-threatening and result in permanent hearing loss or vestibular dysfunction. Serous labyrinthitis represents inflammation of the inner ear without the presence of frank bacterial infection. Though patients with serous labyrinthitis can have severe symptoms, long-term sequelae generally do not occur. Labyrinthitis in both suppurative and serous forms can be further classified as meningogenic or tympanogenic, depending on whether the inner ear inflammation represents extension of intracranial or perilabyrinthine infection. Because of the severity of the acute manifestations and the potentially permanent sequelae that can occur, an awareness of the manifestations and proper management of labyrinthitis is imperative for all involved in the care of patients with otologic and neurologic disease. This chapter focuses on the pathophysiology, manifestations, diagnosis, and treatment of both tympanogenic and meningogenic labyrinthitis. In addition, other forms of inner ear inflammation, such as viral labyrinthitis and labyrinthitis ossificans, are discussed.

■ Inner Ear Pathology in Labyrinthitis

The histopathologic findings in both serous and suppurative labyrinthitis in humans have been well described in postmortem temporal bone studies.[1,2] Merchant et al reviewed the inner ear findings of 41 patients who had died of meningitis.[2] Forty-nine percent of involved temporal bones had inflammatory cells present in the inner ear structures consistent with the diagnosis of suppurative labyrinthitis, while 34% had eosinophilic staining of inner ear fluids with an absence of inflammatory cells, findings consistent with serous labyrinthitis.

In cases of suppurative labyrinthitis, the inflammatory changes affected the scala tympani in all specimens, with the scala vestibuli and vestibular labyrinth affected in only 50% of cases. Notably, the cochlear and vestibular endolymphatic spaces were without inflammatory changes in 95% of the bones. In addition, the neurosensory elements of the inner ear were intact in 75% of the specimens with suppurative labyrinthitis. The remaining 25% of specimens in the suppurative labyrinthitis group had destruction of the organ of Corti and/or the spiral ganglion cells, a finding consistent with previous temporal bone studies.[1]

The inner ears with serous labyrinthitis had a different pattern of inflammatory changes. Eosinophilic staining affected primarily the vestibular labyrinth in both the perilymphatic and endolymphatic spaces. The cochlea was involved in only 40% of cases, with the scala tympani being the most frequently affected fluid compartment. Similar to the temporal bones with suppurative labyrinthitis, the neurosensory elements of the inner ear were intact in nearly all of the cases of serous labyrinthitis. The endolymphatic duct and sac were normal in cases of both serous and suppurative labyrinthitis of meningogenic origin, although the authors did note that labyrinthitis of tympanogenic origin consistently demonstrates findings of endolymphatic hydrops.

Traditionally, it has been thought that suppurative labyrinthitis causes frank destruction of inner ear neurosensory structures while serous inflammation of the inner ear represents a toxic but reversible insult to the cochlea without loss of epithelial elements. Multiple temporal bone studies have challenged this paradigm, as it has been shown that serous labyrinthitis can, in some cases, result in irreversible hearing impairment due to loss of sensory elements in the organ of Corti and neural elements in the spiral ganglion.[3,4] Conversely, some have speculated that mild cases of suppurative labyrinthitis may resolve with appropriate therapy without a resultant hearing loss.[2] Labyrinthitis likely represents a continuum of inflammatory changes of the inner ear producing a range of severity in its manifestations.

■ Tympanogenic Labyrinthitis

Epidemiology

Tympanogenic labyrinthitis represents the spread of inflammation from the middle ear or perilabyrinthine air cells into the inner ear and can occur in the setting of acute or chronic otitis media. In the pre-antibiotic era, tympanogenic labyrinthitis was reported to have occurred in up to 16% of cases of otitis media and was a more common form of labyrinthitis than the meningogenic form.[5] Since the advent and widespread use of antibiotics, tympanogenic labyrinthitis occurs less frequently than the meningogenic form. Clinical labyrinthitis has been found in some studies to occur in 5.37% of cases of chronic otitis media[6] and 5% of cases of acute otitis media.[7] In retrospective studies as recently as 1999, Osma et al[6] and Kangsanarak et al[8] reported that clinical labyrinthitis represented 12% and 34% of all extracranial complications of suppurative otitis media occurring in Turkey and Thailand, respectively. Bluestone et al reported three cases of serous and two cases of suppurative labyrinthitis in a series of 100 pediatric patients with intratemporal complications of otitis media.[7] Correlative temporal bone studies have found that labyrinthitis, whether serous or suppurative, occurs in 38% of patients with purulent otitis media and is more common in children than in adults.[9] Paparella et al[1] found evidence of pathologic labyrinthine changes in 82% of temporal bones with acute otitis media and 77% with chronic otitis media, though this is likely an overestimation of the true incidence secondary to the inherent selection bias of the temporal bone study. The average length of hospital stay in children with tympanogenic labyrinthitis is as long as 8 days in some studies,[7] which underscores the severity of the disease process. Because labyrinthitis is a clinical diagnosis based on a variety of symptoms and signs that occur in the setting of frequently complex otologic disease, a true incidence of the disease may never be clearly delineated.

Pathophysiology of Tympanogenic Labyrinthitis

Tympanogenic labyrinthitis occurs as a result of spread of infection or inflammation from the middle ear, mastoid antrum, or petrous apex. The inflammatory changes can affect the inner ear diffusely or can be localized to a limited portion of the labyrinth—so-called *circumscribed labyrinthitis*.[5] Suppurative labyrinthitis of tympanogenic origin is generally a diffuse infection of the inner ear structures, with some areas more severely affected than others (see above). Serous labyrinthitis can be either a diffuse process, with generally more acute, severe associated symptoms, or a circumscribed process that is often more chronic in nature, with more mild, insidious symptoms. In some cases, the inflammation spreads through an acquired pathway between the inner and middle ear spaces. Examples of this include cholesteatomatous erosion of the bony labyrinth, temporal bone fracture, or after otologic surgery (stapedotomy, fenestration, cochleostomy, etc.). The most common of these is a fistula in the horizontal semicircular canal secondary to erosion by cholesteatoma, often resulting in soft tissue invasion into the labyrinth with a surrounding zone of inflammation within the inner ear.

In many cases of tympanogenic labyrinthitis, there is no known communication between the middle and inner ear spaces. The mechanism of spread of inflammation from the middle to inner ear in these cases has been the subject of many temporal bone and animal investigations over the last century. Though some have entertained the possibility that labyrinthitis could result from direct or embolic spread of inflammation or infection[1] along microscopic vascular channels, there has been little to no evidence to support such a mechanism. Furthermore, because of the different embryologic origins of the middle ear (endoderm and mesoderm) and inner ear (neurectoderm), no direct vascular channels through the otic capsular bone[10] are known to exist. Similarly, the presence of a congenital perilymphatic fistula has been implicated as a potential route of spread in tympanogenic labyrinthitis, although no histopathologic or radiologic evidence exists in the literature to support this mechanism.

The majority of pathologic and experimental studies in tympanogenic labyrinthitis implicate the round window membrane (RWM) as the primary site of spread of middle ear inflammation into the inner ear. The normal RWM is 40 to 70 μm in thickness in humans[11,12] and sits in the round window niche, which measures 1 mm in depth and 2 mm in diameter. The RWM consists of three layers: 1) an outer epithelial layer of nonciliated mucosal cells contiguous with the middle ear epithelium; 2) a middle fibrous layer of fibrocytes with prominent elastic and collagen bundles; and 3) an inner epithelial layer with thin cytoplasmic extensions.[1] The RWM sits adjacent to the sinus tympani, where purulent material can pool in otitis media, particularly when the patient is in the supine position. Multiple RWM pathologic changes are known to occur in otitis media, including vascular hypertrophy and cystic change in the middle layer, with notable thickening of the membrane.[11] Beyond this, many temporal bone studies of patients with tympanogenic labyrinthitis have shown evidence of direct spread of bacteria with associated inflammatory cells through an intact RWM.[12,13,14,15,16,17] Animal studies have shown that thickening of the RWM results in an increase in permeability of the RWM to macromolecules but a decreased incidence of bacterial invasion into the inner ear.[18] Possibly, the thickening of the RWM that occurs in otitis represents a protective mechanism to prevent the direct spread of bacteria from the middle ear, but it may result in an increased susceptibility to influx of inflammatory mediators into the inner ear.

■ Meningogenic Labyrinthitis

Epidemiology

Five to thirty-five percent of patients who survive bacterial meningitis will have bilateral sensorineural hearing loss (SNHL), due to spread of infection or inflammatory mediators to the inner ear, with resultant loss of neurosensory elements.[19,20,21,22,23] In 5% of cases, the damage to the cochlea will result in a profound and permanent loss.[20,22,24,25,26] In children, bacterial meningitis is the leading cause of SNHL (60–90% of all cases) and has significant associated mortality. *Haemophilus influenzae*, *Streptococcus pneumoniae*, and *Neisseria meningitidis* have historically accounted for 64%, 16%, and 10% of cases of meningitis.[27] *S. pneumoniae* has been found to be a particularly virulent organism, with a mortality rate of 19% in children and 20 to 30% in adults.[28,29] In addition, the rate of profound SNHL after *S. pneumoniae* meningitis in children is 31 to 57%, the highest incidence of SNHL among the common pathogens seen in meningitis.[21,30] The introduction of *H. influenzae* and *S. pneumoniae* vaccines has decreased the incidence of bacterial meningitis from these organisms and overall.[21,31]

Pathophysiology

Labyrinthitis in the setting of meningitis, whether suppurative or serous, occurs due to the extension of bacteria or inflammatory byproducts from the meninges to the inner ear. Cochlear pathology in meningitis occurs as a progression of changes, with formation of a serofibrinous exudate initially followed by infiltration of inflammatory cells and ultimately granulation formation.[32] The route of spread has been investigated in both animal and human temporal bone studies, and the cochlear modiolus, with its multiple perineural and perivascular chan-

nels, has been implicated as one of the primary sites involved with transmission of infection in meningogenic labyrinthitis.[5,33,34,35,36] Merchant and Gopen[2] found a high degree of correlation between modiolar inflammation and suppurative labyrinthitis in a human temporal bone study on patients who had died with meningogenic labyrinthitis.

The cochlear aqueduct is another site thought to allow the spread of infection from the meninges to the inner ear.[37,38] This theory of pathogenesis is supported by the frequent involvement of the basal scala tympani, where the aqueduct terminates in the inner ear, in cases of meningogenic labyrinthitis. Furthermore, Merchant and Gopen[2] found inflammatory cells within the lumen of the cochlear aqueduct in 78% of cases of meningogenic labyrinthitis, though the possibility of retrograde involvement of the aqueduct could not be excluded. Interestingly, the presence of labyrinthitis did not correlate with aqueduct patency in this study, raising the possibility that in cases of bony or connective tissue obliteration of the aqueduct, infection may spread through microchannels within the aqueduct not seen on histopathologic examination or through an alternative communication, such as the modiolus.

Another notable finding in the human temporal bone study by Merchant and Gopen[2] is the lack of inflammatory involvement of the vestibular cribrose area and endolymphatic sac, despite their proximity to the meninges. Differences in the ultrastructural anatomy of these structures, leading to a more efficient sealing of the potential communication, are speculated to be responsible for these observations.

Labyrinthitis ossificans (LO) is a process of new bone deposition within the inner ear and occurs most commonly after bacterial meningitis. LO can also occur after tympanogenic labyrinthitis[5] and can be thought of as the end stage of inner ear inflammation. Paparella and Sugiura[5] described the pathology of suppurative labyrinthitis and the subsequent labyrinthine changes that lead to new bone formation within the inner ear. After the acute phase of suppurative labyrinthitis (described previously), wherein a hearing loss can manifest as early as 48 hours after the initial infection, a fibrous stage occurs where granulation tissue, with prominent fibroblasts and vasculature, fills the perilymphatic spaces of the inner ear, with relative sparing of the endolymphatic space.[37,39,40] Disorganized, woven bone is then deposited in the inner ear and with the passage of time, the bone is resorbed and remodeled into dense, lamellar bone that is progressively mineralized.[41] In some cases, complete ossification of the inner ear occurs. The fibrous and osseous stages have been found to occur as early as 2 weeks and 2 months, respectively, after the acute phase of inner ear inflammation.[5] New bone growth was evident as early as 3 weeks after infection and continued for up to 12 months in one animal study.[41]

■ Labyrinthitis: Diagnosis

Symptoms

Labyrinthitis is characterized by vertigo and hearing loss and is to be differentiated from vestibular neuritis by the presence of cochlear symptoms in addition to vestibular complaints. The vertigo seen in suppurative labyrinthitis is often profound and can be associated with nausea and vomiting, whereas patients with serous labyrinthitis tend to have milder vestibular symptoms in general. The vertigo in labyrinthitis can last days to weeks and often has a waxing and waning course. A postural component to the vertigo may be present, causing patients to seek a motionless environment.[10] Patients often have disequilibrium for a period of weeks to months after the acute, fulminant vertigo has diminished.

The hearing loss in suppurative labyrinthitis is profound and generally permanent, whereas serous labyrinthitis often produces a partial loss of hearing, primarily affecting the higher frequencies. Other associated cochlear symptoms, such as tinnitus, aural fullness and otalgia, may be present in patients with labyrinthitis and may be quite severe at times.

Patients with labyrinthitis of tympanic origin may have a history of chronic ear disease, ear surgery, or a draining ear. These patients usually don't have a fever, even when suppurative changes are affecting the inner ear.[42] In contrast, patients with labyrinthitis of meningogenic origin often have fever in addition to the classical symptoms of meningitis, such as nuchal rigidity, photophobia, nausea, vomiting, and mental status changes. Often, the severe symptoms and clinical illness associated with meningitis overshadow those secondary to co-existent labyrinthitis. Because of this, the diagnosis of meningogenic labyrinthitis may not be made until a patient has recovered from meningitis and is found to have hearing loss and persistent vestibular symptoms.

Clinical Findings

The otoscopic findings of acute otitis media (bulging/erythema of tympanic membrane, middle ear purulence) or chronic otitis media (perforation, purulent otorrhea, cholesteatoma) are often evident in patients with tympanogenic labyrinthitis, though not uniformly. Paparella et al[1,43] reported three patients with histologic evidence of tympanogenic labyrinthitis who had minimal or no tympanic membrane pathology visible on otoscopy, which emphasizes the need to maintain clinical suspicion for underlying middle ear or mastoid pathology in cases of labyrinthitis of unknown origin, which often is attributed to an underlying viral etiology by exclusion.

Neurotologic examination in patients with labyrinthitis reveals nystagmus directed toward the uninvolved ear[42,43] after a brief, initial period of nystagmus toward the involved ear.[10] A fistula test may be positive in patients with labyrinthitis resulting from temporal bone trauma or cholesteatomous erosion of the inner ear. Ataxia is often present, and cerebellar examination may reveal past-pointing.[42]

Audiologic evaluation reveals primarily SNHL ranging in severity from a mild loss in cases of serous labyrinthitis to a profound loss in cases with suppurative changes of the inner ear. The higher frequencies are most commonly affected[42] in both tympanogenic[10,44] and meningogenic labyrinthitis. Diplacusis[44] has been reported as a frequent finding. A conductive component to the hearing loss may be present in cases of tympanogenic labyrinthitis.

Caloric testing provides valuable information in cases of labyrinthitis and is an important part of the evaluation. Suppurative labyrinthitis produces a complete loss of labyrinthine function, as manifest by an absent caloric response.[42] In contrast, a preserved, albeit diminished, response is found in cases of serous labyrinthitis. This important difference can help the physician differentiate between the two conditions, enabling appropriate management decisions to be made accurately.

Radiologic Findings

Magnetic resonance imaging (MRI) is the modality of choice in evaluating patients with labyrinthitis. Enhancement of the membranous labyrinth after administration of intravenous contrast is found during the acute phase of both suppurative and serous labyrinthitis on T1 imaging sequences. A hyperintense labyrinthine signal on precontrast T1 imaging is occasionally present and suggests intralabyrinthine hemorrhage secondary to infection of the inner ear structures.[45]

Computed tomography (CT) can provide valuable information in cases of tympanogenic labyrinthitis. When a cholesteatoma is present, CT can help to delineate the extent of disease and erosion of otic capsular bone. In cases of labyrinthitis secondary to temporal bone trauma, acute otitis media, or chronic suppurative otitis media, CT scanning can help to define the site of communication between the middle and inner ear, although in many cases no discrete abnormality is identified.

In the evaluation of SNHL for cochlear implant candidacy, particularly in patients with a history of meningitis, CT and MRI offer complementary information.[46,47,48] The fibrous stage of labyrinthitis ossificans is best evaluated by MRI,[47,49] which will demonstrate a decreased or absent T2 signal intensity in involved portions of the membranous labyrinth.[50] CT is the imaging modality of choice for assessing the extent of bony obliteration of the cochlea affected during the ossifying stage of labyrinthitis ossificans[46,51,52] and for identifying congenital cochlear anomalies in patients being evaluated for cochlear implantation. The radiologic findings in tympanogenic and meningogenic labyrinthitis mirror distribution of the histopathologic changes seen in the two conditions, namely more limited involvement of the cochlea, particularly the basal turn, in the former, with more diffuse labyrinthine involvement in the latter.[50] Information gathered from both CT and MRI can help to determine eligibility for traditional cochlear implantation and aid in planning for a cochlear drill-out procedure in patients with complete bony obliteration of the cochlea.

Differential Diagnosis

In the absence of a history of trauma, vertigo lasting days to weeks associated with peripheral vestibular dysfunction on caloric testing can be due to labyrinthitis, vestibular neuritis, or vestibular schwannoma. The presence of hearing loss or other cochlear symptoms differentiates labyrinthitis from vestibular neuritis. Although vestibular schwannoma can produce a wide spectrum of symptoms, rarely does a retrocochlear lesion present with vertigo and hearing loss of the acuity of that seen in labyrinthitis. MRI clearly and definitively differentiates between labyrinthitis and vestibular neuroma and is indicated in all cases of labyrinthitis without clear evidence of underlying otitis or meningitis.

During the acute phase of symptomatology, it can be difficult to differentiate serous from suppurative labyrinthitis. In examining cases of meningogenic labyrinthitis, Merchant and Gopen found that serous versus suppurative changes cannot be differentiated from each other on the basis of patient age, gender, duration of symptoms, or infecting organism.[2] In general, suppurative labyrinthitis has a rapid onset of symptoms with a more severe clinical course. Notably, a complete loss of cochleovestibular function occurs in suppurative labyrinthitis, manifest by an absent caloric response and a profound SNHL. In contrast, serous labyrinthitis has a somewhat less acute clinical presentation and patients retain a caloric response and some degree of hearing (more often in the lower frequencies).[10,42] Because it can often be difficult prospectively to differentiate between the two conditions and the fact that serous changes can precede the development of frank suppurative involvement of the inner ear, it is important to treat all cases of labyrinthitis as suppurative unless proven otherwise by audiologic and vestibular testing.

■ Treatment

Serous Labyrinthitis

Serous labyrinthitis occurring as a complication of acute otitis media should be treated with antibiotics and myringotomy, possibly tympanostomy.[42] When serous labyrinthitis complicates chronic otitis media, culture-directed parenteral antibiotics should be initiated and tympanomastoidectomy performed to remove underlying cholesteatoma or perilabyrinthine osteitis. Given the inflammatory nature of serous labyrinthitis, treatment with systemic steroids, in combination with antibiotics and surgery, could be entertained but has not been described or validated in the literature.

Suppurative Labyrinthitis

Due to the frequency with which a complete loss of cochleovestibular function occurs in suppurative labyrinthitis, the primary goal of treatment is to prevent the development of meningitis rather than preserve residual inner ear function. Parenteral antibiotics with CSF penetration, and directed toward middle ear pathogens, are the mainstay of treatment in suppurative labyrinthitis. The role and timing of surgery in the treatment of suppurative labyrinthitis are controversial. In 1972, Torok[10] advocated prompt labyrinthectomy for suppurative labyrinthitis in an effort to prevent intracranial extension. Others[42] have reserved labyrinthectomy for cases of suppurative labyrinthitis complicated by lumbar puncture-proven meningitis. Because tympanogenic suppurative labyrinthitis is a rare condition, it is unlikely that further experience will elucidate an evidence-based approach to its treatment. Because of this, each case must be treated with consideration of all pertinent patient factors, with a low threshold for surgical intervention with any signs of intracranial extension unresponsive to appropriate parenteral antibiotics.

Meningogenic Labyrinthitis

Prompt initiation of parenteral antibiotics to treat the underlying meningitis in cases of meningogenic labyrinthitis is of critical importance in preventing mortality and reducing morbidity, including SNHL. Systemic steroids to prevent the development of SNHL after meningitis have proven beneficial in some clinical studies,[53,54,55,56,57,58,59] while other studies[60] have failed to show a clear benefit. Animal models of meningitis have shown that the use of steroids[61] and other anti-inflammatory medications[27] can reduce the incidence of SNHL. Further studies in humans will be needed to better define the role of steroids and anti-inflammatory medications in preventing SNHL in patients with meningitis.

Inpatient audiologic testing of children with bacterial meningitis has shown that SNHL occurs within the first 48 hours of the course of the disease. Whether the SNHL seen in bacterial meningitis is due to serous or suppurative labyrinthitis (or possibly toxic inflammatory effects on the cochlear nerve or blood supply, as has been suggested by some investigators[62]), early identification of hearing impairment is of the utmost importance, especially in children. The ideal method and timing of screening for SNHL after bacterial meningitis are the subject of considerable debate in the literature. Both auditory brainstem response (ABR) testing[56,62] and otoacoustic emission (OAE) testing[63,64,65] have been advocated as sensitive methods for early detection of SNHL in children recovering from bacterial meningitis. Unfortunately, both methods have inherent limitations[66,67] that complicate their routine use as a screening tool in children after meningitis. Further studies are needed to better define the role of ABR, OAE, and routine audiometry as routine screening methods for SNHL in patients with meningitis.

Equally important to the screening methodology used to identify SNHL after bacterial meningitis is the need to initiate early and diligent audiologic follow-up for all patients with bacterial meningitis. Multiple studies have found unacceptably low rates of referral for, and compliance with, audiologic follow-up among pediatric patients with bacterial meningitis.[68,69,70] Furthermore, the neo-osteogenesis that characterizes LO, which occurs as early as 3 weeks after bacterial meningitis, can result in an inability to achieve a full cochlear implant electrode insertion. This can, in turn, result in compromised cochlear implant performance or, in the case of complete cochlear ossification, the need to perform a cochlear drill-out procedure, which is associated with less favorable hearing outcomes.[41,71,72] As a result of this, there is essentially a "window of opportunity" for cochlear implantation after bacterial meningitis that, when missed, results in compromised success rates of the procedure. Because of this, every effort should be made by the treating otolaryngologist to identify SNHL promptly and monitor for the development of labyrinthitis ossificans. Consideration should be given to early cochlear implantation, possibly bilaterally, when imaging identifies impending bony obliteration of the cochlear duct or when auditory deprivation exists for a significant enough period of time that speech and language development may be compromised in any child who has had meningitis.

■ Viral Labyrinthitis

A variety of viruses can infect the human inner ear, most commonly in children, and cause hearing loss and vertigo, including paramyxoviruses (measles and mumps), cytomegalovirus, and herpes zoster virus, among others. Limited viral inner ear infections with cochlear, vestibular, or facial nerve manifestations alone have been described[3] and implicated in many inner ear disorders, such as idiopathic sudden SNHL,[3,73,74,75,76] vestibular neuritis,[77] Meniere's disease,[73,78,79,80] otosclerosis,[81,82,83] and idiopathic facial paralysis.[84,85,86] In cases of viral labyrinthitis, in general there is no associated middle ear or CNS involvement, which makes confirmation of the underlying etiologic agent difficult if not impossible. In some cases, inner ear manifestations occur simultaneously or after an infectious syndrome specific to a particular strain of virus, allowing correlative evidence for labyrinthine infection due to the same agent. Many reports of labyrinthitis without coexistent middle ear or CNS disease have used elevated antibody titers as evidence for infection due to a particular viral agent,[76,87] although this method of investigation cannot definitively establish causality. Temporal bone studies of patients with a suspected viral etiology as a cause for permanent hearing loss and/or vestibular dysfunction have found several characteristic pathologic changes. The clinical manifestations and temporal bone changes seen in some of the better-defined causes of viral labyrinthitis are briefly reviewed below.

Measles

Measles is caused by a paramyxovirus and occurs in children not immunized with the live attenuated vaccine. Clinical manifestations include fever, cough, conjunctivitis, maculopapular rash, and characteristic eruptions on the labial and buccal mucosa. Hearing loss is usually bilateral and moderate to profound in severity. More severe manifestations include encephalitis and subacute sclerosing panencephalitis. Measles infection has been found to cause severe degeneration of the vestibular sense organs and organ of Corti. Characteristically, the organ of Corti is shrunken and devoid of hair cells, with notable atrophy of the stria vascularis. Loss of cochlear neurons with severe degeneration of the spiral ganglion is also found in some cases.[3]

Mumps

Mumps infection is uncommon and occurs in non-immunized adults and children more than 2 years old. The clinical manifestations of mumps infection include sialadenitis, orchitis, meningoencephalitis, myocarditis, nephritis, and prostatitis. Mumps typically causes a unilateral hearing loss, which may go undetected in young children until school age. Temporal bone studies of patients with a history of mumps labyrinthitis have found collapse of Reissner's membrane, with detachment and encapsulation of the tectorial membrane. Atrophy of the organ of Corti and stria vascularis, with loss of cochlear neurons and notable preservation of the saccule, utricle, and semicircular canals, were characteristic findings in mumps infection.[88]

Cytomegalovirus (CMV)

Congenital CMV has a wide variation in severity of clinical manifestations, including abortion and stillbirth. Congenital infection is estimated to result in SNHL in 17% of cases,[89] and the SNHL can be mild to profound in severity. Infection in adults occurs in immunocompromised patients and may represent reactivation of a latent virus rather than newly acquired disease. Cytomegalic intranuclear inclusions are found in the epithelial cells lining the cochlear duct, without obvious damage to the organ of Corti.[90]

As mentioned previously, viral labyrinthitis can be difficult to diagnose and is assigned to patients only after exclusion of tympanogenic or meningogenic causes. Serologic evaluation for antibodies to viral pathogens is generally not performed unless a known, viral-associated syndrome is evident. As with bacterial labyrinthitis, a thorough otologic examination, audiometry, and vestibular testing (if the patient is old enough to tolerate it) should be performed routinely. Treatment is limited to supportive measures. Close otologic and audiologic follow-up are of critical importance to ensure that hearing amplification (and possibly cochlear implantation) is performed without significant delay after a hearing loss has occurred.

References

1. Paparella MM, Oda M, Hiraide F, Brady D. Pathology of sensorineural hearing loss in otitis media. Ann Otol Rhinol Laryngol 1972;81(5):632–647

2. Merchant SN, Gopen Q. A human temporal bone study of acute bacterial meningogenic labyrinthitis. Am J Otol 1996;17(3):375–385

3. Schuknecht H. Pathology of the Ear. 2nd ed. Philadelphia, PA: Lea & Febiger; 1993

4. Wittmaack K. Hydrops labyrinthi (labyrinthitis serosa). In: Henke OLF, ed. Handbuch der Speziellen Pathologischen Anatomie und Histologie. Berlin: Verlag von Julius Springer; 1926

5. Paparella MM, Sugiura S. The pathology of suppurative labyrinthitis. Ann Otol Rhinol Laryngol 1967;76(3):554–586

6. Osma U, Cureoglu S, Hosoglu S. The complications of chronic otitis media: report of 93 cases. J Laryngol Otol 2000;114(2):97–100

7. Goldstein NA, Casselbrant ML, Bluestone CD, Kurs-Lasky M. Intratemporal complications of acute otitis media in infants and children. Otolaryngol Head Neck Surg 1998;119(5):444–454

8. Kangsanarak J, Fooanant S, Ruckphaopunt K, Navacharoen N, Teotrakul S. Extracranial and intracranial complications of suppurative otitis media. Report of 102 cases. J Laryngol Otol 1993;107(11):999–1004

9. Tekin M, Schachern PA, Mutlu C, Jaisinghani VJ, Paparella MM, Le CT. Purulent otitis media in children and adults. Eur Arch Otorhinolaryngol 2002;259(2):67–72

10. Torok N. Tympanogenic labyrinthitis. Otolaryngol Clin North Am 1972;5(1):45–57

11. Sahni RS, Paparella MM, Schachern PA, Goycoolea MV, Le CT. Thickness of the human round window membrane in different forms of otitis media. Arch Otolaryngol Head Neck Surg 1987;113(6):630–634

12. Dean LW. Pathology and routes of infection in labyrinthitis secondary to middle ear otitis. Ann Otol Rhinol Laryngol 1934;43:702–717

13. Altman F, Waltner J. Labyrinthitis due to Pneumococcus: type III histopathologic studies. Arch Otolaryngol 1944;40:75–91

14. Mackenzie G. Suppurative labyrinthitis with report of cases. Ann Otol Rhinol Laryngol 1927;36:1019–1059

15. Druss J. Pathways of infection in labyrinthitis: Report of three different types. Arch Otolaryngol 1929; 9:392–403

16. Sprowl F. Tympanogenous purulent labyrinthitis: report of cases. Ann Otol Rhinol Laryngol 1931; 40:253–258

17. Turner AL. The pathology of labyrinthitis (part II). Journal of Laryngology 1928;43:609–644

18. Schachern PA, Paparella MM, Hybertson R, Sano S, Duvall AJ III. Bacterial tympanogenic labyrinthitis, meningitis, and sensorineural damage. Arch Otolaryngol Head Neck Surg 1992;118(1):53–57

19. Baldwin RL, Sweitzer RS, Freind DB. Meningitis and sensorineural hearing loss. Laryngoscope 1985; 95(7 Pt 1):802–805

20. Berlow SJ, Caldarelli DD, Matz GJ, Meyer DH, Harsch GG. Bacterial meningitis and sensorineural hearing loss: a prospective investigation. Laryngoscope 1980;90(9):1445–1452

21. Dodge PR, Davis H, Feigin RD, et al. Prospective evaluation of hearing impairment as a sequela of acute bacterial meningitis. N Engl J Med 1984;311(14):869–874

22. Keane WM, Potsic WP, Rowe LD, Konkle DF. Meningitis and hearing loss in children. Arch Otolaryngol 1979;105(1):39–44

23. Nadol JB Jr. Hearing loss as a sequela of meningitis. Laryngoscope 1978;88(5):739–755

24. Rosenhall U, Nylén O, Lindberg J, Kankkunen A. Auditory function after Haemophilus influenczae meningitis. Acta Otolaryngol 1978;85(3–4):243–247

25. Finitzo Hiebcr T, Simliadri R, Hleber JP. Abnormalities of the auditory brainstem response in post-meningitic infants and children. Int J Pediatr Otorhinolaryngol 1981;3(4):275–286

26. Eisenberg LS, Luxford WM, Becker TS, House WF. Electrical stimulation of the auditory system in children deafened by meningitis. Otolaryngol Head Neck Surg 1984;92(6):700–705

27. Aminpour S, Tinling SP, Brodie HA. Role of tumor necrosis factor-alpha in sensorineural hearing loss after bacterial meningitis. Otol Neurotol 2005;26(4):602–609

28. Wenger JD, Hightower AW, Facklam RR, Gaventa S, Broome CV; The Bacterial Meningitis Study Group. Bacterial meningitis in the United States, 1986: report of a multistate surveillance study. J Infect Dis 1990;162(6):1316–1323

29. Schlech WF III, Ward JI, Band JD, Hightower A, Fraser DW, Broome CV. Bacterial meningitis in the United States, 1978 through 1981. The National Bacterial Meningitis Surveillance Study. JAMA 1985;253(12):1749–1754

30. Ozdamar O, Kraus N, Stein L. Auditory brainstem responses in infants recovering from bacterial meningitis. Audiologic evaluation. Arch Otolaryngol 1983; 109(1):13–18

31. Novak MA, Fifer RC, Barkmeier JC, Firszt JB. Labyrinthine ossification after meningitis: its implications for cochlear implantation. Otolaryngol Head Neck Surg 1990;103(3):351–356

32. Wellman MB, Sommer DD, McKenna J. Sensorineural hearing loss in postmeningitic children. Otol Neurotol 2003;24(6):907–912

33. Druss J. Labyrinthitis secondary to meningococcic meningitis: a clinical and histopathologic study. Arch Otolaryngol 1936;24:19–28

34. Igarashi M, Schuknecht HF. Pneumococci otitis media, meningitis and labyrinthitis: a human temporal bone report. Arch Otolaryngol 1970;76:126–130

35. Schunknecht HF, Montandon P. Pathology of the ear in pneumococcal meningitis. Arch Klin Exp Ohren Nasen Kehlkopfheilkd 1970;195(3):207–225

36. Crowe S. Pathologic changes in meningitis of the inner ear. Arch Otolaryngol 1930;11:537–568

37. Bhatt S, Halpin C, Hsu W, et al. Hearing loss and pneumococcal meningitis: an animal model. Laryngoscope 1991;101(12 Pt 1):1285–1292

38. Lindsay JR. Deafness acquired in early postnatal childhood. In profound childhood deafess: inner ear pathology. Ann Otol Rhinol Laryngol 1973;82(5):88–102

39. Kaplan SL, Hawkins EP, Kline MW, Patrick GS, Mason EO Jr. Invasion of the inner ear by Haemophilus influenzae type b in experimental meningitis. J Infect Dis 1989;159(5):923–930

40. Rodriguez AF, Kaplan SL, Hawkins EP, Mason EO Jr. Hematogenous pneumococcal meningitis in the infant rat: description of a model. J Infect Dis 1991; 164(6):1207–1209

41. Nabili V, Brodie HA, Neverov NI, Tinling SP. Chronology of labyrinthitis ossificans induced by Streptococcus pneumoniae meningitis. Laryngoscope 1999;109(6):931–935

42. Glasscock ME, Julianna G, George WC. Surgery of the Ear. 5th ed. Hamilton BC Decker; 2003:xvi, 808.

43. Maire R, Van Melle G. Horizontal vestibulo-ocular reflex dynamics in acute vestibular neuritis and viral labyrinthitis: evidence of otolith-canal interaction. Acta Otolaryngol 2004;124(1):36–40

44. Shambaugh G. Diplacusis: a localizing symptom of disease of the organ of Corti. Arch Otolaryngol 1940; 31:160–184

45. Palacios E, Valvassori G. Hemorrhagic labyrinthitis. Ear Nose Throat J 2000;79(2):80

46. Abdullah A, Mahmud MR, Maimunah A, Zulfiqar MA, Saim L, Mazlan R. Preoperative high resolution CT and MR imaging in cochlear implantation. Ann Acad Med Singapore 2003;32(4):442–445

47. Arriaga MA, Carrier D. MRI and clinical decisions in cochlear implantation. Am J Otol 1996;17(4):547–553

48. Nikolopoulos TP, O'Donoghue GM, Robinson KL, Holland IM, Ludman C, Gibbin KP. Preoperative radiologic evaluation in cochlear implantation. Am J Otol 1997; 18(6, Suppl):S73–S74

49. Phelps PD, Annis JA, Robinson PJ. Imaging for cochlear implants. Br J Radiol 1990;63(751):512–516

50. Himi T, Akiba H, Yamaguchi T. Topographic analysis of inner ear lesions in profoundly deafened patients with tympanogenic and meningogenic labyrinthitis using three-dimensional magnetic resonance imaging. Am J Otol 1999;20(5):581–586

51. Phelps PD. The basal turn of the cochlea. Br J Radiol 1992;65(773):370–374

52. d'Archambeau O, Parizel PM, Koekelkoren E, Van de Heyning P, De Schepper AM. CT diagnosis and differential diagnosis of otodystrophic lesions of the temporal bone. Eur J Radiol 1990;11(1):22–30

53. Lebel MH, Freij BJ, Syrogiannopoulos GA, et al. Dexamethasone therapy for bacterial meningitis. Results of two double-blind, placebo-controlled trials. N Engl J Med 1988;319(15):964–971

54. McCracken GH Jr, Lebel MH. Dexamethasone therapy for bacterial meningitis in infants and children. Am J Dis Child 1989;143(3):287–289

55. Kennedy WA, Hoyt MJ, McCracken GH Jr. The role of corticosteroid therapy in children with pneumococcal meningitis. Am J Dis Child 1991;145(12):1374–1378

56. Külahli I, Oztürk M, Bilen C, Cüreoglu S, Merhametsiz A, Cağil N. Evaluation of hearing loss with auditory brainstem responses in the early and late period of bacterial meningitis in children. J Laryngol Otol 1997;111(3):223–227

57. McIntyre PB, Berkey CS, King SM, et al. Dexamethasone as adjunctive therapy in bacterial meningitis. A meta-analysis of randomized clinical trials since 1988. JAMA 1997;278(11):925–931

58. Syrogiannopoulos GA, Lourida AN, Theodoridou MC, et al. Dexamethasone therapy for bacterial meningitis in children: 2- versus 4-day regimen. J Infect Dis 1994;169(4):853–858

59. Odio CM, Faingezicht I, Paris M, et al. The beneficial effects of early dexamethasone administration in infants and children with bacterial meningitis. N Engl J Med 1991;324(22):1525–1531

60. Wald ER, Kaplan SL, Mason EO Jr, et al; Meningitis Study Group. Dexamethasone therapy for children with bacterial meningitis. Pediatrics 1995;95(1):21–28

61. Rappaport JM, Bhatt SM, Burkard RF, Merchant SN, Nadol JB Jr. Prevention of hearing loss in experimental pneumococcal meningitis by administration of dexamethasone and ketorolac. J Infect Dis 1999;179(1):264–268

62. Vienny H, Despland PA, Lütschg J, Deonna T, Dutoit-Marco ML, Gander C. Early diagnosis and evolution of deafness in childhood bacterial meningitis: a study using brainstem auditory evoked potentials. Pediatrics 1984;73(5):579–586

63. Richardson MP, Williamson TJ, Reid A, Tarlow MJ, Rudd PT. Otoacoustic emissions as a screening test for hearing impairment in children recovering from acute bacterial meningitis. Pediatrics 1998;102(6):1364–1368

64. Richardson MP, Reid A, Tarlow MJ, Rudd PT. Hearing loss during bacterial meningitis. Arch Dis Child 1997;76(2):134–138

65. Riordan A, Thomson A, Hodgson J. Hearing assessment after meningitis and meningococcal disease. Arch Dis Child 1995;72(5):441–442

66. Gibson WP, Brown C, Everingham C, Herridge S, Rennie M, Steinberg T. Necessity of early diagnosis and assessment of postmeningitis children in view of cochlear implantation. Ann Otol Rhinol Laryngol Suppl 1995;166:208–210

67. Fortnum H, Farnsworth A, Davis A. The feasibility of evoked otoacoustic emissions as an in-patient hearing check after meningitis. Br J Audiol 1993;27(4):227–231

68. Fortnum HM, Hull D. Is hearing assessed after bacterial meningitis? Arch Dis Child 1992;67(9):1111–1112

69. Riordan A, Thomson A, Hodgson J, Hart A. Children who are seen but not referred: hearing assessment after bacterial meningitis. Br J Audiol 1993;27(6):375–377

70. Drake R, Dravitski J, Voss L. Hearing in children after meningococcal meningitis. J Paediatr Child Health 2000;36(3):240–243

71. Balkany T, Bird PA, Hodges AV, Luntz M, Telischi FF, Buchman C. Surgical technique for implantation of the totally ossified cochlea. Laryngoscope 1998;108(7):988–992

72. Rauch SD, Herrmann BS, Davis LA, Nadol JB Jr. Nucleus 22 cochlear implantation results in postmeningitic deafness. Laryngoscope 1997;107(12 Pt 1):1606–1609

73. Schattner A, Halperin D, Wolf D, Zimhony O. Enteroviruses and sudden deafness. CMAJ 2003;168(11):1421–1423

74. Sando I, Loehr A, Harada T, Sobel JH. Sudden deafness: histopathologic correlation in temporal bone. Ann Otol Rhinol Laryngol 1977;86(3 Pt 1):269–279

75. Yoon TH, Paparella MM, Schachern PA, Alleva M. Histopathology of sudden hearing loss. Laryngoscope 1990;100(7):707–715

76. Veltri RW, Wilson WR, Sprinkle PM, Rodman SM, Kavesh DA. The implication of viruses in idiopathic sudden hearing loss: primary infection or reactivation of latent viruses? Otolaryngol Head Neck Surg 1981;89(1):137–141

77. Davis LE. Viruses and vestibular neuritis: review of human and animal studies. Acta Otolaryngol Suppl 1993;503:70–73

78. Bergström T, Edström S, Tjellström A, Vahlne A. Ménière's disease and antibody reactivity to herpes simplex virus type 1 polypeptides. Am J Otolaryngol 1992;13(5):295–300

79. Adour KK, Byl FM, Hilsinger RL Jr, Wilcox RD. Ménière's disease as a form of cranial polyganglionitis. Laryngoscope 1980;90(3):392–398

80. Williams LL, Lowery HW, Shannon BT. Evidence of persistent viral infection in Ménière's disease. Arch Otolaryngol Head Neck Surg 1987;113(4):397–400

81. Karosi T, Kónya J, Szabó LZ, et al. Codetection of measles virus and tumor necrosis factor-alpha mRNA in otosclerotic stapes footplates. Laryngoscope 2005;115(7):1291–1297

82. McKenna MJ, Mills BG. Immunohistochemical evidence of measles virus antigens in active otosclerosis. Otolaryngol Head Neck Surg 1989;101(4):415–421

83. Arnold W, Friedmann I. Otosclerosis—an inflammatory disease of the otic capsule of viral aetiology? J Laryngol Otol 1988;102(10):865–871

84. Adour KK, Bell DN, Hilsinger RL Jr. Herpes simplex virus in idiopathic facial paralysis (Bell palsy). JAMA 1975;233(6):527–530

85. Adour KK, Byl FM, Hilsinger RL Jr, Kahn ZM, Sheldon MI. The true nature of Bell's palsy: analysis of 1,000 consecutive patients. Laryngoscope 1978;88(5):787–801

86. Morgan M, Moffat M, Ritchie L, Collacott I, Brown T. Is Bell's palsy a reactivation of varicella zoster virus? J Infect 1995;30(1):29–36

87. Van Dishoeck HA, Bierman TA. Sudden perceptive deafness and viral infection; report of the first one hundred patients. Ann Otol Rhinol Laryngol 1957;66(4):963–980

88. Lindsay JR, Davey PR, Ward PH. Inner ear pathology in deafness due to mumps. Ann Otol Rhinol Laryngol 1960;69:918–935

89. Stagno S, Pass RF, Dworsky ME, Alford CA. Congenital and perinatal cytomegalovirus infections. Semin Perinatol 1983;7(1):31–42

90. Strauss M. A clinical pathologic study of hearing loss in congenital cytomegalovirus infection. Laryngoscope 1985;95(8):951–962

11 Superior Semicircular Canal Dehiscence Syndrome

Cameron C. Wick, Cliff A. Megerian, Nauman F. Manzoor, and Maroun T. Semaan

■ Introduction

Inner ear fistulas or areas of bony labyrinthine dehiscence can be associated with vertigo, especially when the affected ear is subjected to external pressure. This so-called "fistula sign" has classically been linked to oval and round window fistulas, cholesteatoma erosion of the horizontal semicircular canal, and syphilitic labyrinthitis. However, as noted by Baloh, any defect in the bony labyrinth can be the source of similar symptomatology: "Because of the rigid bony capsule, the vestibular part of the labyrinth is unaffected by sound or pressure changes in the middle ear and cerebrospinal fluid (CSF). However, a break in the bony capsule renders the vestibular labyrinth sensitive to sound and pressure changes."[1]

In 1998, Minor and colleagues' landmark description of a unique subset of patients in whom sound- and pressure-induced vertigo were found to be due to a dehiscence of the superior semicircular canal (sSCC) led to a new disease entity termed *superior semicircular canal dehiscence syndrome* (SSCD).[2] Interestingly, some of the patients had undergone negative explorations for perilymphatic fistula in the past, but the presence of vertical nystagmus after sound (Tullio phenomenon) or pressure (Hennebert sign) led the group to suspect a defect at the level of the sSCC. This suspected defect was confirmed when computed tomography (CT) revealed a dehiscence of the bone overlying the sSCC in each case. Two of the patients with disabling vertigo experienced improvement in their symptoms after a middle cranial fossa surgical procedure, at which time the affected canals were plugged.

The proposed mechanism by which a defect in the vestibular bony labyrinth renders the vestibular neuroepithelium sensitive to sound or pressure is based on the concept of a "third window" to the inner ear (in addition to the round and oval windows). In the normal setting, sound pressure transduction by the stapes results in only cochlear hair cell deflection due to the round window, which dissipates cochlear vibration by impedence matching. Because the semicircular canals do not have a membrane or release valve to dissipate vibration, their pressure remains constant and the neuroepithelium remains undisturbed. However, if there is a defect in the superior canal bone, the energy typically confined to the cochlea escapes along a path of least resistance toward the defect or "third window." Displaced endolymphatic fluid within the sSCC activates the canal's vestibular apparatus, leading to vertigo after sound or pressure changes.[2,3,4]

In the short time since Minor's landmark paper, SSCD has become a validated disease entity. Superior semicircular canal dehiscence syndrome's clinical presentation overlaps with many other otologic diseases, which has led it to be called the great otologic mimicker. In the modern otology practice, a thorough understanding of SSCD pathophysiology, variable presentations, diagnostic subtleties, and treatment options are critical to prevent patients from unnecessary tests, surgeries, or frustration with diagnostic ambiguity. This chapter discusses the evolution of SSCD, diagnostic pearls, new classification schemes, treatment options, and outcomes data.

■ Historical Background

In 1929, an Italian biologist, Pietro Tullio, introduced the concept of a "third window" as the mechanism behind sound-induced vertigo, imbalance, and eye movements.[5] Tullio created a fistula in the horizontal semicircular canals of pigeons and then exposed the birds to a loud sound, which led to quick deviation of their head away from the damaged ear. Tullio's experiments with pigeons set the stage for the realization that openings in the bony labyrinth can render the semicircular canal sensitive to loud sounds; hence the term *Tullio phenomenon* was coined.

Modern animal studies have further validated Tullio's observations. Using a chinchilla model, Hirvonen et al measured neuronal firing rates in response to pressure from semicircular canal afferents before and after fenestration.[6] Prior to fenestration of the sSCC, only one of nine superior canal afferents responded to pressure, whereas after fenestration, all such afferents were excited by pressure. Also, after fenestration, half of the otolithic and most of the horizontal canal afferents were still unaffected by pressure. These findings were reversed to normal when a rigid seal was applied to the fenestrated superior canal. In a second set of experiments, Carey et al performed an identical study using acoustic stimuli and similarly demonstrated that SSCD lowers the threshold for sound-evoked afferent stimulation of the superior canal.[7] Taken together, these findings support the concept that SSCD creates selectively abnormal endolymphatic flow in the region of the sSCC when there is a dehiscence in that particular canal and provides further insight regarding the mechanisms behind key physical exam findings like the Tullio phenomenon and Hennebert sign.

The Tullio phenomenon was first clinically relevant in patients with congenital syphilis, in which later temporal bone studies revealed gummatous osteomyelitis and fistulas of the labyrinth. Hennebert, who in 1911 described the finding of pressure-induced vestibular changes, had previously linked the syphilis patient population to inner ear dysfunction.[8,9] The elicitation of pressure-induced nystagmus was later termed *Hennebert sign* and was linked to other otologic conditions, such as advanced Meniere's disease and perilymphatic fistula.[10,11] Despite overlap with other disease processes, the presence of concomitant Tullio phenomenon and Hennebert sign provided early insight into the possibility of a bony defect in the labyrinthine defect.[12]

■ Etiology and Pathophysiology

The exact cause of SSCD remains unknown, but generally the theories are grouped into either congenital or acquired mechanisms. The congenital theory of SSCD argues that thin bone overlying the sSCC causes a persistent dehiscence or predisposes a patient to dehiscence later in life. The sSCC is the first semicircular canal to develop in utero but at birth it may still be covered with only a monolayer of periosteal bone. In most cases, a well-formed trilaminar bone does not cover the sSCC until 2 to 3 years of age.[13] Even if bone eventually covers the sSCC, it is unclear if the overlying dura or superior petrosal sinus predisposes certain people to having a thin tegmen and eventual dehiscence later in life, when SSCD is most prevalent. In 2000, Carey et al reviewed temporal bones from 27 deceased infants and children all less than 4 years old whose bones had been donated to the Johns Hopkins Temporal Bone Collection. They found that, at birth, the average bone covering the sSCC measured 0.092 mm and the bone did not reach adult thickness until 32.4 months of age.[13]

On account of the rarity of pediatric temporal bone specimens, attempts have been made to characterize the incidence of congenital SSCD radiographically. Jackson et al in 2015 examined high-resolution temporal bone CT scans, including Pöschl reconstructed images, in 700 patients less than 18 years old. They found a dehiscent sSCC in 1.9% of bones and an additional 15.6% with a thin covering. The prevalence of a thin or dehiscent sSCC was highest among patients less than 12 months old, which supports Carey's observation that bone overlying the sSCC grows postnatally.[13,14] Additionally, in 2011 Nadgir et al reviewed high-resolution temporal bone CT scans from 304 patients with ages ranging from 7 months to 89 years. Their results showed a 93% increase in SSCD prevalence from pediatric to adult populations. They also noted a trend toward tegmen thinning with age. Their findings correlate with SSCD's being diagnosed more commonly in middle-aged or older age groups. Of the 46 patients they studied who were less than 20 years old, only one had SSCD. Their conclusion was that congenital SSCD does exist, but more often is an acquired condition.[15] Despite its being less common than the acquired form, the congenital variant of SSCD is important to recognize for pediatric patients hindered by auditory or vestibular symptoms.[16]

Carey et al's temporal bone survey also examined 1,000 adult temporal bones from 596 adults. In control specimens without dehiscence, they found an average bone thickness of 0.96 ± 0.61 mm between the sSCC and the middle fossa dura, and 1.79 ± 1.2 mm between the sSCC and the superior petrosal sinus. Five of the specimens (0.5%) demonstrated dehiscence, and an additional 14 specimens (1.4%) were markedly thinned (≤ 0.1 mm).[13] The first radiographic correlate to Carey's histologic analysis was performed in 2003 and used coronal reconstructions of temporal bone CT imaging in 442 temporal bones of patients 7 to 87 years old (mean age = 45 years). This radiographic survey identified 39 bones (9%) with a dehiscent sSCC.[17] The overestimation is largely due to the resolution limitations of conventional multislice CT temporal bone imaging, which typically has a slice thickness of 1.0 mm, leading to a resolution limit of 0.324 mm. Additionally, the coronal view is not in the plane of the sSCC, which may or may not impair diagnostic accuracy.[18,19] Since that 2003 study, attention to ultra-high-resolution CT scans with a slice thickness of 0.5 mm or less and orientation in the plane of the sSCC (Pöschl or Stenvers view) has led to improved diagnostic accuracy. Another radiographic survey in 2011 also overestimated the radiographic dehiscence, at 3% of the 164 temporal bones assessed, although only 0.6% had clinical manifestations consistent with SSCD.[20] The diagnosis of SSCD on imaging alone should be avoided, because even modern techniques can overestimate the size of the defect or falsely detect a dehiscence.[21]

Regardless of the true SSCD incidence in the adult population, the vast majority of cases are acquired defects. Some patients may be predisposed to developing SSCD if the bone overlying their sSCC is inherently thin. Other patients may have a dehiscence associated with a traumatic event, such as a car accident, postpartum strain, or barotrauma.[21,22,23] There is growing recognition that obesity can cause thinning of the lateral skull base, which may lead to temporal bone encephaloceles, cerebrospinal fluid leaks, SSCD, or all of the above.[24,25,26]

The presumed mechanism of SSCD symptoms is that a dehiscent segment of the superior canal produces a third window, so that sound- or pressure-evoked changes (either via external stimuli or internal CSF pressure) induce cupular deviation secondary to endolymphatic fluid displacement. Fluid displacement then results in either ampullofugal or ampullopetal displacement of the superior canal cupula and thus excitatory or inhibitory stimuli to the superior vestibular nerve, with resulting upbeating or downbeating torsional nystagmus and vertigo, respectively.[6,7,27]

A clinical example of this pathophysiology would be a patient with a left dehiscent sSCC hearing a loud noise in his left ear. The acoustic energy enters the inner ear via the stapes and oval window. Rather than being confined to the cochlea, a portion of the transmitted energy escapes into the vestibule and then to the ampullated end of the sSCC before being released at the third window. In this example, the energy would push the sSCC cupula away from the vestibule (ampullofugal displacement), thus exciting the left sSCC and causing the brain to think the patient's head is rotating down and to the left. As a result of this excitation, the eyes will rotate upward and to the right (from the patient's perspective, this is a clockwise, torsional, slow-phase nystagmus). The nystagmus-defining fast phase would then be down and to the left (counterclockwise from the patient's perspective). The nystagmus can be reversed if the initiating force comes from an intracranial source, like a Valsalva maneuver, which would result in ampullopetal sSCC cupular displacement and inhibition of the affected canal (**Fig. 11.1**).[27]

The mechanism of the previously mentioned pathway has been studied in both human subjects and animal models. Hirvonen et al's elegant chinchilla study from 2001 is described previously in the introduction. In 2004, Rowsowski et al also used both human subjects with known SSCD and the chinchilla model to investigate the effects of SSCD on inner ear fluid mechanics and how it affects hearing. Acoustic

symptomatology of SSCD includes reduced (hypersensitive) thresholds for bone-conducted stimuli, increased thresholds for air-conducted sounds at low frequencies (< 2 kHz), with a resultant air–bone gap of as much as 30 to 60 dB in the low-frequency range. Rowsowski et al's first experiment used laser-Doppler vibrometry (LDV) to measure the magnitude of tympanic membrane change in response to acoustic stimulation in patients with and without SSCD. They showed that, in the low-frequency range, the LDV magnitudes in four out of five SSCD ears was 0.9 standard deviation larger than mean normal magnitude. This finding suggests a decrease in load on the tympanic membrane, likely due to SSCD-induced

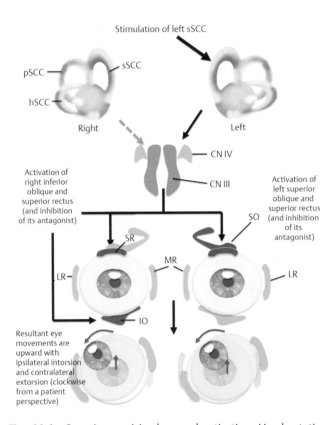

Fig. 11.1 Superior semicircular canal activation. Head rotation down and 45° to the left activates the left superior semicircular canal (sSCC). Excitatory interneurons from the left vestibular nuclei synapse on the oculomotor nucleus (CN III) and trochlear nucleus (CN IV), which excite the ipsilateral superior oblique (SO) and superior rectus (SR) as well as the contralateral inferior oblique (IO) and SR muscles. The slow phase component is upward/clockwise (from patient's perspective) eye deviation. The corrective nystagmus beats downward and counterclockwise (from patient's perspective). In the case of SSCD, acoustic energy and positive middle ear pressure excite the sSCC, whereas Valsalva maneuver and negative middle ear pressure inhibit the sSCC. hSCC, horizontal semicircular canal; LR, lateral rectus; MR, medial rectus; pSCC, posterior semicircular canal. Used with permission from Semaan MT, Wick CC, Megerian CA. Vestibular physiology. In: Pensak ML, Choo DI, eds. Clinical Otology. 4th ed. New York, NY: Thieme; 2015:41.

decrease in cochlear impedance and shunting of the acoustic energy away from the cochlea and toward the dehiscence. In another experiment, bone-conduction-evoked cochlear potentials were studied in the chinchilla model. After induction of SSCD, cochlear potential increased by a factor of 3 over the 200–4,000 Hz range, and this effect was reversed when the dehiscence was plugged. The data also demonstrated that altering the inner ear impedance made the cochlea become more sensitive to bone-conducted sound, particularly at low frequencies.[28]

■ Symptoms and Clinical Presentation

Patients with SSCD can present with vestibular symptoms, auditory symptoms, or both. The mean age at diagnosis is 43 years old.[29,30] The syndrome is rare in pediatrics, but reported examples do exist.[16,31] Up to a third of patients with SSCD will have bilateral defects.[13,29] Most patients will have had symptoms for many years and some even report prior middle ear explorations for perilymphatic fistula or conductive hearing loss. Patients may have had extensive work-ups for Meniere's disease, tests for spirochete-related inner ear conditions with negative Lyme, Venereal Disease Research Laboratory (VDRL) testing, and fluorescent treponemal antibody (FTA)-ABS testing. Most patients have no history of otologic disease, but 25% of Minor's original group of patients had an antecedent history of head trauma.[2]

Vestibular signs and symptoms associated with SSCD include sound- and pressure-induced vertigo and chronic disequilibrium. Sensitivity to sound or pressure can be grouped into four categories: eye movement evoked by external pressure on the ear canal (Hennebert sign), eye movement evoked by internal pressure (Valsalva maneuver, cough, sneeze), eye movement evoked by sound (Tullio phenomenon), or sound-induced head tilt in the plane of the affected canal. Minor's review of 60 patients with vestibular symptoms from SSCD noted a prevalence of 45%, 75%, 82%, and 20%, respectively, for each group. Overall, vestibular symptoms appear to be more commonly triggered by loud noise (90%) than by pressure (73%), but some patients will experience symptoms from both (67%).[30] Chronic disequilibrium is also a common, and often debilitating, complaint affecting up to 76% of patients in one series.[29] Disequilibrium and gait disturbances may worsen when the patient is exposed to loud sounds. Patients with bilateral SSCD may experience oscillopsia.[32] Still, a small subset of patients may experience no vestibular symptoms.[30] In general, the vestibular characteristics can be perplexing for the patient to describe. Some articulate patients, like the one described in Minor's

original report, have provided colorful descriptions of their SSCD experience, such as the environment's appearing to "move like on a clock face" whenever he whistled or hummed a specific tune.[2]

Auditory symptoms are also variable and include: hyperacusis, autophony, aural fullness, hearing loss, and pulsatile tinnitus. As previously described, SSCD causes increased sensitivity to bone-conducted sounds, and bone-conduction thresholds on audiometry can be less than 0 dB normal hearing level (NHL). This suprathreshold bone conduction creates an air–bone gap, particularly at low frequencies, and manifests as a conductive hearing loss.[28,33,34] The conductive hearing loss can mimic otosclerosis, a key difference being preservation of the stapedial reflex in SSCD but not in otosclerosis. It is less common for patients to experience auditory symptoms without vestibular complaints (7.7%).[30,34,35]

Autophony is the increased awareness of hearing one's voice or bodily movements. Patients with SSCD often hear their own voice and may also describe hearing their eyes move. This differs from the autophony associated with a patulous eustachian tube, which is typically amplified by respiration and correlates with direct visualization of tympanic membrane movement.[36]

Other auditory symptoms, such as conductive hyperacusis, defined as hearing or feeling the pulse in the affected ear, occur in 39% of SSCD patients. A smaller subset will experience gaze-evoked tinnitus, presumably due to abnormal neuronal sprouting between the cochlear and vestibular nuclei induced by SSCD.[37]

One report describes a patient who experienced bradycardia and hypotension evoked by sound and ear pressure, which were believed to be related to saccular stimulation. The otolithic receptors are known to have a role in the vestibulosympathetic reflex and play a role in cardiovascular regulation. The fact that the autonomic symptoms in this particular patient improved after plugging of the affected superior canal further supports the concept that, in rare circumstances, cardiac autonomic symptomatology in response to sound or pressure can herald the presence of SSCD.[29]

■ Diagnostic Evaluation

Physical Examination Signs

Patients with SSCD will often demonstrate a conductive hearing loss on physical examination, with the Weber test at 512 Hz lateralizing to the affected ear.[1,2] Brantberg et al, in a series of eight patients, demonstrated that all had Weber test lateralization to the affected side, but stapedial reflex testing was always normal, thus differentiating the audiometric scenario from otosclerosis.[38]

Neurotologic examination will often reveal vertical-torsional movement of the eyes during sound presentation. Offending sound frequencies can range from 250 to 3,000 Hz and are effective in causing nystagmus, usually between 100 and 110 dB. In some cases, only one tone (440 Hz, for example) will elicit symptoms, whereas in most other cases a range of frequencies are equally effective in producing symptoms.[2] Vertical-torsional eye movement induced by loud sounds was seen in 89% of the 28-patient Hopkins group, whereas 82% of the group had such eye findings during a Valsalva maneuver, and only 54% demonstrated these findings with pneumatic otoscopy.[37]

In some rare circumstances, jugular venous compression with pressure to the upper aspect of the neck near the jugular foramen will elicit symptoms and nystagmus, presumably via increased intracranial pressure. Most patients demonstrate the absence of nystagmus after horizontal or vertical head shaking, and head thrust testing typically reveals symmetrical vestibulo-ocular reflexes.[2]

Spontaneous nystagmus is usually not present in SSCD. However, in the rare circumstance that it occurs, it is quite debilitating. Spontaneous pulse-synchronous vertical nystagmus was described in a patient with bilateral SSCD who also presented with complaints of oscillopsia. The spontaneous nystagmus can also assume a vertical-rotatory appearance; both of these scenarios are likely due to large-enough defects in the sSCC to allow pulse-initiated intracranial pressure variations to activate the sSCC.[39]

Audiologic Testing

Most ears affected by SSCD will have an audiogram with at least a 10 to 20 dB low-frequency (250 to 1,000 Hz) conductive hearing loss, with normal speech discrimination score, stapedial reflex, and tympanogram (**Fig. 11.2**).[2,30] The fact that many SSCD patients have decreased (hypersensitive) thresholds to bone-conducted sound helps explain why normal body sounds (heartbeat, eye movement, voice) can become bothersome.[1] Patients with a characteristic low-frequency air–bone gap with an intact acoustic reflex and a lateralizing Weber without evidence of tympanic membrane or ossicular chain abnormality should undergo further testing for SSCD. Prior to the discovery of SSCD, patients with SSCD-related conductive hearing loss were often diagnosed with otosclerosis and incorrectly underwent stapedectomy or middle ear exploration.[34,40] The conductive hearing loss associated with SSCD has been described as an "inner ear conductive hearing loss."[33,34]

Recent studies have attempted to characterize the length and location of the dehiscence and how it relates to audiometric testing. Pisano et al used intracochlear sound pressure measurements to show that, for low-frequency sound (< 600 Hz), more energy was shunted from the cochlea as the defect size increased, thus producing the characteristic low-frequency air–bone gap. Interestingly, small (pinhole) defects created a more pronounced loss at frequencies greater than 1,000 Hz.[41] The literature does have conflict-

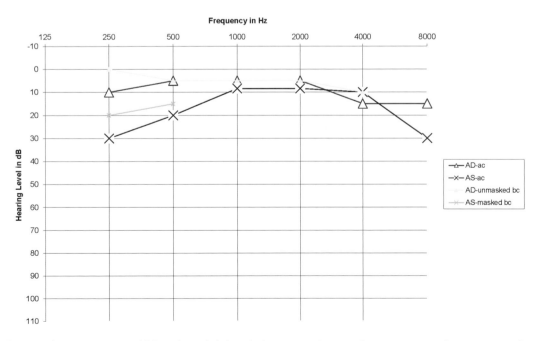

Fig. 11.2 Audiogram from a 39-year-old female with left-sided SSCD syndrome. The patient noted pressure- and sound-induced vertical eye movements. Note the conductive low-frequency hearing loss in the left ear. Although the right ear was not symptomatic, CT scanning revealed not only obvious left-sided SSCD syndrome but also subtle dehiscence of the right superior canal, which is likely reflected in the mild low-frequency loss in the right ear as well.

ing reports on how defect size and location relate to cochleovestibular symptoms.[34,35,42,43] The discrepancies in these studies may relate to small sample sizes and varied methods of measuring the dehiscence length. Additionally, the relationship between defect size and hearing sensitivity may be more complex than a monotonic relationship.[28,41,43,44]

Niesten et al used a novel method of measuring the defect length and location, which included ultra-high-resolution temporal bone CT scans with axial, Pöschl, and Stenvers reconstructions, to create a curved reconstruction of the sSCC.[44] As reported in other studies, they utilized Hounsfield units (HU) to aid in diagnostic accuracy.[21,44] Their analysis of 147 ears in 104 patients identified that patients with auditory symptoms have a larger dehiscence (median length: 4.5 vs 2.7 mm) and their dehiscence is closer to the sSCC ampulla. They did not find a correlation between defect length and location and specific individual SSCD symptoms.[44] Chien et al analyzed 85 patients with SSCD who underwent surgical correction via a middle cranial fossa approach. The defects were measured intraoperatively and a multivariate analysis of defect size and hearing outcome was performed. The. analysis showed a statistically significant association between dehiscence length and maximal air–bone gap, but there was not a significant correlation with pure-tone average, average bone-conduction threshold, or the total number of symptoms.[43]

Vestibular Testing

Vestibular testing can be an important adjunct for confirming the SSCD diagnosis. As previously discussed, physical exam findings like sound-induced or pressure-induced nystagmus may indicate the presence of a third window. The exact prevalence of the Tullio phenomenon and Hennebert sign remains unknown, and absence of these findings does not rule out SSCD. Head thrust test results appear to be affected by dehiscences measuring greater or equal to 5 mm, as the function of the affected canal is impaired enough to produce lower-gain responses for head thrusts that are normally excitatory for the affected canal.[29] Smaller dehiscences do not appear to disturb head thrust responses, likely due to the concept that large dehiscences allow more substantial compression of the membranous superior canal labyrinth and thereby the blockage of normal endolymphatic flow during head movement.[37]

Electronystagmography (ENG) and rotatory chair testing typically do not aid in the diagnosis of SSCD. Five of the eight original Minor et al patients had ENG and their results were all normal, with no localizing findings. Likewise, two of three patients tested with the rotatory chair had normal findings, whereas one did show vestibular hypofunction in the affected ear.[2]

The most widely used vestibular testing adjunct is the vestibular evoked myogenic potential (VEMP) test. VEMP efficacy has been demonstrated in multiple SSCD studies, as well as in patients with an enlarged vestibular aqueduct that also demonstrate a third window phenomenon.[2,3,30,45,46] Patients with SSCD have a low-threshold, high-amplitude response to sound-evoked (i.e., click) VEMP.[45] Halmagyi et al further characterized the SSCD response to click-evoked VEMP as having a short onset latency (~ 10 milliseconds), low threshold of activation (80 dB), and a largely torsional-vertical vestibular ocular reflex, with a velocity of up to 25°/s. In contrast, normal subjects show a threshold of activation between 100 and 110 dB and a velocity of only 2°/s.[12,47] VEMPs in response to skull-taps (i.e., bone conduction) tend to show a less robust response in SSCD patients.[3,12]

The clinical validation of VEMP findings in SSCD patients has been replicated in multiple studies. In one study of eight patients with SSCD, VEMP recordings revealed lowered thresholds at 72 ± 8 dB NHL, compared with 96 ± 5 dB in control subjects.[45] Minor reviewed VEMP data from 51 ears with confirmed SSCD and compared the results against 30 unaffected ears in patients with SSCD as well as 60 control ears. He found that the threshold of 81 ± 9 dB in the SSCD ears was significantly lower than the thresholds in the unaffected ears (99 ± 7 dB) and control ears (98 ± 4 dB) (**Fig. 11.3**).[30]

Attempts to correlate dehiscent size and location with the VEMP findings have yielded mixed results. Niesten et al found that larger dehiscences and a location closer to the ampulla corresponded with lowered VEMP thresholds, while Chien et al did not find a correlation between defect length and VEMP threshold.[43,44] VEMP testing can also be used to distinguish the conductive hearing loss associated with a third window defect and that of ossicular chain disease. Rather than the typical lowered VEMP threshold associated with a dehiscence, ossicular chain disease may show an absent or elevated threshold.[48] Conversely, a normal VEMP response in the setting of a mild to moderate conductive hearing loss suggests a "third window." Ocular VEMP, which has been proposed to test utricular function and is measured at the contralateral eye, has also shown ability to diagnose SSCD.[49]

Electrocochleography (ECoG) has also shown promise as a diagnostic tool for SSCD. Arts et al in 2008 reported an elevated SP/AP ratio (> 0.4) in 14 out of 15 ears with known SSCD, and the remaining ear had a borderline elevation at 0.4. Five of these patients underwent sSCC obliteration and had postoperative normalization of their SP/AP ratio.[50] The ECoG test may be useful for real-time confirmation of effective plugging of the sSSC. A follow-up study identified ECoG as having an 89% sensitivity and 70% specificity for SSCD, with affected ears having a mean SP/AP ratio of 0.62, compared with 0.29 in unaffected ears.[51]

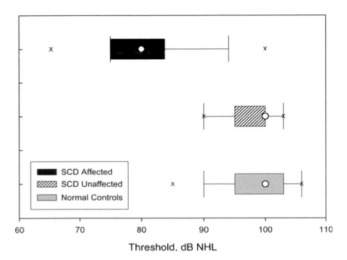

(legend inside figure)
- ■ SCD Affected
- ▨ SCD Unaffected
- ▦ Normal Controls

Threshold, dB NHL

Fig. 11.3 Thresholds for evoking a vestibular evoked myogenic potential (VEMP) response in ears affected with superior canal dehiscence (SCCD), unaffected ears in patients with SCCD of the contralateral ear, and normal control ears. Each box represents the 25th to 75th percentile range, the vertical bars represent the 10th to 90th percentile range. The two outer Xs represent the 5th and 95th percentile range, and the middle circle denotes the median value. Used with permission from Minor LB. Clinical manifestations of superior semicircular canal dehiscence. Laryngoscope. 2005;115:1717–1727.

Radiologic Findings

Radiographic findings can be an important adjunct for making the SSCD diagnosis but they must be interpreted with vigilance, paying attention to the slice thickness, axis of orientation, and correlation with clinical symptoms. CT is the gold standard for its ability to visualize bony anatomy. CT imaging with 0.5 mm collimation and projection of the images into the plane of the superior canal is used to most accurately confirm the presence of a dehiscence of the superior canal.[37] CT scanning in the standard coronal plane with thin images (0.5 to 0.6 mm) can give a good indication that one is dealing with a likely dehiscent superior canal (**Fig. 11.4**). However, thin collimation with reformatting into the plane of the superior canal gives the most accurate information regarding the radiographic validity of the diagnosis of SSCD (**Fig. 11.5**).

The two most common reformatted views are the Pöschl and Stenvers planes.[31] The Pöschl plane is 45° from both the sagittal and coronal views, thus creating sections that are perpendicular to the long axis of the petrous bone. This enables the entire sSCC arch to be visualized in one image. The Stenvers plane is perpendicular to that of Pöschl; therefore, sections are parallel to the long axis of the petrous bone. The Stenvers plane enables cross-section cuts of the sSCC.

Belden et al performed CT scans with either 1.0 or 0.5 mm collimation in 50 patients with SSCD symptomatology and 50 controls. They found that the positive predictive value of an apparent dehiscence in the diagnosis of SSCD improves from 50% with 1.0 mm collimation using transverse and coronal imaging to 93% using 0.5 mm collimation with reformatting the CT in the plane of the sSCC.[52]

Hirvonen et al studied 27 known SSCD patients and 88 controls using CT (0.5 mm collimation and sSCC plane reformatting) to determine whether variations in thickness in the bone overlying the sSCC is suggestive of an abnormality in development in cases of SSCD. They found that the thickness of bone over the superior canal in controls measured 0.67 ± 0.38 and that the thickness correlated with the contralateral side (r = 0.43, $p < 0.0001$). In those with documented SSCD unilaterally, the contralateral side measured 0.31 ± 0.23 mm, demonstrating that the intact side on those with SSCD is thinner than in normal controls ($p < 0.0001$) and suggesting that a developmental predisposition exists for SSCD by virtue of bone thickness.[53]

It is important to make the SSCD diagnosis based on clinical symptoms and signs on physical examination, especially when dealing with CT images obtained using standard 1 mm cuts, which may mislead the clinician with regard to the presence of SSCD. Williamson et al reviewed temporal bone CTs with 1 mm slices obtained for general otologic issues over a 2-year period and noted that 9% of the studies revealed a dehiscent-appearing sSCC. Upon review, none of the patients with suspicious CT scans were being worked up for SSCD and none had historical or audiologic findings suggestive of SSCD.[17] This report

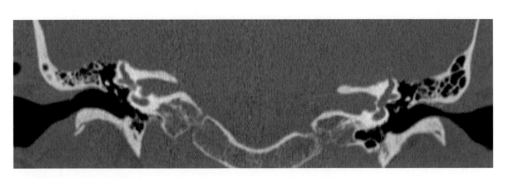

Fig. 11.4 Coronal CT scan images (0.6 mm) from the same patient as in **Fig. 11.2**. Note the appearance of dehiscence that is more pronounced on the left side.

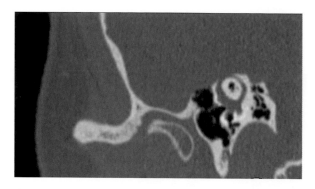

Fig. 11.5 Reformatted (0.6 mm) CT scan of the temporal bone, with formatting into the plane of the left superior semicircular canal. Note the obvious dehiscence, which corresponds with the conductive low-frequency hearing loss in the patient in **Fig. 11.2**.

points out the need for careful assessment of patients prior to embarking on surgical therapy and the need to use the 0.5 mm collimation with reformatting to the plane of the sSCC.

Magnetic resonance imaging (MRI) is typically normal in SSCD syndrome. MRI may be of diagnostic value if a concomitant CSF leak or meningoencephalocele exists.[54] As radiographic technology continues to improve, new protocols and techniques continue to push the diagnostic envelope. Some authors have recently advocated for digital volume tomography (also called cone-beam CT) for its higher resolution and reduced artifact.[55,56]

Radiographic Classification

A recent publication has proposed a comprehensive radiologic classification system for SSCD based on dehiscence location and adjacent tegmen topography.[57] Standardization of the dehiscence type may provide future insight into the variable symptomatology and treatment options. Lookabaugh et al characterized sSCC defects into six categories: (1) intact sSCC, (2) dehiscence on the lateral upslope of the sSCC, (3) dehiscence of the arcuate eminence, (4) dehiscence on the medial downslope of the sSCC, (5) superior petrosal sinus–associated SSCD, and (6) arcuate eminence defect with near-dehiscent superior petrosal sinus. Among the 202 patients they reviewed who had SCCD, they found the most common defects to be at the arcuate eminence (59.5%) and medial downslope (28.8%).

■ Differential Diagnosis

Because SSCD is heralded as the great otologic mimicker, numerous conditions have to be considered as differentials when patients present with SSCD symp-

toms. Other common etiologies of nonpositional vertigo, including Meniere's disease, vestibular neuritis, viral or syphilitic labyrinthitis, and perilymphatic fistula, should all be considered. Otosclerosis can yield low-frequency conductive hearing loss but can be differentiated from SSCD by acoustic reflexes as well as VEMP testing. Cholesteatoma-induced or iatrogenic horizontal canal erosion can be the cause of pressure- or sound-induced vertigo.

High-resolution imaging can identify less common anatomic causes that may mimic SSCD. Contact of superior petrosal sinus (SPS) with the sSCC can cause exercise- and exertion-related dizziness.[31] Jugular bulb diverticula can create a defect of the posterior semicircular canal and can cause hearing loss and unsteadiness.[58] Imaging should show a high jugular bulb and diverticulum, with encroachment and erosion of the posterior semicircular canal. Other rare causes include venous malformations and temporal bone fibrous dysplasia involving the superior canal wall.

Congenital dehiscences have been described between the middle and inner ear, which may also create a third window and induce symptoms of SSCD due to defects not along the semicircular canals but at other sites along the bony labyrinth. For example, a bony dehiscence between the round window niche and the cribrose area of the singular canal has been described in human temporal bone studies.[59] Such conditions may be considered when radiographic studies fail to confirm clinical suspicion of SSCD.

Finally, careful attention must be paid to the CT appearance of a suspected SSCD prior to assuming idiopathic SSCD. The potential for the sSCC to be eroded by a brain or dural neoplasm must be considered when extensive erosion of the sSCC and surrounding petrous bone is visualized on CT. Magnetic resonance imaging in such cases will be necessary to rule out the rare occurrence of transdural infiltration and erosion of the sSCC and middle fossa floor by tumors like glioblastoma and meningioma.[60,61]

■ Treatment

Medical Treatment

Many patients have only mild to moderate symptoms from SSCD. Treatment options should be considered on the basis of the severity of the symptoms. Many patients can achieve control of their symptoms through avoidance of the offending stimuli. In six of the eight original Minor et al patients, diagnosis and avoidance of offending stimuli were sufficient treatment.[2] Placement of a pressure-equalizing tube in the offending ear may be beneficial in some patients, especially those complaining of pressure-induced symptoms.[29,30,36]

Surgical Treatment

Preoperative Considerations

Surgical therapy is reserved for the patient whose combination of physical exam findings and audiologic, vestibular, and radiographic testing results confirms the SSCD diagnosis. Some symptomatic patients may not demonstrate the full spectrum of sound- and pressure-induced findings and in some cases may even fail to reveal confirmatory nystagmus, despite debilitating symptoms. In other patients with bilateral dehiscence, it may be difficult to target which ear is the more symptomatic. These issues make surgery an undertaking that should be embarked on after nonsurgical measures have failed. Informed consent regarding the potential complications of the surgical approach of choice should be obtained. It is also important to have a frank preoperative discussion on the unpredictability of the procedure's ability to eliminate all of the patient's bothersome symptoms. For example, surgery may provide relief from autophony and Tullio phenomenon but postoperatively there may be persistent disequilibrium or new vestibular complaints, such as oscillopsia.[36]

The surgical approaches to SSCD have evolved since Minor's first description of a middle cranial fossa approach in 1998. Approaches now include the classic middle cranial fossa, endoscopic-assisted middle cranial fossa, transmastoid plugging, transmastoid resurfacing, endoscopic resurfacing, and round window patching. Regardless of the approach, the common objective remains to close the third window and to prevent aberrant energy passage throughout the labyrinth. The ideal approach to SSCD remains controversial and likely depends on many patient and surgeon factors (**Video 11.1**).[62]

Surgical Technique: Middle Cranial Fossa Approach

A Foley catheter is placed and 50 to 100 g of mannitol and 20 mg of furosemide are given to induce a brisk diuresis. This allows for relaxed dura and permits easier retraction of the temporal lobe. The head is shaved to facilitate a 4 cm × 4 cm craniotomy in a similar manner as a middle fossa craniotomy performed for acoustic neuroma removal or facial nerve decompression. A facial nerve monitor is employed to help avoid injury to a dehiscent geniculate ganglion during dural elevation. Dura is elevated medially until the arcuate eminence is reached and further medially toward the petrous ridge. Bone may be thin or absent over the tegmen, and care must be taken to avoid aspiration of perilymph that may be exposed by "tearing" the membranous labyrinth as dura is peeled from the dehiscent superior canal. A House-Urban middle fossa retractor is helpful at this point to keep the arcuate eminence exposed during preparation for occlusion of the sSCC (**Fig. 11.6**).

Next, bone wax is pushed into the dehiscence with neurosurgical patties or sterile cotton applicators. Minor et al, as well as Mikulec et al, have noted the relative inability of canal "resurfacing" with fascia and bone to produce satisfactory results.[2,36] Thus the "plugging" of the superior canal is analogous to that performed during posterior canal ablation with bone wax or bone dust as described for intractable benign paroxysmal positional vertigo.[63] Any large bony defects over the middle ear or mastoid should be repaired with split calvarial bone grafts harvested from the bone flap to avoid the risk of postoperative dural herniation and meningocele. After the canal is plugged, dura is allowed to relax and the bone can be replaced with self-tapping screws and titanium plating. Care is taken to avoid epidural hematoma by ensuring the absence of bleeding under the bone flap. The reattachment of the temporalis muscle and fascia will help secure the bone flap. Skin and subcutaneous tissue closure in two more layers is then performed, and a drain is not normally necessary. In the event of a cerebrospinal fluid leak from a dural defect created during dissection of the middle fossa floor, primary dural repair, fascia grafting, and/or fibrin glue products can be employed to prevent postoperative CSF-related complications.

Minor's description of the middle cranial fossa approach in 1998 has yielded successful and reproducible results. The approach allows direct access to the defect and may bypass anatomic variations, such as a low-lying tegmen, that make a transmastoid approach more difficult. Additionally, the approach allows the surgeon to address other tegmen defects, like CSF leak or meningoencephalocele, with limited additional dissection.[26] Some have advocated for the

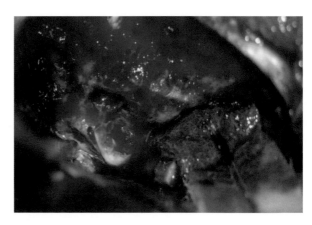

Fig. 11.6 Middle cranial fossa approach. Intraoperative photo of a superior semicircular canal dehiscence at the arcuate eminence as seen through a middle cranial fossa approach. Courtesy of J. Walter Kutz Jr., MD.

use of 0° and 30° endoscopes for better visualization of the dehiscence with less brain retraction.[64] A modified endoscopic middle cranial fossa approach has been described using a postauricular incision and a 2-cm craniotomy. Still, the downside to any middle fossa approach is the need for a craniotomy as well as the inherent risks and the high-acuity care they require.[63]

Surgical Technique: Transmastoid Approach

In an effort to reduce the surgical morbidity associated with a craniotomy, a less invasive approach via a transmastoid route was developed. In 2008, Agrawal and Parnes were the first to describe identification and plugging of the sSCC through a mastoidectomy for SSCD.[65] In 2009, Kirtane described performing a mastoidectomy and sSCC plugging under local anesthesia with resolution of SSCD symptoms.[66] That same year, Deschenes et al reported the feasibility of performing the transmastoid approach as an outpatient procedure, which provides a stark contrast to the postoperative care required for a middle cranial fossa approach.[67] Early detractors of the transmastoid approach cited the inability to visualize the sSCC defect, risk of sensorineural hearing loss, difficulty repairing other tegmen defects, and lack of resurfacing. Since then, transmastoid techniques for repairing temporal bone meningoencephaloceles and resurfacing sSCC dehiscences have been described.[68,69]

The surgical setup for the transmastoid approach is identical to a standard mastoidectomy and typically includes facial nerve monitoring. A postauricular incision is made 2 to 3 mm behind the postauricular sulcus. Skin flaps are elevated along the plane of the temporalis fascia, temporalis fascia is harvested, and the pericranium is elevated to expose the mastoid cortex. A cortical mastoidectomy is performed, with identification of the sSCC. Under constant irrigation, a small diamond bur is used to blue-line the ampullated end of the sSCC. The ampullated end is then fenestrated and immediately plugged with a free muscle graft. Bone wax is then used to seal the plug. This fenestration technique is repeated at the non-ampullated end of the sSCC. Care is taken to avoid suction or manipulation of the membranous labyrinth. Conchal cartilage is harvested. Blunt instrumentation is used to elevate an intracranial epidural pocket from the mastoid cavity. The conchal cartilage is placed into the epidural pocket as an overlay graft covering the sSCC. Temporalis fascia is also placed on top of the repair site to cover the canal (**Fig. 11.7**). The attic is plugged with Gelfoam (Pfizer) and the mastoid cavity is filled with tissue sealant.[67] Other technique variants include dissecting the epidural pocket with a Buckingham mirror in an attempt to visualize the sSCC defect.[69]

Surgical Technique: Transcanal Approach

The newest and least invasive approach for SSCD attempts to fix the third window phenomenon by closing or reinforcing one of the other windows. Through the external auditory canal, a tympanomeatal flap is elevated and the round window niche is visualized. The round window is then occluded or obliterated with tissue, often a free fascia graft. A multi-institutional review has demonstrated early symptomatic control but long-term data are still lacking for this novel techinque.[70]

Surgical Outcomes

Both the middle cranial fossa and transmastoid approaches have had success in relieving symptoms associated with SSCD. Most patients will report an immediate postoperative cessation of pressure- or sound-induced nystagmus.[36] Symptomatic recovery, however, takes weeks to months, in part due to the need for compensation of a new peripheral defect after ablation of the superior canal. Symptomatic recovery may also vary depending on the specific symptom of interest. For instance, Mikulec et al noted that only half of their patients with the preoperative complaint of chronic disequilibrium noted resolution, and one patient developed this complaint postoperatively, whereas autophony and associated conductive hearing loss improved in most cases.[36] Minor reported complete resolution of vestibular symptoms in eight of nine patients after canal plugging and seven of eleven patients after resurfacing, both via a middle cranial fossa approach.[30] In subsequent review of 43 patients who underwent sSCC plugging via the middle cranial fossa, Ward et al found that low-frequency air–bone gap decreased, partially due to elevated bone conduction and partially due to decreased air conduction. They also found that a mild high-frequency sensorineural hearing loss without significant decline in word discrimination score persisted in 25% of patients.[71] Other groups have also reported the relative safety of canal plugging for postoperative hearing.[72] The safety and efficacy have also been reported for the transmastoid approach.[65,66,67,69,73] Beyea et al in 2012 reported on 16 patients who underwent transmastoid plugging for SSCD. Vestibular symptoms were greatly improved or completely resolved in 15 of the 16 patients and hearing was preserved or improved in all 16 patients.[73]

Serious complications of SSCD surgery are rare, but the potential for iatrogenic injury to critical structures or decline in function warrants a frank preoperative discussion with the patient on the risks, benefits, and alternative therapies. In addition to facial nerve risks inherent to any ear surgery, additional discussion should address the possibility of postoperative decline in hearing, the production of new vestibular complaints, such as chronic imbalance, or new vestibular hypofunction-related problems, including oscillopsia.

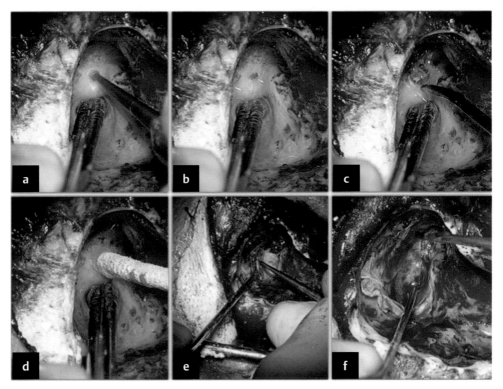

Fig. 11.7 Transmastoid approach: intraoperative photos of superior semicircular canal dehiscence plugging and resurfacing via a transmastoid approach. **(a)** Superior semicircular canal is identified with a small diamond bur. **(b)** The canal is fenestrated, first at the ampullated end. **(c)** The fenestration is plugged with a free muscle graft. **(d)** The muscle plug is secured with bone wax. These steps are repeated at the non-ampullated end of the canal. **(e)** Cartilage is placed over the canal in an epidural pocket from the mastoid cavity. **(f)** Fascia is also used to overlie the canal.

Questions

Q1: A 33-year-old female presented with dizziness and sound-induced vertigo for 1 year. As part of her work-up, an audiogram revealed left-sided conductive hearing loss in low frequencies, and radiographically she had a dehiscent left SCC. The mechanism for hearing loss in this patient is:

A. Decreased bone conduction thresholds only.

B. Stapes fixation.

C. Decreased bone-conduction thresholds and increased air-conduction thresholds.

D. Increased air-conduction thresholds only.

Q2: VEMP characteristics of SSCD are best characterized as:

A. Short onset latency and low threshold of activation.

B. Short onset latency and high threshold of activation.

C. Long onset latency and high threshold of activation.

D. Long onset latency and low threshold of activation.

Q3: A patient has radiographic evidence of right-sided SCCD and is clinically symptomatic. The nystagmus-defining fast phase can be best characterized as:

A. Down and to the right.

B. Down and to the left.

C. Up and to the left.

D. Up and to the right.

Q4: Positive predictive value for diagnosis of SSCD using 0.5 mm collimation with reformatting CT scan is:

A. 93%

B. 76%

C. 50%

D. 33%

Q5: The most common radiographic SSCD deformity observed on standard CT imaging is:

A. Dehiscence of the lateral upslope of the SCC.

B. Dehiscence of the medial downslope of the SCC.

C. Superior petrosal sinus associated SCC.

D. Dehiscence of the arcuate eminence.

Answers

A1: C

A2: A

A3: A

A4: A

A5: D

References

1. Baloh RW. Superior semicircular canal dehiscence syndrome: Leaks and squeaks can make you dizzy. Neurology 2004;62(5):684–685

2. Minor LB, Solomon D, Zinreich JS, Zee DS. Sound- and/or pressure-induced vertigo due to bone dehiscence of the superior semicircular canal. Arch Otolaryngol Head Neck Surg 1998;124(3):249–258

3. Brantberg K, Bergenius J, Tribukait A. Vestibular-evoked myogenic potentials in patients with dehiscence of the superior semicircular canal. Acta Otolaryngol 1999;119(6):633–640

4. Mong A, Loevner LA, Solomon D, Bigelow DC. Sound- and pressure-induced vertigo associated with dehiscence of the roof of the superior semicircular canal. AJNR Am J Neuroradiol 1999;20(10):1973–1975

5. Tullio P. Das Ohr und die Enstehung der Sprache und Schrift. Berlin: Urban & Schwartzenberg; 1929

6. Hirvonen TP, Carey JP, Liang CJ, Minor LB. Superior canal dehiscence: mechanisms of pressure sensitivity in a chinchilla model. Arch Otolaryngol Head Neck Surg 2001;127(11):1331–1336

7. Carey JP, Hirvonen TP, Hullar TE, Minor LB. Acoustic responses of vestibular afferents in a model of superior canal dehiscence. Otol Neurotol 2004;25(3):345–352

8. Hennebert C. A new syndrome in hereditary syphilis of the labyrinth. Presse Med Belg Brux. 1911;63:467

9. Mayer O, Fraser JS. Pathological changes in the ear in late congenital syphilis. J Laryngol Otol 1936;51:683–714

10. Nadol JB Jr. Positive Hennebert's sign in Meniere's disease. Arch Otolaryngol 1977;103(9):524–530

11. Daspit CP, Churchill D, Linthicum FH Jr. Diagnosis of perilymph fistula using ENG and impedance. Laryngoscope 1980;90(2):217–223

12. Halmagyi GM, Curthoys IS, Colebatch JG, Aw ST. Vestibular responses to sound. Ann N Y Acad Sci 2005; 1039:54–67

13. Carey JP, Minor LB, Nager GT. Dehiscence or thinning of bone overlying the superior semicircular canal in a temporal bone survey. Arch Otolaryngol Head Neck Surg 2000;126(2):137–147

14. Jackson NM, Allen LM, Morell B, et al. The relationship of age and radiographic incidence of superior semicircular canal dehiscence in pediatric patients. Otol Neurotol 2015;36(1):99–105

15. Nadgir RN, Ozonoff A, Devaiah AK, Halderman AA, Sakai O. Superior semicircular canal dehiscence: congenital or acquired condition? AJNR Am J Neuroradiol 2011;32(5):947–949

16. Lee GS, Zhou G, Poe D, et al. Clinical experience in diagnosis and management of superior semicircular canal dehiscence in children. Laryngoscope 2011; 121(10):2256–2261

17. Williamson RA, Vrabec JT, Coker NJ, Sandlin M; RA. Coronal computed tomography prevalence of superior semicircular canal dehiscence. Otolaryngol Head Neck Surg 2003;129(5):481–489

18. Bremke M, Luers JC, Anagiotos A, et al. Comparison of digital volume tomography and high-resolution computed tomography in detecting superior semicircular canal dehiscence—a temporal bone study. Acta Otolaryngol 2015;135(9):901–906

19. Branstetter BF IV, Harrigal C, Escott EJ, Hirsch BE. Superior semicircular canal dehiscence: oblique reformatted CT images for diagnosis. Radiology 2006; 238(3):938–942

20. Masaki Y. The prevalence of superior canal dehiscence syndrome as assessed by temporal bone computed tomography imaging. Acta Otolaryngol 2011; 131(3):258–262

21. Tavassolie TS, Penninger RT, Zuñiga MG, Minor LB, Carey JP. Multislice computed tomography in the diagnosis of superior canal dehiscence: how much error, and how to minimize it? Otol Neurotol 2012; 33(2):215–222

22. Watters KF, Rosowski JJ, Sauter T, Lee DJ. Superior semicircular canal dehiscence presenting as postpartum vertigo. Otol Neurotol 2006;27(6):756–768

23. Remenschneider A, Santos F. Pneumocephalus, hearing loss, and vertigo after airline flight in a patient with superior canal dehiscence. Otol Neurotol 2014;35(1):e60–e61

24. Stevens SM, Lambert PR, Rizk H, McIlwain WR, Nguyen SA, Meyer TA. Novel radiographic measurement algorithm demonstrating a link between obesity and lateral skull base attenuation. Otolaryngol Head Neck Surg 2015;152(1):172–179

25. Schutt CA, Neubauer P, Samy RN, et al. The correlation between obesity, obstructive sleep apnea, and superior semicircular canal dehiscence: a new explanation for an increasingly common problem. Otol Neurotol 2015;36(3):551–554

26. Allen KP, Perez CL, Isaacson B, Roland PS, Duong TT, Kutz JW. Superior semicircular canal dehiscence in patients with spontaneous cerebrospinal fluid otorrhea. Otolaryngol Head Neck Surg 2012;147(6):1120–1124

27. Semaan MT, Wick CC, Megerian CA. Vestibular physiology. In: Pensak ML, Choo DI, eds. Clinical Otology. New York, NY: Thieme; 2015:35–44

28. Rosowski JJ, Songer JE, Nakajima HH, Brinsko KM, Merchant SN. Clinical, experimental, and theoretical investigations of the effect of superior semicircular canal dehiscence on hearing mechanisms. Otol Neurotol 2004;25(3):323–332

29. Minor LB. Superior canal dehiscence syndrome. Am J Otol 2000;21(1):9–19

30. Minor LB. Clinical manifestations of superior semicircular canal dehiscence. Laryngoscope 2005; 115(10):1717–1727

31. McCall AA, McKenna MJ, Merchant SN, Curtin HD, Lee DJ. Superior canal dehiscence syndrome associated with the superior petrosal sinus in pediatric and adult patients. Otol Neurotol 2011;32(8):1312–1319

32. Deutschländer A, Strupp M, Jahn K, Jäger L, Quiring F, Brandt T. Vertical oscillopsia in bilateral superior canal dehiscence syndrome. Neurology 2004;62(5):784–787

33. Minor LB, Carey JP, Cremer PD, Lustig LR, Streubel SO, Ruckenstein MJ. Dehiscence of bone overlying the superior canal as a cause of apparent conductive hearing loss. Otol Neurotol 2003;24(2):270–278

34. Mikulec AA, McKenna MJ, Ramsey MJ, et al. Superior semicircular canal dehiscence presenting as conductive hearing loss without vertigo. Otol Neurotol 2004;25(2):121–129

35. Chi FL, Ren DD, Dai CF. Variety of audiologic manifestations in patients with superior semicircular canal dehiscence. Otol Neurotol 2010;31(1):2–10

36. Mikulec AA, Poe DS, McKenna MJ. Operative management of superior semicircular canal dehiscence. Laryngoscope 2005;115(3):501–507

37. Minor LB, Cremer PD, Carey JP, Della Santina CC, Streubel SO, Weg N. Symptoms and signs in superior canal dehiscence syndrome. Ann N Y Acad Sci 2001; 942:259–273

38. Brantberg K, Bergenius J, Mendel L, Witt H, Tribukait A, Ygge J. Symptoms, findings and treatment in patients with dehiscence of the superior semicircular canal. Acta Otolaryngol 2001;121(1):68–75

39. Tilikete C, Krolak-Salmon P, Truy E, Vighetto A. Pulse-synchronous eye oscillations revealing bone superior canal dehiscence. Ann Neurol 2004;56(4):556–560

40. Halmagyi GM, Aw ST, McGarvie LA, et al. Superior semicircular canal dehiscence simulating otosclerosis. J Laryngol Otol 2003;117(7):553–557

41. Pisano DV, Niesten ME, Merchant SN, Nakajima HH. The effect of superior semicircular canal dehiscence on intracochlear sound pressures. Audiol Neurootol 2012;17(5):338–348

42. Pfammatter A, Darrouzet V, Gärtner M, et al. A superior semicircular canal dehiscence syndrome multicenter study: is there an association between size and symptoms? Otol Neurotol 2010;31(3):447–454

43. Chien WW, Janky K, Minor LB, Carey JP. Superior canal dehiscence size: multivariate assessment of clinical impact. Otol Neurotol 2012;33(5):810–815

44. Niesten MEF, Hamberg LM, Silverman JB, et al. Superior canal dehiscence length and location influences clinical presentation and audiometric and cervical vestibular-evoked myogenic potential testing. Audiol Neurootol 2014;19(2):97–105

45. Streubel SO, Cremer PD, Carey JP, Weg N, Minor LB. Vestibular-evoked myogenic potentials in the diagnosis of superior canal dehiscence syndrome. Acta Otolaryngol Suppl 2001;545(Suppl):41–49

46. Sheykholeslami K, Schmerber S, Habiby Kermany M, Kaga K. Vestibular-evoked myogenic potentials in three patients with large vestibular aqueduct. Hear Res 2004;190(1-2):161–168

47. Halmagyi GM, McGarvie LA, Aw ST, Yavor RA, Todd MJ. The click-evoked vestibulo-ocular reflex in superior semicircular canal dehiscence. Neurology 2003;60(7):1172–1175

48. Gopen Q, Zhou G, Poe D, Kenna M, Jones D. Posterior semicircular canal dehiscence: first reported case series. Otol Neurotol 2010;31(2):339–344

49. Manzari L, Burgess AM, McGarvie LA, Curthoys IS. Ocular and cervical vestibular evoked myogenic potentials to 500 Hz fz bone-conducted vibration in superior semicircular canal dehiscence. Ear Hear 2012;33(4):508–520

50. Arts HA, Adams ME, Telian SA, El-Kashlan H, Kileny PR. Reversible electrocochleographic abnormalities in superior canal dehiscence. Otol Neurotol 2009; 30(1):79–86

51. Adams ME, Kileny PR, Telian SA, et al. Electrocochleography as a diagnostic and intraoperative adjunct in superior semicircular canal dehiscence syndrome. Otol Neurotol 2011;32(9):1506–1512

52. Belden CJ, Weg N, Minor LB, Zinreich SJ. CT evaluation of bone dehiscence of the superior semicircular canal as a cause of sound- and/or pressure-induced vertigo. Radiology 2003;226(2):337–343

53. Hirvonen TP, Weg N, Zinreich SJ, Minor LB. High-resolution CT findings suggest a developmental abnormality underlying superior canal dehiscence syndrome. Acta Otolaryngol 2003;123(4):477–481

54. Suryanarayanan R, Lesser TH. 'Honeycomb' tegmen: multiple tegmen defects associated with superior semicircular canal dehiscence. J Laryngol Otol 2010;124(5):560–563

55. Eibenberger K, Carey J, Ehtiati T, Trevino C, Dolberg J, Haslwanter T. A novel method of 3D image analysis of high-resolution cone beam CT and multi slice CT for the detection of semicircular canal dehiscence. Otol Neurotol 2014;35(2):329–337

56. Bremke M, Luers JC, Anagiotos A, et al. Comparison of digital volume tomography and high-resolution computed tomography in detecting superior semicircular canal dehiscence—a temporal bone study. Acta Otolaryngol 2015;135(9):901–906

57. Lookabaugh S, Kelly HR, Carter MS, et al. Radiologic classification of superior canal dehiscence: implications for surgical repair. Otol Neurotol 2015;36(1):118–125

58. Wadin K, Thomander L, Wilbrand H. Effects of a high jugular fossa and jugular bulb diverticulum on the inner ear. A clinical and radiologic investigation. Acta Radiol Diagn (Stockh) 1986;27(6):629–636

59. Sato H, Takahashi H, Sando I. Bony dehiscence between singular canal and round window niche. Laryngoscope 1993;103(1 Pt 1):78–81

60. Licht AK, Schulmeyer F, Allert M, Held P, Woenckhaus M, Strutz J. Vertigo and hearing disturbance as the first sign of a glioblastoma (World Health Organization grade IV). Otol Neurotol 2004;25(2):174–177

61. Crane BT, Carey JP, McMenomey S, Minor LB. Meningioma causing superior canal dehiscence syndrome. Otol Neurotol 2010;31(6):1009–1010

62. Shaia WT, Diaz RC. Evolution in surgical management of superior canal dehiscence syndrome. Curr Opin Otolaryngol Head Neck Surg 2013;21(5):497–502

63. Agrawal SK, Parnes LS. Human experience with canal plugging. Ann N Y Acad Sci 2001;942:300–305

64. Carter MS, Lookabaugh S, Lee DJ. Endoscopic-assisted repair of superior canal dehiscence syndrome. Laryngoscope 2014;124(6):1464–1468

65. Agrawal SK, Parnes LS. Transmastoid superior semicircular canal occlusion. Otol Neurotol 2008; 29(3):363–367

66. Kirtane MV, Sharma A, Satwalekar D. Transmastoid repair of superior semicircular canal dehiscence. J Laryngol Otol 2009;123(3):356–358

67. Deschenes GR, Hsu DP, Megerian CA. Outpatient repair of superior semicircular canal dehiscence via the transmastoid approach. Laryngoscope 2009; 119(9):1765–1769

68. Manjila S, Wick CC, Cramer J, et al. Meningoencephalocele of the temporal bone: pictorial essay on transmastoid extradural-intracranial repair. Am J Otolaryngol 2013;34(6):664–675

69. Amoodi HA, Makki FM, McNeil M, Bance M. Transmastoid resurfacing of superior semicircular canal dehiscence. Laryngoscope 2011;121(5):1117–1123

70. Silverstein H, Kartush JM, Parnes LS, et al. Round window reinforcement for superior semicircular canal dehiscence: a retrospective multi-center case series. Am J Otolaryngol 2014;35(3):286–293

71. Ward BK, Agrawal Y, Nguyen E, et al. Hearing outcomes after surgical plugging of the superior semicircular canal by a middle cranial fossa approach. Otol Neurotol 2012;33(8):1386–1391

72. Goddard JC, Wilkinson EP. Outcomes following semicircular canal plugging. Otolaryngol Head Neck Surg 2014;151(3):478–483

73. Beyea JA, Agrawal SK, Parnes LS. Transmastoid semicircular canal occlusion: a safe and highly effective treatment for benign paroxysmal positional vertigo and superior canal dehiscence. Laryngoscope 2012; 122(8):1862–1866

12 Autoimmune Vestibular Dysfunction, Perilymph Fistulas, Mal de Debarquement Syndrome, and Alcohol-Related Dizziness

Louis M. Hofmeyr

■ Introduction

Little has changed in these subject areas since the 2008 publication of the first edition of this book, except perhaps some aspects of the management of some of the conditions.[1] Despite advances in vestibular assessment over the last decade, the impact on these conditions has yet to be appreciated.

■ Autoimmune Vestibular Dysfunction

Autoimmune vestibular dysfunction is an immunologically mediated attack on the vestibular system. Autoimmune inner ear disease (AIED)—as the name implies—refers to the involvement of the inner ear. AIED can occur in isolation or in association with systemic autoimmune disease. AIED is uncommon and accounts for less than 1% of all cases of hearing loss and dizziness.[2]

Apart from the inner ear, the nervous system and other body systems can have immunologic involvement that causes dizziness and disequilibrium. The focus in this section, however, is on the vestibular system, and more specifically the inner ear. Because it is less likely that autoimmune vestibular dysfunction will occur without hearing loss, AIED is reviewed first.

AIED is characterized by rapidly progressive, often fluctuating, bilateral sensorineural hearing loss (SNHL). Tinnitus and aural fullness are often present. Dizziness occurs in 50% of patients with active AIED. Patients are more likely to complain of episodic lightheadedness and mild ataxia than true vertigo.[3] Spells of vertigo occur in less than a third of patients. The rapid progression of the hearing loss over weeks to months helps to distinguish it from that attributable to other causes, such as sudden bilateral hearing loss from ototoxicity or noise-induced hearing loss that develops over years. AIED is more common in females between 20 and 50 years old, especially if a systemic autoimmune disease (e.g., rheumatoid arthritis or multiple sclerosis) is present. In 30% of patients with AIED, a systemic autoimmune disorder is present. AIED is rare in children.

There are four theories of how AIED arises: cross-reactions, bystander damage, intolerance, and genetic factors. The inner ear, which is not exposed to many antigens, possesses only some active cells, and has no lymphatic drainage, is nevertheless able to generate cellular and humoral immunity. The cochlea has its own innate immunity and the endolymphatic sac can process antigen and produce its own antibody response.[4] Leukocytes enter the cochlea via the spiral modiolar vein. In AIED, it is believed that the damage due to antibodies or immune cells occurs in certain genetically susceptible patients when they are exposed to unknown environmental pathogens. The damage to the inner ear causes cytokines (e.g., tumor necrosis factor [TNF] and interleukin-1 [IL-1]) to be released in the cochlea. This may also provoke a delayed, additional immune reaction and might explain the attack and remission cycle of disorders like Meniere's disease. TNF-α expressed by the sac may be one way in which Meniere's disease is linked to AIED.

Examination of the ear is usually normal. Tuning fork testing may support a diagnosis of SNHL. Patients with dizziness may demonstrate abnormalities, none of which is really diagnostic. In some patients, systemic autoimmune disease may be present. Audiologic testing will reveal progressive bilateral SNHL over time. The hearing may be asymmetric at first and may fluctuate. Otoacoustic emissions (OAE) are likely to support cochlear involvement and electrocochleography (ECoG) may support endolymphatic hydrops. Vestibular testing, including rotatory chair, vestibular evoked myogenic potentials, and platform posturography, may all be used to assess vestibular function. Findings depend on the degree and location of the involvement of the vestibular system.

Imaging does not contribute to the confirmation of the diagnosis in AIED, but MRI should nevertheless be done to rule out bilateral vestibular schwannoma in neurofibromatosis type 2, an unlikely cause for bilateral hearing and vestibular loss.

Serological testing is not essential to make the diagnosis. Anticochlear antibody (also called anti-heat shock protein 70 or anti-HSP 70) also occurs in other disorders, such as Lyme disease. It is also present in up to 5% of the general population. Western blot analysis for this protein may support the diagnosis, but with a sensitivity of ~ 50%, its value is questionable.[5] The migration inhibition and lymphocyte transformation tests are not readily available and have not really proved helpful. Other blood tests that may indicate systemic autoimmune disease include erythrocyte sedimentation rate, C-reactive protein, antinuclear antibodies, to rheumatoid factor, anti-thyroid antibodies, complement C1Q, smooth muscle antibody, antigliadin and antiendomysial antibodies (for celiac disease), HLA testing, and Raji cell assay. Syphilis, diabetes, HIV infection, and Lyme disease may mimic AIED and appropriate tests should be ordered if indicated.

The initial treatment of AIED is the same whether dizziness is present or not. Systemic steroids (prednisone or dexamethasone) are the first line of treatment. A clinical history of rapidly progressive bilateral SNHL over weeks to months and an unrevealing clinical examination, as well as a positive response to systemic steroids, are considered diagnostic for AIED. Prednisone is usually taken daily for 1 month, with repeat audiograms performed after 14 days and 1 month. Regardless of whether or not a patient responds, it is not advisable to continue with a high dose of steroids beyond 1 month. If the steroid is ineffective, it is tapered down and stopped. Patients need to adjust their maintenance dose depending on disease activity; to avoid potential side effects the lowest dose possible should be prescribed.

Since long-term control with systemic steroids is usually not feasible due to side effects, intratympanic administration, especially of dexamethasone, has been considered as an alternative. This route of administration may reach adequate levels in the perilymph but it is unpredictable and depends on the permeability of the round window membrane. Direct intracochlear administration through a cochleostomy is under investigation. Unfortunately, it needs to be administered on numerous occasions in both ears, necessitating many office visits, which is not practical. Its use in AIED is still off label. Placing ventilation tubes for repeat administration carries a higher risk for permanent tympanic membrane perforation.

After 1 month of systemic steroids, cytotoxic chemotherapeutic drugs are often prescribed, but they have mixed success. Methotrexate is still used either for steroid sparing in responders or as an alternative in nonresponders, despite the fact that it was shown to be ineffective in a large multicenter study.[6] Cyclophosphamide, a powerful immunosuppressive agent with fast therapeutic activity but with more risks than steroids and methotrexate, should not be used without the help of a clinical immunologist. Plasmapheresis removes humoral and cellular immunopathogens from the circulation, but its potential benefit is relatively short-term. It should be reserved for adjuvant therapy when acute, fulminant AIED associated with systemic immune disease is not responsive to more traditional therapy.

Anti-TNF drugs, such as etanercept and infliximab, show some promise and are currently under investigation.[7] Ustekinumab is a monoclonal antibody used in the treatment of psoriasis; as an anti-TNF agent, it is directed against IL-12 and IL-23. In general, it seems likely that drugs that work for psoriasis, rheumatoid arthritis, and ulcerative colitis may also be helpful for AIED. Anti-TNF drugs suppress the immune system and may increase the risk of developing lymphoma and other malignancies.

As with other causes of cochlear hearing loss, the goal of replacing the lost and defective cells has stimulated research into stem cell implantation and gene therapy. Fortunately, patients who do not benefit from conventional hearing aids can do well after cochlear implantation. The vestibular dysfunction is usually mild and improves with standard immunotherapy.

It is suggested that 16% of bilateral and 6% of unilateral Meniere's disease may be caused by immune dysfunction. Bilateral Meniere's disease may be a clinical variant of AIED. In patients who present with fluctuating hearing loss, aural pressure, tinnitus, and episodic dizziness suggestive of endolymphatic hydrops, a possible autoimmune disorder should be considered.[8] Another clinical variant of AIED is delayed endolymphatic hydrops. To complicate matters further, the opposite ear can be affected, a phenomenon that has also been described after endolymphatic surgery where an underlying immune-mediated response has been postulated.

The standard treatment regimens for Meniere's disease are used to treat suspected immune-mediated endolymphatic hydrops (Meniere's disease); they are discussed in Chapter 7 of this book. The aim is to minimize the dose of systemic steroids required to maintain hearing and to prevent dizziness. Drop attacks are luckily rare in autoimmune disease but often may respond only to surgery. Caution is needed when deciding on a surgical option that destroys vestibular function, as failure of the vestibular function in the nonoperated ear due to the disease process may lead to permanent oscillopsia (Dandy syndrome).

Bilateral vestibular failure (BVF) is a rare condition and in 50% of patients a specific cause cannot be identified. Ototoxicity, Meniere's disease, and meningitis are the most common identifiable causes. Autoimmune mechanisms are suspected in ~ 5% of cases. Due to low specificity, autoimmune testing is not advised, and in patients with normal hearing, steroids do not improve oscillopsia. Vestibular rehabilitation is currently the only option. Vibrotactile rehabilitative systems may improve general balance but do not restore the vestibulo-ocular reflex (VOR). Vestibular implantation to restore the VOR is currently under investigation.

■ Perilymph Fistulas

A perilymph fistula (PLF) is a defect of the oval or round window that produces abnormal communication between the perilymph surrounding the membranous labyrinth and the middle ear space. In his review, Hornibrook highlights the controversy surrounding PLF over the past 50 years.[9] Spontaneous fistulas are very rare and controversial and seemingly occur without any obvious antecedent event, but it is now known that the antecedent event is often forgotten and sometimes deliberately not mentioned. Using the most stringent criteria, Meyerhoff and Pollock could not identify any event in at least 2% of proven PLF during surgical exploration in 212 patients.[10] The term "idiopathic fistula" may be a better description for this group.

Acquired fistulas due to an antecedent event also include those iatrogenically created during surgery. The pressure force at the oval and round membrane creating the tear can be implosive or explosive. Implosive fistulas arise from increased pressure in the middle ear due to barotrauma, which can be caused by events like rapid airplane descent, blunt trauma to the ear, whiplash, acoustic trauma, and scuba diving. Implosive forces drive the membranes of the oval or round windows inward, tearing them and permitting escape of perilymph into the middle ear space. Explosive fistulas arise from increased intracranial pressure resulting from activities like weight lifting, vigorous coughing, straining, or the Valsalva maneuver. Increased intracranial pressure is theorized to communicate with the perilymphatic space by way of the internal auditory canal or cochlear aqueduct. Explosive forces drive the membranes of the oval and round windows outward, tearing them and permitting escape of perilymph into the middle ear space. Barotraumatic "implosive" forces are most likely to cause a round window fistula, and head trauma is most likely to cause an oval window fistula. The distinction between implosive and explosive is not particularly important, since symptoms and management are similar. In some cases, a "double membrane break" occurs when, in addition to oval and round window membrane rupture, the intralabyrinthine membrane of the cochlear duct also ruptures.

PLF can result from ear surgery, including stapes surgery, chronic ear surgery, and cochlear implantation (CI). Temporal bone anomalies and inner ear malformations increase the likelihood of fistula formation.[11] PLF should be distinguished from a "gusher," which is a term used for the sudden drainage of profuse clear fluid on making an opening into the inner ear. This fluid is CSF and is due to a defect of variable size between the malformed inner ear and the internal auditory canal (IAC). The onset of the CSF drainage can be delayed after surgery.

Because of indistinct, nonspecific features of the history and physical examination, PLF often represents a diagnostic challenge. Other disorders can present in a similar way and therefore it is important to establish a possible precipitating event in the history. The most common complaints include dizziness, imbalance, chronic positional disequilibrium, and episodic vertigo. Nausea and vomiting may accompany intermittent spells lasting anything from a few seconds to hours. Motion intolerance can occur.

Permanent or fluctuating hearing loss, tinnitus, and aural pressure can occur without vestibular complaints. The evidence that PLF is a cause of sudden hearing loss is poor, unless it is preceded by a distinct traumatic event.

The otoscopic examination can be normal, although tympanic membrane perforation, middle ear effusion, and signs of ossicular dislocation may be present. An office fistula test should be performed by gently applying positive-pressure insufflation followed by negative-pressure insufflation of the ear canal with a pneumatic endoscope. The test is positive when the patient complains of increased dizziness (or induced nystagmus with Frenzel glasses). In the absence of clinical middle ear or mastoid disease, a positive fistula test is referred to as the Hennebert sign. Unfortunately, the test is positive in only half of patients with presumed fistula. The Romberg and Fukuda stepping test may demonstrate unilateral hypofunction on the affected side.

Audiometric testing is nonspecific and may reveal a conductive, sensorineural, or mixed hearing loss. The hearing can be normal. Sensorineural hearing loss may fluctuate.

Nystagmography may show spontaneous nystagmus or positional nystagmus, as well as reduced caloric function in the affected ear, or it may be normal. A fistula test performed with impedance audiometry and recorded with nystagmography is more objective than office testing. Valsalva and Tullio testing used in the diagnosis of superior semicircular canal dehiscence (SSCD) may also be positive. Sheppard and others showed a diagnostic specificity of 56% for PLF in patients who demonstrated postural sway with sinusoidal ear canal pressure stimulation on platform posturography (**Video 12.1**).[12]

The role of vestibular evoked myogenic potentials (VEMP) in PLF has not been established. Electrocochleography (ECoG) has been reported to aid in the diagnosis; in that regard, a change on the intraoperative ECoG is considered the most unequivocal evidence that a window fistula is present.[13] Unfortunately, it requires special equipment that is not widely available.

High-resolution computed tomography (CT) of the temporal bone is recommended if labyrinthine fistula or congenital anomaly is suspected, but it is of little help in PLF. Air visualized in the vestibule on CT (pneumolabyrinth), has been described with round window fistulas but is not confirmatory of an active leak.

The indications for, and urgency of, surgical exploration are questioned, since over 90% of PLF heal spontaneously. This creates an ethical dilemma about whether or not to surgically verify with prospective clinical trials the current poor predictability of all preoperative tests.

Stable hearing, resolving dizziness, and sudden hearing loss without an antecedent event usually do not require surgery. In the majority of patients, a trial of rest at home is sufficient, with strict bed rest not really required. Any form of increased pressure should be avoided. Symptomatic relief can be expected from vestibular suppressants, mild sedation, steroids, and laxatives. Since PLF is a rare example of an unstable peripheral organ, vestibular rehabilitation is not effective, and in long-standing cases, contradictory of an active leak.

Many agree that the ear should be explored if dizziness persists or increases or if bone conduction falls on serial audiometry. In an only hearing ear, early exploration can be strongly debated. Poststapedectomy and penetrating trauma fistulas usually require surgery. After cochlear implantation, vertigo usually settles, and if persistent dizziness occurs, exploration should be considered with care.

Transcanal explorative tympanotomy can be performed under general or local anesthesia with sedation. The use of fiberoptic and rigid endoscopes has been described.

Oval window leaks are usually found anterior to the footplate in relation to the fissula ante fenestram. Round window leaks are more common on the inferior attachment and in some cases the bony overhang must be removed with a diamond drill for optimal visualization. After stapedotomy, the round window should also be visualized. Bearing in mind that there are only 75 µL of perilymph, time should be taken to look for a leak. With a more profuse leak, CSF should be suspected. Only a change in the light reflex may be indicative of a leak. If leakage is suctioned away, a drop may not immediately reappear. Packing of absorbable hemostatic gelatin sponge around the windows may limit contamination from other fluid and local anesthetic. Thick mucosal adhesions that obscure the view should be removed.

With the patient under general anesthesia, the anesthetist can be asked to increase the intrathoracic pressure, and positioning the patient in the head-down position can make the leak easier to visualize.

Due to low sensitivity, intraoperative analysis of middle ear fluid in an attempt to confirm perilymph is not advised. The same is true of preoperative lavage of the middle ear in an attempt to avoid unnecessary surgical exploration. Cochlin-tomoprotein (CTP) is a novel perilymph-specific protein, not found in CSF, saliva, or serum. Beta transferrin does not occur in serum and the concentration in perilymph is only 50% of that in CSF. A typical clinical sample of PLF fluid is 0.5 µL and this is often contaminated with plasma or local anesthetic. Visualization of fluorescein in the middle ear after intravenous and intrathecal administration has not really proved beneficial; it can be harmful and is therefore not recommended.

Defects are repaired by connective tissue packing of the involved window and sealed with fibrin glue if available. In 1989, a questionnaire on PLF management was sent to members of the American Otological Society and the American Neurotological Society; 75% of respondents said they would graft a window even if a fistula were not found.[14] This is probably still true today.

The House Ear Clinic reported on the exploration of 86 ears over a 12-year period.[15] When a fistula was found, 68% had an improvement in their major symptom; but when a fistula was not found, 29% felt better anyway, suggesting a placebo effect. In patients in whom a fistula was found, one-third had no history of ear surgery or trauma. Based on this, the House Clinic advocated a very cautious approach to the diagnosis of PLF, especially for sudden hearing loss and in children. When the predominant symptom of suspected PLF is hearing loss, recovery of hearing after surgery is rare.

■ Mal de Debarquement Syndrome

Mal de debarquement (MDD), also known as "sickness of disembarkment," is a disorder characterized by a persistent feeling of dizziness and disequilibrium that usually follows an ocean cruise. It can also occur after air travel, prolonged train rides, space flight, and even skiing. It is rare, with a prevalence estimated at 0.05%, and it can be very distressing.[16] MDD should be distinguished from other forms of motion sickness, such as land sickness. Land sickness is common and occurs in between 47% and 73% of persons disembarking from seagoing voyages.[17] The persistence of motion, however, is short-lived and resolves spontaneously within 2 days, whereas MDD lasts longer than 1 month, and may persist for more than a year.

In 1796, Erasmus Darwin described some of the symptoms of MDD after travelling by boat and stagecoach.[18] MDD has always been considered a variant of motion sickness. Motion sickness or "mal de mer" is commonly experienced while traveling by boat, but in the majority of patients with MDD, symptoms are not experienced until after disembarking.[6] On the contrary, it is often reported that travelling afterward reduces the symptoms of MDD.

Patients with MDD complain mainly of a persistent sensation of swaying, rocking, or bobbing immediately or shortly after cessation of the voyage. Spinning vertigo is uncommon. In severe cases, patients may complain of disorientation, impaired cognition, fatigue, ataxia, insomnia, headache, anxiety, and depression. In a case series of 27 individuals, Hain et al reported that 93% of subjects indicated rocking and 81% indicated swaying, with imbalance less common (74%).[19] They further indicated that the mean duration of symptoms was 3.5 years, with a range of 1 to 10 years. Symptoms were constant in 85% and intermittent in 15%. MDD mainly affects women: according to a 2014 survey of the Chicago Dizziness and Hearing database, 93 out of 109 patients (85%) were females between 30 and 50 years old.[16]

The pathomechanism of MDD is still controversial. The predominant opinion is that it is a variant of motion sickness. On the other hand, motion sickness does not really explain the female and age predominance in MDD; therefore, some experts believe that it is related to migraine. The female preponderance has also raised the question whether genetics (the two X chromosomes) and female hormones can perhaps contribute.

Some experts still believe that MDD is a somatization disorder or a form of anxiety. There are some reports of MDD following use or withdrawal from serotonergic medications. Serotonin may inhibit glutamate, which is an excitatory transmitter in the vestibular nucleus. The data supporting the hypothesis that MDD is caused by reweighting of visual, vestibular, or somatosensory input are contradictory. Nachum et al hypothesized that there is an increased reliance on somatosensory input after motion exposure, and a reduced weighting of vision and vestibular input.[20] In contrast to this, Peterka suggested an increased reliance on visual and vestibular information (and thus decreased somatosensory weighting).[21] This occurs in normal subjects who are exposed to situations where somatosensory feedback is distorted.

Currently the two most attractive proposed mechanisms for the development of MDD are the inappropriate internal predictive model and maladaptation of the VOR to the roll of the head during rotation. An internal predictive model is a method whereby someone reacts to an event before it happens.[22] It appears that after a few days on a boat, a person develops an internal model of the periodic motion in his brain. With this model, he predicts and cancels out visual or somatosensory input that is phase-locked to pitch rotation, and enhances responses due to surge that is not. This predictive model of boat motion is selected and applied to avoid falling. When back on land, this model is usually disposed of within hours to days; but in patients with MDD, it takes months and even years to disappear. Patients then benefit from this model only when in motion, for instance when driving in a car. The rest of the time they are symptomatic.

Dai et al recently proposed that MDD was caused by maladaptation of the VOR to roll of the head during rotation.[23] This maladaptation was previously produced in humans in NASA space flight experiments.[24] In monkeys, it was shown that only those with long VOR time-constants developed abnormalities, implying that the maladaptation of the VOR depends on the velocity storage mechanism. Velocity storage is the central vestibular mechanism that allows peripheral labyrinthine responses that fatigue with sustained rotational stimulation to be prolonged. It ultimately allows the ability of the VOR to transduce the low-frequency component of head rotation. Maladaptation adds vertical and horizontal components to ocular torsion induced by head roll and body oscillations at a frequency centered on 0.2 Hz.

The diagnosis of MDD is based on the development of symptoms after a sea voyage or prolonged exposure to motion, an improvement when driving, and the exclusion of other vestibular pathology. Motion exposure is on the order of 7 days, with 2 hours being a minimum. The clinical examination, audiometry, and imaging studies are usually unremarkable. If symptoms occur after a flight, perilymphatic fistula should be considered.

There are no vestibular test findings specific to MDD. In a case series by Baloh, quantitative vestibular testing in patients with MDD revealed no consistent abnormality, although a static direction-changing positional nystagmus was noted in 50%.[25]

Treatment of MDD is still predominantly medical and is mostly ineffective. As stated by Hain, it is merely aimed at making the patient comfortable while awaiting spontaneous remission.[16] Despite potentially being addictive, benzodiazepines, such as low-dose clonazepam, seem to help the majority of patients. Antidizziness and motion-sickness drugs, including meclizine, Dramamine (Prestige), scopolamine, betahistine, baclofen, and verapamil, are of little to no benefit. Anecdotal reports supported the use of some antimigraine drugs, such as gabapentin, amitriptyline, and venlafaxine. SSRI-type antidepressants, dopamine agonists, phenytoin, carbamazepine, and even nonsteroidal anti-inflammatories have been reported to be helpful in selected cases. In 2013, Cha et al, in a pilot study, proposed repetitive transcranial magnetic stimulation (TMS) over the dorsolateral prefrontal cortex to offer short-term symptom improvement.[26] Evidence supporting the benefit of physical (balance) therapy is lacking. Although movement by self-motion or driving is often beneficial, it is not advised as treatment and may even prolong symptoms. Surgery plays no role.

Dai et al reported that re-adaptation of the VOR relieves the symptoms in MDD.[23] Using a full-field optokinetic stimulus, given while the head was rolled at the frequency of the subjects' rocking (usually around 0.2 Hz), reversed the MDD in 23 out of

24 patients. Unfortunately, the treatment effects regressed in six patients. In the other 17 (70%), the MDD was cured or substantially reduced for prolonged periods (mean follow-up = 11.6 months). This approach is currently under further investigation.

Patients who suffered with MDD previously and who need to travel may benefit from small dosages of clonazepam before and during the voyage. It is also advised that they walk on deck only when the sea is calm and the horizon is clearly visible.

■ Alcohol-Related Dizziness

Alcohol is a common cause of dizziness. The relationship between the timing and quantity of alcohol ingestion and onset of symptoms is important when analyzing the effects of alcohol. The social and economic effects of alcohol-related injuries as a result of dizziness and disequilibrium are far reaching and beyond the scope of this chapter.

Acute alcohol intoxication is associated with gait imbalance, slurring of speech, and, at times, vertigo. Nausea and vomiting often accompany a sensation of impending doom. The stereotypical gait ataxia and dysarthria are suggestive of cerebellar involvement, although vestibular pathways are probably involved as well. The direct effect of alcohol on vestibular nuclei has been noted in animal studies, where synaptic transmission was impaired.[27] Vestibular testing in patients with alcohol intoxication has revealed normal vestibulo-ocular reflex (VOR) gain, albeit with impaired fixation suppression of vestibular nystagmus. This is consistent with cerebellar dysfunction.[28] With moderate alcohol ingestion, slowing of saccades and smooth pursuit eye movement is consistently observed.

Gaze-evoked nystagmus is commonly observed with alcohol ingestion. This nystagmus is predominantly observed with horizontal eye movements, with the fast phase of the nystagmus in the same direction as the direction of gaze. This is a reliable sign of intoxication, the magnitude of which is highly correlated with blood alcohol concentration.[29]

Positional nystagmus, and the associated vertigo, is another effect of alcohol on the vestibular system. This phenomenon has been well studied, particularly with regard to amount, type, and rate of alcohol ingestion.[30] In 1911, Barany described the direction-changing characteristics of positional alcohol nystagmus (PAN) in humans with changes in head position.[31] The specific gravity of alcohol is less than that of endolymph. When alcohol blood levels approach 40 mg/dL, alcohol diffuses into the cupula via its adjacent vascular supply. This makes the cupula lighter than endolymph, transforming the semicircular canals into receptors that are sensitive to gravity. Vertigo and nystagmus then occur in the supine position. In the first phase of alcohol induced nystagmus (PAN I or resorptive phase), start-ing ~ 30 minutes after ingestion of alcohol, a geotropic nystagmus is seen, with the fast phase of nystagmus toward the lower ear. This phase may last 3 to 4 hours. The nystagmus is suppressed by visual fixation. This is an important point, as centrally mediated nystagmus is not fixatable, supporting that this phenomenon is peripheral in nature. After PAN I, there is a "silent intermediate period" where there is neither positional nystagmus nor vertigo. This takes place 3 to 5 hours after alcohol ingestion and occurs as alcohol diffuses into the endolymph, with the specific gravities of the cupula and endolymph approaching one another.

The next phase, referred to as the reduction phase or PAN II, occurs 5 to 10 hours after alcohol ingestion, and the direction of nystagmus is opposite that of PAN I, with nystagmus toward the upper ear. This is the case because the specific gravity differential is such that the endolymph becomes "heavier" than the cupula with alcohol moving out of the cupula and into the endolymph. This period is when "hangover vertigo" may be experienced. Positional vertigo may persist until the alcohol completely leaves the endolymph but may not occur until hours after the blood alcohol level has reached zero. PAN II is usually associated with motion sickness and is a major contributor to the hangover. The "morning after" drink thus may have a physiological basis, transiently lessening the intensity of the hangover. The practical implication of PAN is recognized and respected in the aviation industry, where airline pilots are not permitted to fly within 8 to 12 hours of consuming alcohol. The question is whether this "throttle to the bottle" rule should not be extended to 48 hours, in light of PAN.

Chronic alcohol intake leads to cerebellar atrophy and Purkinje cell loss, particularly in the anterior vermis.[32] The Purkinje cells regulate and coordinate motor movements by means of inhibition of certain neurons. Wernicke's encephalopathy, which occurs in alcoholics, is due to a thiamine deficiency. It consists of a triad of acute confusion, ataxia, and ophthalmoplegia and may be fatal if untreated. The ataxia is predominantly related to acute vestibular hypofunction. This syndrome may progress to Korsakoff's syndrome, which is characterized by a memory deficit in which the person is unable to establish new memories. Patients are noted to confabulate, and this behavior may be used to cover up gaps in memory.[33]

Some patients may report a temporary improvement in their dizzy symptoms after consuming small amounts of alcohol.[34] In these cases, the possibility of phobic postural vertigo (PPV), chronic subjective dizziness (CSD), or what is nowadays classified as persistent postural perceptual dizziness (PPPD) should be considered.[35] In these conditions, alcohol acts as an anxiolytic with which patients self-medicate.

Alcohol is highly toxic to the inner ear when absorbed through the round window, a fact to be taken into account with local application of alcohol-containing eardrops and solutions.

AutoImmune Vestibular Dysfunction

Q1: The hallmarks of AIED are rapidly progressive bilateral sensorineural hearing loss, normal clinical examination, and a positive response to oral steroids.

Q2: Anti-heat shock protein 70 (anti-HSP 70) is diagnostic for AIED.

Q3: Positional vertigo occurs in 90% of patients with AIED.

Q4: Vertigo in AIED should be managed by early surgical intervention, the only effective way to avoid falls.

Q5: In patients with BVF and normal hearing, antibodies attack the ampullae of the semicircular canals.

Perilymph Fistulas

Q6: Perilymph fistulas (PLF) are common after trauma, and early surgical intervention is required to prevent permanent hearing loss.

Q7: Fluctuating hearing loss after scuba diving is diagnostic of a PLF.

Q8: The endoscopic approach to confirmation and closure of a PLF is preferred above explorative tympanotomy because it is less traumatic, easier, and safer.

Q9: A fistula test performed with nystagmography and impedance audiometry is more objective than office testing.

Q10: When conservative management fails and a PLF does not close, vestibular rehabilitation is successful and is the treatment of choice.

Mal de Debarquement Syndrome

Q11: Mal de debarquement syndrome (MDD) is a common condition in deep-sea fisherman during rough seas.

Q12: MDD should be considered in patients with new-onset vertigo after 1 week of disembarking.

Q13: Patients with MDD often report disappearance of symptoms while travelling in a motor vehicle.

Q14: Research supports the idea that an abnormal velocity storage system may be responsible for MDD.

Q15: Benzodiazepines (e.g., clonazepam) are an excellent choice for treating MDD and usually cure the problem after continuous use for 3 months.

Alcohol-Related Dizziness

Q16: Gaze nystagmus is commonly observed with alcohol intoxication.

Q17: Positional alcohol nystagmus (PAN) occurs due to the higher specific gravity of alcohol than that of endolymph.

Q18: The cerebellum is not affected by alcohol.

Q19: Chronic alcohol use can lead to thiamine deficiency, which can be fatal if untreated.

Q20: Moderate alcohol consumption may improve dizziness in patients with phobic postural vertigo (PPV) due to suppression of the vestibulo-ocular reflex (VOR).

Answers

A1: True

A2: False

A3: False

A4: False

A5: False

A6: False

A7: False

A8: False

A9: True

A10: False

A11: False

A12: False

A13: True

A14: True

A15: False

A16: True

A17: False

A18: False

A19: True

A20: False

References

1. Hughes GB, Cherian N. Autoimmune vestibular dysfunction, perilymph fistula, mal de debarquement syndrome and alcohol-related dizziness. In: Weber PC, ed. Vertigo and Disequilibrium. A Practical Guide to Diagnosis and Management. 1st ed. New York, NY: Thieme Medical Publishers Inc; 2008

2. Bovo R, Ciorba A, Martini A. Vertigo and autoimmunity. Eur Arch Otorhinolaryngol 2010;267(1):13–19

3. Yukawa K, Hagiwara A, Ogawa Y, et al. Bilateral progressive hearing loss and vestibular dysfunction with inner ear antibodies. Auris Nasus Larynx 2010; 37(2):223–228

4. Harris JP. Immunology of the inner ear: evidence of local antibody production. Ann Otol Rhinol Laryngol 1984;93(2 Pt 1):157–162

5. Matsuoka AJ, Harris JP. Autoimmune inner ear disease: a retrospective review of forty-seven patients. Audiol Neurootol 2013;18(4):228–239

6. Harris JP, Weisman MH, Derebery JM, et al. Treatment of corticosteroid-responsive autoimmune inner ear disease with methotrexate: a randomized controlled trial. JAMA 2003;290(14):1875–1883

7. Hain TC. Autoimmune Inner Ear Disease (AIED) [Internet]. 2015 [updated 2015 Feb 4; cited 2015 Jun 22]. Available from: http://dizziness-and-balance.com/disorders/central/aied.html

8. Greco A, Gallo A, Fusconi M, Marinelli C, Macri GF, de Vincentiis M. Meniere's disease might be an autoimmune condition? Autoimmun Rev 2012; 11(10):731–738

9. Hornibrook J. Perilymph fistula: fifty years of controversy. ISRN Otolaryngol 2012;2012:281248

10. Meyerhoff WL, Pollock KJ. A patient-oriented approach to perilymph fistula. Arch Otolaryngol Head Neck Surg 1990;116(11):1317–1319

11. Sennaroglu L. Cochlear implantation in inner ear malformations—a review article. Cochlear Implants Int 2010;11(1):4–41

12. Shepard NT, Telian SA, Niparko JK, Kemink JL, Fujita S. Platform pressure test in identification of perilymphatic fistula. Am J Otol 1992;13(1):49–54

13. Gibson WPR. Electrocochleography in the diagnosis of perilymphatic fistula: intraoperative observations and assessment of a new diagnostic office procedure. Am J Otol 1992;13(2):146–151

14. Hughes GB, Sismanis A, House JW. Is there consensus in perilymph fistula management? Otolaryngol Head Neck Surg 1990;102(2):111–117

15. Rizer FM, House JW. Perilymph fistulas: the House Ear Clinic experience. Otolaryngol Head Neck Surg 1991;104(2):239–243

16. Hain TC. Mal de Debarquement Syndrome (MDD or MdDS) [Internet]. 2015 [updated 2015 May 27; cited 2015 Jun 10]. Available from: http://dizziness-and-balance.com/disorders/central/mdd.html

17. Gordon CR, Shupak A, Nachum Z. Mal de debarquement. Arch Otolaryngol Head Neck Surg 2000;126(6):805–806

18. Darwin E. Zoonomia. London: J. Johnson; 1796.

19. Hain TC, Hanna PA, Rheinberger MA. Mal de debarquement. Arch Otolaryngol Head Neck Surg 1999;125(6):615–620

20. Nachum Z, Shupak A, Letichevsky V, et al. Mal de debarquement and posture: reduced reliance on vestibular and visual cues. Laryngoscope 2004; 114(3):581–586

21. Peterka RJ. Sensorimotor integration in human postural control. J Neurophysiol 2002;88(3):1097–1118

22. Blakemore SJ, Goodbody SJ, Wolpert DM. Predicting the consequences of our own actions: the role of sensorimotor context estimation. J Neurosci 1998;18(18):7511–7518

23. Dai M, Cohen B, Smouha E, Cho C. Readaptation of the vestibulo-ocular reflex relieves the mal de debarquement syndrome. Front Neurol 2014;5:124

24. Guedry FE Jr, Graybiel A. Compensatory nystagmus conditioned during adaptation to living in a rotating room. J Appl Physiol 1962;17:398–404

25. Brown JJ, Baloh RW. Persistent mal de debarquement syndrome: a motion-induced subjective disorder of balance. Am J Otolaryngol 1987;8(4):219–222

26. Cha YH, Cui Y, Baloh RW. Repetitive transcranial magnetic stimulation for mal de debarquement syndrome. Otol Neurotol 2013;34(1):175–179

27. Kashii S, Ito J, Matsuoka I, Sasa M, Takaori S. Effects of ethanol applied by electrosmosis on neurons in the lateral and medial vestibular nuclei. Jpn J Pharmacol 1984;36(2):153–159

28. Umeda Y, Sakata E. Alcohol and the oculomotor system. Ann Otol Rhinol Laryngol 1978;87(3 Pt 1):392–398

29. Goding GS, Dobie RA. Gaze nystagmus and blood alcohol. Laryngoscope 1986;96(7):713–717

30. Aschan G, Bergstedt M. Positional alcoholic nystagmus (PAN) in man following repeated alcohol doses. Acta Otolaryngol Suppl 1975;330:15–29

31. Barany R. Experimentelle Alkoholintoxikation. Mschr Ohrenheilk 1911;45:959–962

32. Andersen BB. Reduction of Purkinje cell volume in cerebellum of alcoholics. Brain Res 2004;1007(1-2):10–18

33. Victor M, Adams RD, Collins CH. The Wernicke-Korsakoff Syndrome. Philadelphia, PA: FA Davis;1971

34. Brandt T. Phobic postural vertigo. Neurology 1996; 46(6):1515–1519

35. Staab JP. Chronic subjective dizziness. Continuum (Mineapp. Minn.). Neurotology 2012;18:1118–1141

13 Allergy and Autonomic Dizziness

Louis M. Hofmeyr and Marcelle Groenewald

■ Introduction

Vertigo and disequilibrium have many causes. Allergy and autonomic dysfunction are well recognized in the literature as two of these causes. However, in clinical practice they are often overlooked or even missed by general practitioners. If the prevalence in the general population is taken into account, it would suggest that more patients may be suffering from vertigo or disequilibrium due to these causes than is presently thought to be the case. Health care practitioners should be more aware of these two possible causes.

■ Allergy

Allergy-associated dizziness refers to vertigo and disequilibrium mediated primarily by the allergic involvement of the vestibular system. In general, symptoms of allergic disease, side effects of medication used in the management of allergy, and anaphylactic reactions all may include nonspecific dizziness and lightheadedness of varying severity. The end-organ targeted by the allergic response may include not only the vestibular system but also the other systems responsible for image stabilization, spatial orientation, and balance control.

The prevalence of allergic diseases has been on the increase in the industrialized world for more than 60 years, affecting 10 to 30% of the population[1] and more than 1 billion people worldwide. This is expected to reach 4 billion by the 2050s.[2] The increase in allergic rhinitis, asthma, and atopic eczema is defined as the "allergic epidemic."[1] Food allergy is becoming more prevalent in the westernized world and has doubled in the last decade, with a sevenfold increase in hospital admissions for severe reactions (anaphylaxis) in Europe. This is known as the "second wave" of the allergic epidemic.[3] Sensitization rates to one or more common allergens among school children are currently approaching 40 to 50%.[4]

The terminology used to describe allergic and allergy-like reactions is confusing. Therefore, the World Allergy Organization Nomenclature Review Committee[5] revised the nomenclature, which now states that the term *hypersensitivity* should be used for "all reactions" that result in objectively reproducible symptoms and signs initiated by exposure to a defined stimulus that is tolerated by normal persons. *Allergy* is a hypersensitivity reaction initiated by immunologic mechanisms and can be antibody- or cell-mediated. It can be either IgE-mediated (IgE antibodies) or non-IgE-mediated (IgG antibodies, immune complexes, allergen-specific lymphocytes). *Atopy* is a genetic (inherited) tendency to produce IgE antibodies, usually to protein allergens in childhood or adolescence, and can produce typical symptoms of eczema, rhinoconjunctivitis, or asthma. Allergy symptoms in a typical atopic individual can be referred to as *atopic*, as in atopic asthma. *Non-allergic hypersensitivity* describes hypersensitivity reactions in which immunologic mechanisms cannot be proven (e.g., aspirin hypersenistivity). *Sensitivity* is an alternative term for special circumstances within the field of environmental medicine (e.g., total drug sensitivity, multiple chemical sensitivity, and symptomatic reactions attributed to amalgam in tooth fillings and electrical waves) that do not fill the criteria to be called hypersensitivity. An *allergen* is an antigen causing allergic disease.

The allergic diseases are one of the most chronic diseases and involve many organs, such as the eyes, respiratory tract, gastrointestinal tract, and skin. The diseases include rhinoconjunctivitis, asthma, eczema, urticaria, and angioedema, as well as drug and food allergies and anaphylaxis, and they vary in severity and clinical course.[1] Allergic conjunctivitis (AC—acute or perennial) is the most common allergic eye disorder and affects ~ 25% of the population.[6] Allergic rhinitis (AR) is the most chronic noncommunicable disease, affects 10 to 20% of the total population, and may be a predisposing factor for development of disease in the adjacent structures, such as the paranasal sinuses, middle ear, nasopharynx, and larynx. Failing to diagnose sensitization to inhalant allergens could result in inadequate management of rhinosinusitis, tubal dysfunction, middle ear problems, laryngopharyngeal disorders, and dysphonia. The upper and lower airways are viewed as one entity and AR and allergic asthma are considered part of the airway allergy syndrome.[6] Asthma is a global and chronic inflammatory disease affecting 1 to 18% of the population, depending on the country.[6] The global prevalence of asthma ranges from 4.5% in young adults to 14% in children.[7] In the industrialized countries, atopic eczema has increased two- to threefold and now affects up to 20% of children and 2 to 10% of adults. This increase in prevalence may be linked to the Western lifestyle.[6] Food allergy (FA) is an adverse reaction to food, caused by an overreaction of the immune system, and affects ~ 3 to 8% of children and 1 to 5% of adults. These responses can be mediated by IgE antibodies, by immune cells, or by a combination of both.[8] Drug allergy affects 7% of the general population and has doubled in the last decade.[6]

The *inhalant allergens* mainly involved are grass pollens, house dust mites, tree pollen, animal dander, and molds and vary according to geographic region. The most common *food allergens* in children are milk, hen's eggs, peanuts, tree nuts, soya, and wheat. In adults, the most common food allergens are fish, shellfish, peanuts, tree nuts, fruits, and vegetables. Usually, peanuts, tree nuts, and seafood allergies are seldom outgrown. Other foods may be more prevalent in certain countries. Allergic reactions can be triggered by food, sometimes in very small amounts or even by inhalation and skin contact.[8] The most common cause of anaphylaxis in children is food; in adults, drugs and *Hymenoptera* venom. In drug allergy, the most common allergen in children is penicillin; in adults, nonsteroidal anti-inflammatory drugs (NSAIDs), penicillin and related antibiotics, and sulfonamides.

The atopic (allergic) march is defined as the progression of atopic diseases, generally during childhood, and the first steps are usually atopic eczema and food allergies, followed later by respiratory allergies, including asthma and AR.[6] With early onset of eczema in the first few weeks or months of life, ~ 30% of children will suffer from AR and/or asthma, and if the eczema is more severe, this increases to 50%. In infancy, FA is often seen with eczema, especially in boys, and children with multiple FAs have a higher risk of developing asthma.[8] Milk, egg, and peanut allergens account for 80 to 90% of all eczema in the infant in the first year of life. Milk protein is the first allergen the infant encounters and milk allergy is the most common FA in infants (2–5%), inducing a larger spectrum of allergic diseases (eczema, asthma, and AR) and possibly heralding the start of a long-last-ing atopic disease. Associated hypersensitivity reactions to other foods develop in ~ 50% and allergy to inhalants in 50 to 80% before puberty. Egg-specific IgE, with a positive family history (FH) of atopy, is a highly specific and predictive marker for sensitization to inhalant allergens at 3 to 4 years of age, and the child will develop either upper airway (AR) or lower airway disease (asthma).[6] Clinical FA and IgE sensitization to food often precede the development of asthma.[8] About 80% of asthma patients have associated AR and/or rhinosinusitis and 40% of AR patients develop asthma later.[9]

The head and neck are the most commonly affected areas in an allergic response. Lasisi and Abdullahi found ear symptoms in 66% of patients with nasal allergy.[10] Vertigo was found in 13% and peripheral vestibular signs of imbalance were seen in 9%. The scientific basis for the involvement of the inner ear is poorly understood. The endolymphatic sac and duct are considered to be the immunoactive parts of the inner ear that secrete immunoglobulins and immunocompetent cells, and they may be the target of mediators released from the systemic inhalant or food reactions.[11] Furthermore, the deposition of circulating immune complex can produce inflammation and interference with the sac's filtering capability, and a predisposing viral infection may interact with allergies in adulthood and cause the endolymphatic sac to decompensate, resulting in endolymphatic hydrops.[12]

In 1923, Duke was the first to report on a suspected allergic etiology for Meniere's disease (MD). Derebery has suggested that 30% of patients with MD have food allergy.[12] The prevalence of allergy in patients with MD was established as ~ 41.6% for inhalants and 26.6% for food. The prevalence of type I hypersensitivity reactions to inhalants and food in the MD population evaluated was greater than in the general population. Allergy is believed to be one of the possible extrinsic factors that combine with underlying intrinsic factors to lead to MD.[13]

Electrocochleography (ECoG) has been shown to document changes in inner ear function objectively after intranasal challenge of patients with inhalant allergy (with no prior immunotherapy) and MD, using antigen to which they were most sensitive.[14] Whether immunotherapy is able to reduce symptoms in patients with MD needs further clarification. Although some authors question the role of the sac and hydrops in the development of MD, a significant proportion of patients with cochlear hydrops showed improvement in their symptoms following treatment of inhalant and food allergy.[12] Eustachian tube (ET) dysfunction with blockage may be due to underlying inhalant or food allergies.[15] With or without a middle-ear effusion, ET dysfunction has been considered one of the most common causes of balance disturbances in young children. Balance problems are found in 50% of children with chronic serous otitis media (CSOM) and serous otitis media (SOM) may be associated with both hearing loss and vertigo.[16] Mostafa and coworkers found that in adults with CSOM, 54% complained of vertigo. Rotatory chair abnormalities were found in 70% of the cases, caloric hypofunction in 61.6%, and abnormal vestibular evoked myogenic potentials in 25%.[17] These findings implied the involvement of both the semicircular canals and the saccule. Possible mechanisms of inner ear involvement may include pressure changes with restricted movement at the oval and round windows and the spread of toxins, inflammation, and immunocompetent particles to the inner ear.

Alternobaric vertigo is a condition that occurs in scuba divers. Up to 25% of divers may experience it at some time.[18] The dizziness results from unequal pressure changes being exerted between the ears during especially ascent, descent, or immediately after surfacing. It is believed to happen when the two ETs do not function in tandem, with one opening slower or later than the other. Perilymph fistula (PLF) of the oval and round windows is a more serious cause of audiovestibular symptoms and occurs due to rapid pressure changes, especially with underlying ET dysfunction. Since the function of the ET may be influenced by allergy, allergy can therefore contribute to a higher incidence of alternobaric vertigo and PLF.

The existing medical literature supports a correlation between allergy and migraine.[19] Allergy occurs more often in migraine patients with vertigo and motion sickness than in those without. In general, food allergy presents more specifically with migraine headaches, gastrointestinal upset, or chronic colitis. Headaches are otherwise not associated with MD. It is possible that the success of dietary control in the management of migraine with or without vestibular symptoms may be related to the avoidance of an underlying food allergen. Nonallergic (nonimmunological) mechanisms may also be involved for food-related migraine. Additives and chemicals have all been implicated, for example ethanol, sodium nitrate, caffeine, monosodium glutamate, sodium metabisulfite, theobromine, and benzoic acid. This may also depend on the direct effect of the vasoactive amines naturally found in foods, for example histamine, tyramine, phenylethylamine, and serotonin. The largest amount of histamine and tyramine are found in fermented foods such as cheese, alcoholic beverages, canned fish, tuna, sauerkraut, and also in chocolate, peanuts, tree nuts, and coffee, for example. The latter are called "trigger foods," but milk and wheat have also been implicated. Some patients have symptoms after eating a very small amount of food containing one or more amines, while others react after an accumulative effect of a few days.

Allergy is a major contributor in the development and management of asthma. Individuals with asthma demonstrated a greater area for the center of pressure

(CoP) displacement under somatosensory perturbations and a higher velocity in the forward-backward direction on a mobile balance platform when vestibular information only was made available, in comparison to a control group.[20] The relationship between asthma and anxiety has consistently been described in the literature. Up to a third of patients with anxiety may experience dizziness and balance disorders.[21] The strong correlation between anxiety-asthma and anxiety-balance disorders suggests that balance abnormalities may also be present in asthmatic patients.

Balance disorders and ataxia are common with cerebellar disease. Acute cerebellar ataxia has been reported after administration of the human papilloma virus (HPV)-16/18 vaccine, with the short temporal association strongly suggesting an allergic reaction to the vaccine.[22] Some patients with celiac disease, the classic form of wheat allergy, develop cerebellar ataxia. This is believed to be due to an immune reaction of the human body to gluten, the protein responsible for wheat allergy, causing damage to the cerebellum.[23] A detailed history should be taken of the indoor and outdoor allergens, the food ingested, environmental factors, and a personal and family history of atopy, to help determine the possible association with the symptom of dizziness. Allergy should be considered in all dizzy patients, especially with bilateral ear involvement, with a history of seasonal or weather-related symptoms, other allergic symptoms, atopic eczema, asthma, and allergic rhinosinusitis, or in patients refractory to usual medical therapy. Lightheadedness and dizziness are common symptoms of food allergies. It can occur immediately after eating the offending food but also hours later, often disguising the relationship between trigger and symptoms. In young children who present with balance problems, unsteady gait, pulling at the ear(s), banging the head against the cot, trouble hearing (especially when spoken to from behind), and restless sleep, CSOM should be considered and the child should be investigated for food allergies. Older children and adults may complain of a "popping" sensation in the ear, earache, or deafness.

Although the bedside neurotologic examination may be normal, the clinician is more likely to observe some symptoms and signs of the specific disease(s) involved. *Allergic rhinoconjunctivitis* presents with the classical symptoms of rhinorrhea, sneezing, itchy nose and eyes, and watery, red, bloodshot eyes. There is a marked "allergic facies"; twitching of the nose and mouth to relieve itching; a broad nasal bridge together with a nasal crease (Darrier's line) due to the "allergic salute," when the patient rubs the nose upward to relieve itching and nasal congestion; mouth breathing due to the blocked nose; and lower lid eye creases (Denne-Morgan lines) together with periorbital edema and bluish-black discoloration under the lower eyelids ("allergic shiners").[9] The comorbid condition of *rhinosinusitis* presents with blocked nose, with or without polyps, a chronic postnasal drip, enlarged lymphoid tissue of the pharynx (cobblestone appearance), and a cough that is often mistaken for asthma. Evidence of wheezing and eczema may be found. However, eczema lesions around the mouth are an indication that a culprit food or drink has been ingested, as eczema is sparing of the perioral region in the young child. In children with SOM, pneumatic otoscopy and immitance of the middle ear may support the diagnosis.

Allergy diagnosis depends mainly on the clinical history and physical examination and is supported by some tests. Two tests commonly used to determine IgE antibodies are skin prick tests (SPTs) and allergen-specific IgE in the serum (ImmunoCAP). For food allergen SPTs, standardized commercial extracts and fresh extracts can be used. Positive SPTs and allergen-specific serum IgE results for specific food and inhalant allergens indicate sensitization to the allergen, but not necessarily clinical symptoms. Negative results do not indicate that the patient is not allergic, because the reaction may be by other immunologic pathways; for example, milk allergy may be either IgE-mediated or non-IgE-mediated. Elimination of the suspected food(s) or oral food challenges may be necessary to confirm the diagnosis of FA. Generally, the stronger the positive reaction, the more likely the patient is allergic to the allergen. CAST testing (cellular allergen stimulation test) is indicated in certain food allergies, reactions to additives (colorants, flavorants, preservatives), and drug allergies, because these allergens have a small molecular structure and reactions are mainly non-IgE-mediated. CAST testing sensitivity is ~ 80%. Iron-deficiency anemia is common in children with food allergies and recurrent upper respiratory tract infections. Therefore, a full blood count and iron studies should always be done.

Imaging, such as chest X-rays in asthma or computed tomography (CT) of the nose and paranasal sinuses, may support target organ involvement in general allergic disease, but it is usually not helpful in assessing the involvement of the inner ear and vestibular system. In small children with imbalance that persists after management of SOM, magnetic resonance imaging (MRI) with gadolinium is indicated to rule out a posterior fossa tumor. A vestibular test is only requested to support a specific diagnosis, but should not be requested to prove the presence of an allergy. In cases where allergies have been identified as the root cause, the specific treatment can improve the dizziness. However, it is important to first determine the reason for the dizziness and then to treat accordingly, before assuming allergy is the cause. Based on a strong history and clinical findings, treatment can be started empirically for the dizziness.

Allergic rhinoconjunctivitis is mainly a clinical diagnosis and the management is mainly threefold:

1. *Environmental control:* Avoiding known triggers, such as foods and indoor and outdoor inhalants, as far as possible, together with avoiding the adjuvant triggers, such as cold air, tobacco, and wood smoke.

2. *Pharmacotherapy:* Second-generation nonsedating antihistamines should be used, such as cetirizine, levoceterizine, fexofenadine, loratidine, and desloratidine, because they have greater selectivity for the peripheral H_1 receptors. Intranasal steroids (INS) are first-line drugs to reduce the inflammation and congestion in the nose and for moderate to severe AR. The main INS are budesinide, beclomethasone, fluticosone propionate, and mometasone. They are often combined with antihistamines. Leukotriene antagonists (e.g., montelukast) are indicated in seasonal AR, in preschool children with AR, and in comorbid asthma and AC. Combination with antihistamines appears to be beneficial.[9] Topical nasal and ocular antihistamines, together with mast cell stabilizers, are also very effective.

3. *Allergen immunotherapy (AIT)* is the only disease-modifying treatment with long-lasting effects. The two most common routes are subcutaneous injections (SCIT) and sublingual drops or tablets (SLIT). However, as AIT is given as a treatment for 3 to 5 years, compliance is poor, especially with SLIT, as it requires a daily maintenance dose. Unlike pharmacotherapy, the effects of AIT persists once discontinued and can prevent new allergen sensitizations or progression to asthma. Oral immunotherapy is being investigated for food allergy at present and may prove to be useful in the future.[6]

Although the timing of drainage and placement of ventilation tubes is still debated, it should be seriously considered if a child has SOM or CSOM with balance problems. Peripherally acting histamines, such as loratidine, fexofenadine, and cetirizine, should be used in patients taking betahistine for MD.[24] Betahistine is a histamine analogue that has a central effect and is neutralized by centrally acting antihistamines and antidepressants with antihistaminergic properties, such as amitriptyline.

■ Autonomic Dizziness

Autonomic dizziness is any form of dizziness that follows or is caused by dysfunction of the autonomic nervous system. The attacks in Meniere's disease

(MD) are often accompanied by autonomic manifestations, such as increased heart rate, vomiting, sweating, hyperventilation, and even diarrhea. In this section, however, the focus is on vertigo and disequilibrium caused by autonomic dysfunction.

The autonomic nervous system is part of the nervous system that functions mostly on a subconscious level. It helps to regulate functions like heart rate, blood pressure, digestion, and respiratory rate, etc. It can be divided into the sympathetic "fight or flight" system and the parasympathetic "rest and digest" system. The hypothalamus regulates and maintains the constant dynamic balance between the two. If the sympathetic system prevails, it is referred to as the adrenergic state, which is characterized by increased heart rate, elevated blood pressure, and an exaggerated response to a stimulus that usually provokes a normal adrenergic response, such as standing up. An increase in the parasympathetic tone, referred to as a hypervagal state, leads to slowing of the heart rate, lowered blood pressure, and an exaggerated response to normal stimuli, such as urination and digestion. It is also possible that the regulation of both systems may be impaired.

A functional autonomic system relies on the structural and functional integrity of all its components. The autonomic reflex is generated in receptor organs that respond to specific stimuli (e.g., the baroreceptors respond to blood pressure). Functional nerve tracts and central nervous system regulation are required to affect the different systems throughout the body in an organized manner. Should there be a disruption of these pathways, numerous symptoms can arise, including dizziness and disequilibrium. Other autonomic symptoms include palpitations, anxiety, headache, sweating, fatigue, gastrointestinal upset, and syncope.

The incidence of autonomic dysfunction is unknown. Pappas found that 5% of patients presenting with vertigo in his series had autonomic dysfunction.[25] Females predominated, with a 15:1 ratio, similar to figures found in other autonomic dysfunction studies. In a series of 1,291 patients presenting with complaints of vertigo, dizziness, or disequilibrium, Ohashi and coworkers found a 10% incidence of orthostatic hypotension (OH).[26] Although dysautonomia and OH are well described in the literature, autonomic vertigo is seldom mentioned. Vertigo associated with autonomic dysfunction, OH, or mitral valve prolapse may represent one of several forms of dizziness experienced by the dysautonomic individual. True vertigo may be more common than previously anticipated. OH is defined as dizziness and lightheadedness due to a prolonged drop in blood pressure after standing up and has many potential causes, including heart conditions, dehydration, certain drugs, and heat exposure. Diabetes causes microangiopathy, affecting nerve function, and is an example of a metabolic cause for dysautonomia and OH. Underlying diseases of the brain, spinal cord, or nervous system, such as

Parkinson's disease, multiple system atrophy, pure autonomic failure, and certain neuropathies, cause neurogenic dysautonomia and neurogenic OH. An iatrogenic form of dysautonomia leading to OH is often seen in elderly patients, in whom chronic use of certain medications impairs the reflexive normal autonomic response to changes in body position.[27]

Patients with autonomic vertigo can present with symptoms similar to those of MD. Autonomic dysfunction has been postulated to play a role in the pathophysiology of MD. In his study of 113 patients with autonomic and vestibular dysfunction, Pappas found that half of the patients presented with spontaneous attacks of rotational vertigo.[25] Many had nausea, and in the majority of patients, the attacks occurred daily and lasted for hours. Nearly all the patients had at least one associated otologic symptom. There were also important distinctions from MD in his study. Light-headedness was almost universal (97%), and an additional postural component to the dizziness was present in 50% of patients. Unlike in MD, vertigo worsened with a low-sodium diet or diuretic usage. From the time of onset, a large number had bilateral symptoms, which are not consistent with MD, and although 41% complained of hearing loss, it could actually be shown in only 4%.

It is not known whether autonomically induced vertigo is mediated centrally or peripherally. Impaired cerebral autoregulation is believed to be the mechanism behind central mediation. The peripheral mechanisms include possible autonomic influence of labyrinthine microcirculation or direct modulation of the vestibular neuroepithelium. Pappas supports a peripheral mechanism and believes that the symptom complex of episodic, spontaneous vertigo, ringing or roaring tinnitus, and aural fullness is generally the result of peripheral end-organ involvement. Although hearing loss was rarely measured in his study, electrocochleography (ECoG) findings were consistent with endolymphatic hydrops in 40% of those tested. The long-term improvement in 88% of patients and achievement of high-level function in 74% would not be expected with vertigo of central origin. Another theory is that hyporesponsiveness of the sympathetic nervous system to stress and asymmetric activity of the sympathetic system induce asymmetric blood flow in the vertebral arteries. This may lead to asymmetric activity in the inner ear and/or vestibular nuclei, resulting in the development of vertigo.[28]

Lightheadedness and postural dizziness are common complaints in addition to vertigo. Any previous episode of syncope is highly suspect. Patients may complain of exertional dizziness (**Video 13.1**).[29] Residual dizziness after successful management of benign paroxysmal positional vertigo (BPPV) has been linked to autonomic dysfunction.[30] Otologic symptoms occur bilaterally but unilateral involvement is possible, with one ear being more susceptible or reacting independently from the other.

The neurotologic examination, which is often unrevealing, should include testing for OH. After the resting blood pressure (which may be low) is obtained in the seated position, the patient is requested to stand up. A positive result is defined as a drop of 20 mm Hg in the systolic blood pressure or 10 mm Hg in the diastolic blood pressure within 2 to 5 minutes. If the change in position causes symptoms, it is also considered positive and the onset may be delayed. With a drop in blood pressure, the heart rate usually increases; if it does not, a neurologic cause should be expected. Postural orthostatic tachycardia syndrome (POTS) is characterized by an abnormally long increase in heart rate on getting up. Auscultation of the chest may reveal an abnormal rhythm or a heart murmur suggestive of mitral valve prolapse. Anemia and hypoglycemia should be ruled out. In cases of abnormal findings or if an autonomic disorder is still suspected, a cardiologist who specializes in autonomic dysfunction should be consulted. The test battery will likely include a resting and stress electrocardiogram (ECG), ultrasound of the heart, and 24-hour ambulatory blood pressure and rhythm assessment. The tilt-table test is a reliable test to demonstrate orthostatic intolerance and may be combined with hyperventilation.[31] The Valsalva maneuver may help to distinguish between adrenergic and hypervagal autonomic dysfunction. The baroreflex arc mediates both. The handgrip test assesses parasympathetic tone and the echo stress test assesses central and efferent sympathetic function. Depending on the findings, a neurologist's opinion may be warranted if a neurogenic cause is suspected.

The treatment of autonomic related vertigo is aimed at improving overall autonomic function. Explanation helps to relieve anxiety and postural education may help to reduce symptoms. Hypovolemia caused by anemia, fluid loss, and diuretic use should be addressed. The effects of chronic medication should be critically assessed, especially in the elderly, and if there is uncertainty, the help of a physician should be sought. Intravascular volume expansion for hypotensive patients can be accomplished with increased fluid intake and added salt in the diet. Fludrocortisone causes renal sodium retention and increases the sensitivity of arterioles to norepinephrine. Factors that can aggravate volume depletion and should best be avoided include alcohol, excessive heat exposure, sweating, dehydration, and vasoactive medication, such as certain cold remedies and diet pills. Regular moderate exercise increases the blood-pumping effect of skeletal muscles that could increase venous return and possibly improve vascular tone. Compression stockings improve venous return but are uncomfortable to wear. Peripheral- and central-acting medications that elevate blood pressure include sympathomimetics, β-blockers with negative inotropic effects, dopamine antagonists, prostaglandin inhibitors, and selective serotonin reuptake inhibitors. Anticholinergic drugs can be used to treat unstable autonomic regulation or hypervagal responsiveness. Depending on the condition, caffeine intake can either help or worsen symptoms. Insertion of a pacemaker may help regulate heart rate in some patients. A correct diet and eating regularly helps to avoid insulin spikes and fluctuations in blood glucose. This prevents fatigue and avoids triggering additional autonomic symptoms.

Questions (answer is "True" or "False")

Allergy

Q1: Atopy is a genetic tendency to produce IgE antibodies to proteins.

Q2: Clinical food allergy and IgE sensitization to food often precede development of asthma.

Q3: Drug allergy is the most common cause of anaphylaxis in children.

Q4: First-generation antihistamines are the first line of treatment in allergic rhinitis.

Q5: Allergen immunotherapy is a disease-modifying treatment and it is long-lasting.

Autonomic Dizziness

Q6: True vertigo is not due to autonomic dysfunction.

Q7: In the elderly, autonomic dysfunction may be due to medication.

Q8: The tilt-table test can demonstrate orthostatic intolerance.

Q9: When a patient experiences dizziness and low blood pressure when standing up and the heart rate does not increase, the cause is mitral valve prolapse.

Q10: Caffeine is very effective in the treatment of dysautonomia.

Answers

A1: True

A2: True

A3: False

A4: False

A5: True

A6: False

A7: True

A8: True

A9: False

A10: False

References

1. Ring J, Akdis C, Behrendt H, et al. Davos declaration: allergy as a global problem. [editorial] Allergy 2012;67(2):141–143

2. World Allergy Week 2015. Allergy: an increasing burden for all Europeans [Internet] 2015 April 16 [cited 2015 June 12]. Available from: http://www.eaaci.org/images/EAACI_PressRelease-WorldAllergyWeek2015-FINAL.pdf

3. Allergy F. a burden carried by more than 17 million of Europeans [Internet] 2015 March 9 [cited 2015 June 08]. Available from: http://www.eaaci.org/images/pdf.files/PressRelease-AwarenessCampaign-FOOD_ALLERGY_EAACI_EFA_FINAL-2.pdf

4. Allergy statistics [Internet] 2015 [cited 2015 June 15]. Available from: http://www.aaaai.org/about-the-aaaai/newsroom/allergy-statistics.aspx

5. Johansson SGO, Bieber T, Dahl R, et al. Revised nomenclature for allergy for global use: Report of the Nomenclature Review Committee of the World Allergy Organization, October 2003. J Allergy Clin Immunol 2004;113(5):832–836

6. Akdis CA, Agache I, eds. Global Atlas of Allergy. Zurich: European Academy of Allergy and Clinical Immunology; 2014

7. The global asthma report. [Internet] 2014 [cited 2015 June 15]. Available from: http://www.globalasthmareport.org/burden/burden.php

8. Akdis CA, Agache I, eds. Global Atlas of Asthma. Zurich: European Academy of Allergy and Clinical Immunology; 2013

9. Sukumaran TU. Allergic Rhinitis and Co-morbidities Training Module (ARCTM). Indian Pediatr 2011;48(7):511–513

10. Lasisi AO, Abdullahi M. The inner ear in patients with nasal allergy. J Natl Med Assoc 2008;100(8):903–905

11. Ruckenstein MJ. Immunologic aspects of Meniere's disease. Am J Otolaryngol 1999;20(3):161–165

12. Derebery MJ. Allergic and immunologic features of Ménière's disease. Otolaryngol Clin North Am 2011;44(3):655–666, ix

13. Banks C, McGinness S, Harvey R, Sacks R. Is allergy related to Meniere's disease? Curr Allergy Asthma Rep 2012;12(3):255–260

14. Gibbs SR, Mabry RL, Roland PS, Shoup AG, Mabry CS. Electrocochleographic changes after intranasal allergen challenge: A possible diagnostic tool in patients with Meniere's disease. Otolaryngol Head Neck Surg 1999;121(3):283–284

15. Derebery MJ, Berliner KI. Allergic eustachian tube dysfunction: diagnosis and treatment. Am J Otol 1997;18(2):160–165

16. Kolkaila EA, Emara AA, Gabr TA. Vestibular evaluation in children with otitis media with effusion. J Laryngol Otol 2015;129(4):326–336

17. Mostafa BE, Shafik AG, El Makhzangy AM, Taha H, Abdel Mageed HM. Evaluation of vestibular function in patients with chronic suppurative otitis media. ORL J Otorhinolaryngol Relat Spec 2013;75(6):357–360

18. Alternobaric vertigo [Internet] 2015 [cited 2015 June 15]. Available from: http://www.diversalertnetwork.org/health/ears/alternobaric-vertigo

19. Mehle ME. Migraine and allergy: a review and clinical update. Curr Allergy Asthma Rep 2012;12(3):240–245

20. Cunha ÂG, Nunes MP, Ramos RT, et al. Balance disturbances in asthmatic patients. J Asthma 2013; 50(3):282–286

21. Staab JP, Ruckenstein MJ. Expanding the differential diagnosis of chronic dizziness. Arch Otolaryngol Head Neck Surg 2007;133(2):170–176

22. Yonee C, Toyoshima M, Maegaki Y, et al. Association of acute cerebellar ataxia and human papilloma virus vaccination: a case report. Neuropediatrics 2013;44(5):265–267

23. Bushara KO, Goebel SU, Shill H, Goldfarb LG, Hallett M. Gluten sensitivity in sporadic and hereditary cerebellar ataxia. Ann Neurol 2001;49(4):540–543

24. Hain TC. Serc (betahistine) [Internet]. 2014 [updated 2014 Dec 20; cited 2015 April 10]. Available from: http://dizziness-and-balance.com/treatment/drug/serc.

25. Pappas DG Jr. Autonomic related vertigo. Laryngoscope 2003;113(10):1658–1671

26. Ohashi N, Yasumura S, Nakagawa H, Shojaku H, Mizukoshi K. Cerebral autoregulation in patients with orthostatic hypotension. Ann Otol Rhinol Laryngol 1991;100(10):841–844

27. McFeely WJ, Bojrab DI. Taking the history: associated symptoms. In: Goebel JA, ed. Practical Management of the Dizzy Patient. 2nd ed. Philadelphia, PA: Lippincott Williams & Wilkins; 2008

28. Takeda N. Autonomic dysfunction in patients with vertigo. JMAJ 2006;49(4):153–157

29. Staab JP, Ruckenstein MJ, Solomon D, Shepard NT. Exertional dizziness and autonomic dysregulation. Laryngoscope 2002;112(8 Pt 1):1346–1350

30. Kim HA, Lee H. Autonomic dysfunction as a possible cause of residual dizziness after successful treatment in benign paroxysmal positional vertigo. Clin Neurophysiol 2014;125(3):608–614

31. Staab JP, Ruckenstein MJ. Autonomic nervous system function in chronic dizziness. Otol Neurotol 2007;28(6):854–859

14 Aging: Balance and Vestibular Disorders

Yael Raz

■ Introduction

Dizziness is a very common complaint among older adults. In the over-60 population, 18.2% of community-dwelling adults have a 1-year prevalence of dizziness sufficient to interfere with activity and require a doctor visit or medication.[1] At age 70, 36% of women and 29% of men report a balance problem. This increases to 51% and 45%, respectively, in 88- to 90-year-old individuals.[2] Among patients more than 75 years old presenting to a physician's office, dizziness was the most common complaint, and for patients over 85, dizziness accounts for 7% of all visits to primary care physicians.[3,4] Dizziness is associated with an increased risk of falls and associated morbidity and mortality. Moreover, there are multiple insidious effects, such as decreased physical activity due to fear of falling, decreased quality of life, and a high rate of depression.

Age-related decline in vestibular function is referred to by various terms, including presbystasis, presbylibrium, and disequilibrium of aging. Studies have revealed age-related changes in vestibular organs, including changes in the overall cell number and ultrastructure of vestibular hair cells and vestibular ganglia, degeneration of otoconia, decrease in blood flow to the cristae, and decrease in volume of the crista.[5,6,7,8,9,10] Vestibular dysfunction, determined using a modified Romberg test, increases significantly with age.[11] Comorbidities, such as decreased visual function and peripheral neuropathy, as well as decreased neuroplasticity and impaired executive control, pose obstacles to successful vestibular compensation in the older patient. While aging is inevitable, it is important to note that even individuals with age-related changes in vestibular function can still benefit from interventions. The misconception that dizziness is a part of aging and is therefore not treatable contributes to delays in diagnosis for older patients with treatable causes of dizziness (i.e., benign paroxysmal positional vertigo [BPPV]).[12]

Older dizzy patients sometimes suffer an inverse version of the tale of the blind men, each feeling a different part of an elephant and declaring the object before them to be a rope, a fan, or a tree branch. Patients are sometimes passed from specialist to specialist, each declaring that the dizziness is "not cardiac," "not central," etc., and the patient is left frustrated, without a diagnosis, and without a treatment plan. When the appropriate evaluations do not yield an inner ear source, it is important for the otolaryngologist to go beyond the declaration that the problem is "not peripheral" and to initiate practical interventions (i.e., exercise program, fall risk-reduction program, vestibular physical therapy) aimed at restoring function and reducing the risk of falls. Simple steps, such as asking about falls, can lead to valuable interventions, even if the dizziness is not secondary to inner ear pathology.

■ Etiology

Studies on the etiology of dizziness in the older patient yield widely varying results, depending on the patient population, whether in the community, in a primary care setting, or in a specialty clinic. A large cross-sectional population study from Australia reveals that nonvestibular sources of vertigo are more common than vestibular sources of vertigo.[13] In a large study of patients presenting to a primary care clinic in the Netherlands with dizziness, 57% were found to have a cardiovascular disease as the major cause of their symptoms.[14] However, in a large study of patients referred to ENT clinics in Denmark with a chief complaint of dizziness, the majority of patients had BPPV.[15] Within otolaryngology specialty clinics, common causes of dizziness in the general population are also common in the older population (i.e., BPPV). A retrospective review of more than 1,000 patients over 70 years old presenting to a dizziness clinic revealed that 39% had confirmed or strongly suspected BPPV.[16] Besides BPPV, other neurotologic diagnoses to be considered include vestibular neuritis, Meniere's disease, vestibular hypofunction, and vestibular schwannomas. Multisensory deficits (i.e., a combination of vestibulopathy, peripheral neuropathy, and vision loss) are also common causes of disequilibrium in the older population.

Neurologic causes, such as stroke, need to be considered. Vertebrobasilar insufficiency, multiple sclerosis, Parkinson's disease, cerebellar ataxia, and Arnold-Chiari malformation can present with vertigo, disequilibrium, and/or gait disorder.[17] Migraine-associated dizziness occurs with less frequency in the older population.[16] In patients with cervical disease, cervicogenic dizziness should be considered.[18] There is some evidence that white matter abnormalities (T2 hyperintensities on MRI) may account for symptoms in patients with no other identifiable cause.[19] Cardiovascular issues, such as orthostatic hypotension, are common causes of lightheadedness. Other cardiac issues to consider, particularly in the context of lightheadedness, include arrhythmias (i.e., bradycardia), valvular disease (i.e., aortic stenosis), and other cardiac conditions that result in decreased blood flow to the brain.

Etiologies encountered with greater frequency in the older population include medication side effects, particularly in the setting of polypharmacy. Initiation or change in dosage of antihypertensive medications can lead to postural hypotension and lightheadedness. Other medications often associated with dizziness include anticonvulsants, antidepressants, anxiolytics, sedatives, strong analgesics, muscle relaxants, and anti-arrhythmics.[17] General medical issues, such as anemia or hypoglycemia, must also be considered. Multifactorial etiologies (i.e., multisensory disequilibrium, polypharmacy, and hypoglycemia) are common in older patients. Psychological issues as a primary factor are unusual in the older patient.[20]

■ History, Physical, and Laboratory Examination of the Older Dizzy Patient

While the history, physical, and laboratory examination of the dizzy patient are covered extensively in other chapters of this book, there are unique issues that are important to consider when approaching the older patient. While younger patients are often quite concerned about symptoms like vertigo or imbalance, some older patients may not complain of dizziness. They may assume, for example, that it is normal at their age to have some dizziness when turning to get out of bed. A study of patients in a geriatric clinic, none of whom complained of dizziness to their primary care physicians, revealed that 61% had dizziness.[21] Of the 100 patients who were included in the study, 9% had undiagnosed BPPV. Given the underreporting of dizziness in the older population, symptoms should be solicited with direct questions, such as "Do you get dizzy when you roll over in bed?" or the like.

Polypharmacy is a particularly important issue in the older population, and a detailed review of medications is necessary. It is not uncommon for patients to be placed on vestibular suppressants, such as meclizine, indefinitely and without regard for their effectiveness. Discontinuing the inappropriate use of chronic vestibular suppressants can facilitate vestibular compensation. Particularly when there is memory impairment or cognitive decline, it can be worthwhile to have a family member or friend assist with eliciting the history or filling out a dizziness questionnaire.

Given the high prevalence and underreporting of symptoms, Dix-Hallpike testing should be included in the physical examination of all older dizzy patients. It is also worthwhile to include orthostatic vitals. Observation of gait is vital, as gait deficit is one of the most common risk factors for falls.[22]

On oculomotor testing, it is not uncommon to find some degree of bilateral end-gaze nystagmus as well as limitation in upgaze in the older patient. Difficulty with tandem walking can also be expected. Bedside vestibular tests, as well as more formal measures of vestibular function, should be interpreted in light of normative data that is emerging for healthy older adults. A majority of older adults with no self-reported handicap as measured by the Dizziness Handicap Inventory failed a modified Romberg test (standing on a foam pad with eyes closed to eliminate both visual and proprioceptive input).[23] This same population exhibited a high prevalence of abnormal head impulse testing (30–40%), particularly in the plane of the horizontal semicircular canal. Some authors report a modest age-related decline in canal function (as measured using caloric tests) in comparison to a more marked reduction in vestibular evoked myogenic potential (VEMP) responses.[24] Others report significant declines in both semicircular canal and otolith function (as measured using head thrust dynamic visual acuity, cervical VEMP, and ocular VEMP) in an age-dependent fashion.[25]

■ Benign Paroxysmal Positional Vertigo

The incidence of BPPV increases with age[15] and BPPV is often unrecognized in older adults.[21] Even with directed questions, the reporting of symptoms is not straightforward. Patients may not recognize that a turn to the side triggered the vertigo and will report the complaint as dizziness when they get out of bed—a symptom that can be mistaken for postural hypotension. Given the very high prevalence of BPPV in the older population,[15,16] Dix-Hallpike testing should be included in the assessment of every older dizzy patient.

Decreased neck range of motion, limited trunk mobility, and kyphosis are potential factors that may affect both Dix-Hallpike testing and Epley repositioning maneuvers in the older patient population. The literature is divided on this topic. Some authors did not find a significant association between age and recurrence rate of BPPV.[26,27] Other studies suggest that effectiveness of repositioning maneuvers is age dependent. A study of 86 patients treated for BPPV found that 4% of patients had persistent symptoms after four repositioning maneuvers—all were older women.[28] Another study of 47 patients age 70 and above found that 64% of patients improved with Epley repositioning maneuvers. Those who did not improve were referred for vestibular rehabilitation, which boosted the improvement rate to 77%.[29]

When performing Epley maneuvers in the older patient, an assessment of kyphosis and cervical spine range of motion should precede treatment. It can be helpful to have an assistant in the room. A slow and gentle maneuver, letting the patient recline only as quickly as they are comfortable with, rather than jerking the head back, can still be effective. It is not necessary to hyperextend the neck, since successful repositioning depends on the orientation of the head relative to gravity not relative to the rest of the body. Placing the exam chair in Trendelenburg position can help to overcome anatomic challenges stemming from kyphosis or limited neck range of motion.

Many otolaryngologists provide patients with postrepositioning instructions that include the recommendation to avoid sleeping in a fully reclined position for 24 to 48 hours. However, sleeping in a partially reclined chair or using extra pillows is likely to disturb sleep, and poor sleep presents yet another fall risk.[30] Eliminating these positional restrictions does not seem to affect the success rate of the Epley maneuver.[31,32]

A prospective study of postural stability (using dynamic posturography) revealed that older patients were less likely to show improvements in postural stability after treatment even though the vertigo resolved. It is unclear whether this is a causative phenomenon or whether there is coexistent vestibular pathology.[33] Others have reported an increased fall risk in patients with BPPV.[21] Mild horizontal canal BPPV has been implicated as a possible cause of chronic dizziness.[34]

■ Meniere's Disease

De novo presentation at age 65 and above was noted in 9% of patients with definite Meniere's disease.[35] Among 66 older patients with Meniere's, 41% were found to have reactivation of long-standing disease, as opposed to 59% with de novo appearance of symptoms.[35] Drop attacks are noted more commonly in older patients.[35,36]

A difficult treatment dilemma arises in the older Meniere's patient who fails conservative management. There is a dogma that vestibular compensation is impaired in older individuals, raising the concern that older patients may be more prone to experience chronic disequilibrium after vestibular ablation. The older Meniere's patient with recalcitrant vertigo attacks may be denied chemical or surgical vestibular ablation on this basis. However, there have been challenges to this conventional dogma. It has been demonstrated that older individuals are able to receive the same degree of benefit from vestibular rehabilitation as their younger cohorts.[37] Additionally, recent work examining vestibular compensation after acoustic neuroma surgery has revealed that older patients do compensate successfully and that the degree of preoperative physical activity, more so than age, is a predictor of the ability to regain normal balance function.[38,39] It is worthwhile to consider the patient's "biologic" or functional age rather than their chronologic age. Access to ablative procedures should not be denied purely on the basis of age. Instead, an assessment of comorbidities that present additional insults to equilibrium provides a more useful approach. An otherwise completely healthy 70-year-old is more likely to compensate well than a 50-year-old with peripheral neuropathy and poor vision. It is helpful to have input from a vestibular therapist before ablation, particularly when there are concerns about a patient's ability to successfully compensate.

■ Fall Prevention

The fall risk for an individual over 65 is ~ 30%. This increases to 50% in individuals over 80. A fall in an older person is more likely to result in significant injury: 95% of hip fractures are caused by falls. Adjusting for inflation, the Centers for Disease Control and Prevention (CDC) estimate the direct medical costs of falls at $34 billion.[40,41] Individuals who complain of dizziness and demonstrate vestibular dysfunction (abnormal modified Romberg) have an eightfold increase in the odds of sustaining a fall.[11] Multifactorial fall risk assessment, as well as exercise programs, have been shown to decrease fall risk.[42] Given these figures, providers who evaluate patients with dizziness and vestibular dysfunction are poised to reduce fall risk for their patients. Often, particularly in otolaryngology, training focuses on diagnostics and treatment, and less on prevention. A quick and practical preventative approach aimed at identifying fall risk factors should be included in the assessment of every older dizzy patient (see **Box 14.1**).

Box 14.1   Assessment for fall risk

History

- History of falls
- Ask about imbalance
- Assess use of an assistive device
- Ask about visual deficits
- Check medications, particularly drugs that increase fall risk
- Identify musculoskeletal issues

Physical Exam

- Assess for muscle weakness
- Observe gait
- Assess for cognitive impairment

Asking about previous falls and imbalance identifies two of the top four risk factors for falls: a previous history of falls and a balance deficit.[22] Including an assessment of a patient's gait and muscle strength in the physical exam allows identification of the other two out of the top four risk factors for a fall: muscle weakness and gait deficit. The use of an assistive device should be noted, as this confers a significantly increased odds ratio for a fall.

The older dizzy patient should be questioned regarding any visual deficits. Fall rates decrease after cataract surgery. Multifocal lenses result in decreased depth perception and impaired edge-contrast sensitivity, leaving patients predisposed to falls, particularly on stairs.[43,44,45] Ensure that vision has been recently assessed and that glasses are up to date. An additional visual challenge in older patients is decreased adaptation to darkness. A rapid transition from well-lit to dark areas results in initially very limited vision and can present a high fall risk. Night lights are a simple intervention that can reduce this risk.

Addressing polypharmacy and reducing or eliminating medications that have dizziness as a side effect are effective interventions to decrease fall risk. Fall-risk-increasing drugs (FRIDs) include cardiovascular drugs (antihypertensives, nitrates, anti-arrhythmics), psychotropic drugs (sedatives, antidepressants, anxiolytics, antipsychotics), analgesics, and hypoglycemics. A recent study reported a 40% prevalence of FRID use among patients presenting to a neurotology clinic, with 34% of patients using two or more FRIDs.[46] Discontinuing the use of FRIDs or reducing the dosage has been demonstrated to decrease fall risk.[47] Collaboration with the patient's primary care provider or a geriatric specialist can help to streamline medications and reduce or eliminate FRIDs when possible.

Ask about the patient's environment. Many falls occur in the home, probably simply as a result of the extensive time spent there. Encourage practical steps, such as removing throw rugs and other tripping hazards, installing handrails on both sides of staircases, installing grab bars by the bath and toilet, and installation of night lights.

Patients who are deemed at a high risk for a fall will benefit from referral for an exercise program. Exercise has repeatedly been demonstrated to be effective in reducing fall risk. Encourage exercise that develops strength and balance, such as yoga or tai chi, but anything that the patient enjoys (e.g., dancing, Silver Sneakers, walking) can help. Referral to a vestibular physical therapist who has an interest in working with older patients can provide a coordinated team approach that is more effective at decreasing fall risk.

References

1. Sloane P, Blazer D, George LK. Dizziness in a community elderly population. J Am Geriatr Soc 1989; 37(2):101–108
2. Jönsson R, Sixt E, Landahl S, Rosenhall U. Prevalence of dizziness and vertigo in an urban elderly population. J Vestib Res 2004;14(1):47–52
3. Sloane PD. Dizziness in primary care. Results from the National Ambulatory Medical Care Survey. J Fam Pract 1989;29(1):33–38
4. Koch HKS, Mickey C. Office-based ambulatory care for patients 75 years old and over. In: Smith MC, ed. National Ambulatory Medical Care Survey, 1980 and 1981. Hyattsville, Maryland: U.S. Dept. of Health and Human Services, Public Health Service, National Center for Health Statistics; 1985
5. Jang YS, Hwang CH, Shin JY, Bae WY, Kim LS. Age-related changes on the morphology of the otoconia. Laryngoscope 2006;116(6):996–1001

6. Anniko M. The aging vestibular hair cell. Am J Otolaryngol 1983;4(3):151–160

7. Lyon MJ, Wanamaker HH. Blood flow and assessment of capillaries in the aging rat posterior canal crista. Hear Res 1993;67(1-2):157–165

8. Lyon MJ, King JM. Aging rat vestibular ganglion: II. Quantitative electron microscopic evaluation. Ann Otol Rhinol Laryngol 1997;106(9):753–758

9. Velázquez-Villaseñor L, Merchant SN, Tsuji K, Glynn RJ, Wall C III, Rauch SD. Temporal bone studies of the human peripheral vestibular system. Normative Scarpa's ganglion cell data. Ann Otol Rhinol Laryngol Suppl 2000;181:14–19

10. Rauch SD, Velazquez-Villaseñor L, Dimitri PS, Merchant SN. Decreasing hair cell counts in aging humans. Ann N Y Acad Sci 2001;942:220–227

11. Agrawal Y, Carey JP, Della Santina CC, Schubert MC, Minor LB. Disorders of balance and vestibular function in US adults: data from the National Health and Nutrition Examination Survey, 2001-2004. Arch Intern Med 2009;169(10):938–944

12. Lawson J, Johnson I, Bamiou DE, Newton JL. Benign paroxysmal positional vertigo: clinical characteristics of dizzy patients referred to a falls and syncope unit. QJM 2005;98(5):357–364

13. Gopinath B, McMahon CM, Rochtchina E, Mitchell P. Dizziness and vertigo in an older population: the Blue Mountains prospective cross-sectional study. Clin Otolaryngol 2009;34(6):552–556

14. Maarsingh OR, Dros J, Schellevis FG, et al. Causes of persistent dizziness in elderly patients in primary care. Ann Fam Med 2010;8(3):196–205

15. Lüscher M, Theilgaard S, Edholm B. Prevalence and characteristics of diagnostic groups amongst 1034 patients seen in ENT practices for dizziness. J Laryngol Otol 2014;128(2):128–133

16. Katsarkas A. Dizziness in aging: a retrospective study of 1194 cases. Otolaryngol Head Neck Surg 1994;110(3):296–301

17. Lawson J, Bamiou D-E. Dizziness in the older person. Rev Clin Gerontol 2005;15(3–4):187–206

18. Karlberg M, Johansson R, Magnusson M, Fransson PA. Dizziness of suspected cervical origin distinguished by posturographic assessment of human postural dynamics. J Vestib Res 1996;6(1):37–47

19. Ahmad H, Cerchiai N, Mancuso M, Casani AP, Bronstein AM. Are white matter abnormalities associated with "unexplained dizziness"? J Neurol Sci 2015;358(1-2):428–431

20. Davis LE. Dizziness in elderly men. J Am Geriatr Soc 1994;42(11):1184–1188

21. Oghalai JS, Manolidis S, Barth JL, Stewart MG, Jenkins HA. Unrecognized benign paroxysmal positional vertigo in elderly patients. Otolaryngol Head Neck Surg 2000;122(5):630–634

22. Guideline for the prevention of falls in older persons. American Geriatrics Society, British Geriatrics Society, and American Academy of Orthopaedic Surgeons Panel on Falls Prevention. J Am Geriatr Soc 2001;49(5):664–672

23. Davalos-Bichara M, Agrawal Y. Normative results of healthy older adults on standard clinical vestibular tests. Otol Neurotol 2014;35(2):297–300

24. Maes L, Dhooge I, D'haenens W, et al. The effect of age on the sinusoidal harmonic acceleration test, pseudorandom rotation test, velocity step test, caloric test, and vestibular-evoked myogenic potential test. Ear Hear 2010;31(1):84–94

25. Agrawal Y, Zuniga MG, Davalos-Bichara M, et al. Decline in semicircular canal and otolith function with age. Otol Neurotol 2012;33(5):832–839

26. Nunez RA, Cass SP, Furman JM. Short- and long-term outcomes of canalith repositioning for benign paroxysmal positional vertigo. Otolaryngol Head Neck Surg 2000;122(5):647–652

27. Korkmaz M, Korkmaz H. Cases requiring increased number of repositioning maneuvers in benign paroxysmal positional vertigo. Brazilian J Otorhinolaryngology 2015

28. Ruckenstein MJ. Therapeutic efficacy of the Epley canalith repositioning maneuver. Laryngoscope 2001;111(6):940–945

29. Angeli SI, Hawley R, Gomez O. Systematic approach to benign paroxysmal positional vertigo in the elderly. Otolaryngol Head Neck Surg 2003;128(5):719–725

30. Stone KL, Blackwell TL, Ancoli-Israel S, et al; Osteoporotic Fractures in Men Study Group. Sleep disturbances and risk of falls in older community-dwelling men: the outcomes of Sleep Disorders in Older Men (MrOS Sleep) Study. J Am Geriatr Soc 2014;62(2):299–305

31. Fife TD, Iverson DJ, Lempert T, et al; Quality Standards Subcommittee, American Academy of Neurology. Practice parameter: therapies for benign paroxysmal positional vertigo (an evidence-based review): report of the Quality Standards Subcommittee of the American Academy of Neurology. Neurology 2008;70(22):2067–2074

32. Marciano E, Marcelli V. Postural restrictions in labyrintholithiasis. Eur Arch Otorhinolaryngol 2002;259(5):262–265

33. Blatt PJ, Georgakakis GA, Herdman SJ, Clendaniel RA, Tusa RJ. The effect of the canalith repositioning maneuver on resolving postural instability in patients with benign paroxysmal positional vertigo. Am J Otol 2000;21(3):356–363

34. Johkura K, Momoo T, Kuroiwa Y. Positional nystagmus in patients with chronic dizziness. J Neurol Neurosurg Psychiatry 2008;79(12):1324–1326

35. Ballester M, Liard P, Vibert D, Häusler R. Menière's disease in the elderly. Otol Neurotol 2002;23(1):73–78

36. Lee H, Yi HA, Lee SR, Ahn BH, Park BR. Drop attacks in elderly patients secondary to otologic causes with Meniere's syndrome or non-Meniere peripheral vestibulopathy. J Neurol Sci 2005;232(1-2):71–76

37. Whitney SL, Wrisley DM, Marchetti GF, Furman JM. The effect of age on vestibular rehabilitation outcomes. Laryngoscope 2002;112(10):1785–1790

38. Parietti-Winkler C, Lion A, Frère J, Perrin PP, Beurton R, Gauchard GC. Prediction of balance compensation after vestibular schwannoma surgery. Neurorehabil Neural Repair 2015

39. Gauchard GC, Lion A, Perrin PP, Parietti-Winkler C. Influence of age on postural compensation after unilateral deafferentation due to vestibular schwannoma surgery. Laryngoscope 2012;122(10):2285–2290

40. Stevens JA, Corso PS, Finkelstein EA, Miller TR. The costs of fatal and non-fatal falls among older adults. Inj Prev 2006;12(5):290–295

41. Centers for Disease Control and Prevention, National Center for Injury Prevention and Control, Division of Unintentional Injury Prevention. 2015. Available from: http://www.cdc.gov/homeandrecreationalsafety/falls/adultfalls.html

42. Chang JT, Morton SC, Rubenstein LZ, et al. Interventions for the prevention of falls in older adults: systematic review and meta-analysis of randomised clinical trials. BMJ 2004;328(7441):680

43. Jack CI, Smith T, Neoh C, Lye M, McGalliard JN. Prevalence of low vision in elderly patients admitted to an acute geriatric unit in Liverpool: elderly people who fall are more likely to have low vision. Gerontology 1995;41(5):280–285

44. Brannan S, Dewar C, Sen J, Clarke D, Marshall T, Murray PI. A prospective study of the rate of falls before and after cataract surgery. Br J Ophthalmol 2003;87(5):560–562

45. Lord SR, Dayhew J, Howland A. Multifocal glasses impair edge-contrast sensitivity and depth perception and increase the risk of falls in older people. J Am Geriatr Soc 2002;50(11):1760–1766

46. Harun A, Agrawal Y. The use of fall risk increasing drugs (FRIDs) in patients with dizziness pPresenting to a neurotology clinic. Otol Neurotol 2015;36(5):862–864

47. van der Velde N, Stricker BH, Pols HA, van der Cammen TJ. Risk of falls after withdrawal of fall-risk-increasing drugs: a prospective cohort study. Br J Clin Pharmacol 2007;63(2):232–237

15 Congenital and Pediatric Vestibular Disorders

Kathryn Y. Noonan and James E. Saunders

■ Introduction

The evaluation of a vertiginous child poses unique challenges due in part to the vast differential of congenital and pediatric vestibular disorders. Many factors, such as delayed presentation and progression of disease, vestibular compensation of congenital disease, and incomplete penetrance of genetic disorders, add to the complexity of the evaluation. Additionally, diseases commonly seen in the adult population have lower prevalence rates in children. Nevertheless, the appreciation of these disorders and their functional limitations is important for appropriate counseling of the family.

Although it is impossible to know the exact incidence, inborn defects of the vestibular system are rare. Congenital defects may involve the bony labyrinth or functional defects of the epithelial sensory component. Disorders that involve the vestibular epithelium may be apparent only in postmortem histologic studies and may not be radiographically detectable. Therefore, they are not well studied in the clinical setting.

A wide prevalence range (0.45–15.0%) is reported for dizziness in the pediatric population. The variation can be attributed to different inclusion criteria and varying data collection methods (chart review versus survey results) as well as the difficulty of characterizing symptoms in this population.[1,2,3] Disorders common in the adult population (benign paroxysmal positional vertigo [BPPV] and Meniere's disease) are uncommon in children. In contrast, some diseases seen in children (benign paroxysmal vertigo) are relatively unheard of in adults. The following is a brief account of congenital and pediatric vestibular abnormalities.

■ Embryology of the Vestibular System

It is important to understand the embryologic development of the vestibular system and how various insults to this process result in vestibular dysfunction. The development of the inner ear begins at approximately the third week of gestation, earlier than that of the middle and external ear. It starts with the formation of the otic placode on the lateral surface of the neural tube.[4,5] Gradual invagination of the otic placode to form the otic pit and then the otocyst occurs during the fourth week. As development enters the fifth week, otocyst folds begin to give rise to the primordial cochlea/saccule ventrally, the utricle/vestibule dorsally, and the endolymphatic sac/duct. Elongation and helical formation of the cochlea to its full two and three-quarter turns occurs in the sixth through tenth weeks. The round window and cochlea reach final size around 24 weeks.[6] Three immature semicircular canals (SCCs) develop as half disks from the primordial vestibular portion. Mesenchyme then fills in the central core of the half disks to create well-differentiated SCCs. Richards et al postulate that the canals undergo a progressive unfolding process, reaching adult size by weeks 17 to 25 of gestation.[6,7] However, a recent imaging study of human fetuses found no correlation of the SCC angles with gestational age. The authors concluded the variation in SCC angles is an adaptation to physiologic vestibular function.[8]

Ossification of the otic capsule progresses from 14 ossification centers forming between weeks 16 and 21, with the SCCs ossifying relatively late in gestation.[9] Ossification of the superior SCC occurs around 23 weeks, followed by the posterior and lateral canals, at 24 and 25 weeks, respectively.[6] The last ossification center to form lies over the posterior SCC. Early histologic studies suggest isolated regions of incomplete ossification occur in up to 65% of fetal temporal bones and in children up to 3 years old, but no particular distribution was seen[10] Thus, the vestibular labyrinth is completely formed by halfway through the second trimester, but full ossification with mineralized bone may continue until birth and even into infancy. Incomplete ossification may lead to apparent dehiscences in the SCC in pediatric patients, but the pathophysiology and clinical significance of pediatric SCC dehiscence is not well understood. Chen et al reviewed 131 pediatric CT scans and found an incidental 14% dehiscence rate among patients with hearing loss.[11] The majority involved the superior canal (14 patients) and the remaining involved the posterior canal. If dehiscence is caused by arrested development, one would expect defects in the lateral SCC to be common, yet this has not been the case. Chen et al did find threefold higher rates of posterior SCC dehiscence in a pediatric population than were found in a recent study including adults by Russo et al.[11,12] Of interest, Chen et al did not find a correlation between the CT findings and either hearing results or symptoms. Thus, the pathophysiology and clinical significance of the developmental variations remain unclear.

The vestibular aqueduct, a bony canal extending from the vestibule to the sigmoid sinus, encloses the endolymphatic sac, a small artery, and a vein. It has been theorized that the canal is proportionately larger in early development, with decrease in size of the vestibular aqueduct as the inner ear continues to mature, but more recent studies present conflicting data.[5] Pyle studied the histopathology of 48 developing temporal bones, measuring various points of the vestibular aqueduct during development. He found continued nonlinear growth throughout embryonic life, which contradicts the theory that enlarged vestibular aqueduct syndrome originates from arrested prenatal development.[13]

Although the bony labyrinth is formed early in gestation, the vestibular ganglion cells continue to remodel and mature throughout fetal development. They are present in various shapes after 13 weeks of gestation, reaching a uniform shape at 24 weeks, with continued development until 39 weeks. They are thought to reach maturity around birth.[14] Myelination begins around week 20 of gestation and continues until puberty.[15] Therefore, neonatal and pediatric vestibular reflexes are in varying stages of development and need to be interpreted with appropriate reference standards.

■ Clinical Evaluation of Congenital and Pediatric Vestibular Disorders

History and Physical Exam

A comprehensive history and physical exam are critical to ascertaining the correct diagnosis of pediatric patients with vestibular dysfunction. Young patients may have great difficulty describing their symptoms. The onset, progression, and timing of symptoms are important features to note. The clinician should ask about aggravation of vestibular symptoms in response to minor head trauma or loud sounds. Additionally, vestibular symptoms may be associated with an increase in hearing loss, tinnitus, headaches, seizures, and other associated ear symptoms that may be difficult for a young person to relate. A vestibular anomaly could be masked as general clumsiness and delay presentation for years; therefore, specific note of the age of ambulation should be made. Delayed onset of ambulation beyond 18 months of age should be considered abnormal and may be an indicator of early vestibular disease. Vestibular dysfunction may be induced by recent infections or various toxic insults, and thus it is critical to ask about infections or exposure to ototoxic medications. Congenital infections, such as toxoplasmosis, syphilis (other), rubella, cytomegalovirus, and herpes (TORCH), may hinder development.

The evaluation should also include a thorough history to search for accompanying characteristics of hereditary syndromes. Examples of this would be night-blindness (Usher's syndrome), family history of male-only involvement (X-linked deafness with perilymphatic gusher), and family history of a white forelock (Waardenburg's syndrome). If the history includes hereditary features, construction of a family pedigree is the next step in the diagnostic process.

A comprehensive physical exam is essential. The exam typically starts with micro-otoscopy with pneumatic insufflation. The examiner should observe for vertigo or nystagmus (Hennebert sign) during pneumatic otoscopy. Testing for Tullio phenomenon (vertigo in response to a loud sound) may be performed with a Barany noise box or tuning fork. Additionally, a complete head and neck exam, eye exam, and cranial nerve exam need to be performed. A full-body exam should be performed to search for any dysmorphic features. The child's cardiopulmonary condition should be assessed and abnormal musculoskeletal findings that may cause unsteadiness and gait disorders should be evaluated.

The vestibular system should be evaluated with consideration for developmental milestones. Clearly, there are age-related limitations to the vestibular exam. The exam can be tailored to each child's ability and willingness to follow instructions and ambulate. The vestibular exam of an infant requires some specific exam techniques. Extraocular movements and gaze-evoked nystagmus can be assessed in a small child by using a small toy to draw the child's attention to the four visual quadrants (**Fig. 15.1**).

The presence of an intact vestibulo-ocular reflex (VOR) may be assessed in an infant by holding the child at arm's length and spinning in circles (**Fig. 15.2**; **Video 15.1**). At less than 3 weeks of age, the eyes will deviate away from the direction of acceleration ("doll's eye" phenomenon), but by 3 weeks of age, the eyes should deviate toward the direction of acceleration, as would an adult's eyes. This doll's eye phenomenon may persist in premature infants for up to 3 months. Other inherent reflexes, such as the Moro reflex, parachute reflex, and righting reflex, may also be helpful in evaluating the infant's neurologic development. The presence of the VOR may also be elicited in older children by spinning them in the exam chair for 20 to 30 seconds and looking for normal postrotary nystagmus.

If possible, the full exam, including gait, Fukuda stepping test, eyes-closed Romberg, tandem Romberg, tandem gait, cerebellar testing, and positional testing, should be performed. There are no clear-cut normative data for these clinical examination findings in young children; however, some general age-related milestones are important to consider. Children should be able to ambulate by 18 months of age. By 5 years of age, most children should be able to walk a straight line with minimal errors, but even 7-year-olds may have a few errors on this task. Most school-age children will be able to maintain an eyes-closed Romberg for 15 seconds and a tandem Romberg for 6 seconds (**Fig. 15.3**; **Video 15.2**).

The balance exam in older children may be augmented with the use of a foam pad.[16] Specific physical findings, such as post-head-shake nystagmus and head thrust exam, may be helpful in detecting vestibular weakness. The Bruininks-Oseretsky Test of Motor Proficiency, second edition (BOT-2) includes a subtest for balance with normative data down to 4 years of age. The test scores a series of tasks (**Table 15.1**; **Video 15.3**) and then applies an age adjustment for a final score. Such quantitative assessment is critical for research studies and similar assessment tools may be useful in practice.

Additional audiometric and vestibular testing should be tailored to each child. Age-appropriate audiologic evaluation is required in every patient. In selected patients, the examination can be further augmented with videonystagmography to search for vestibular loss or hypofunction. The VOR

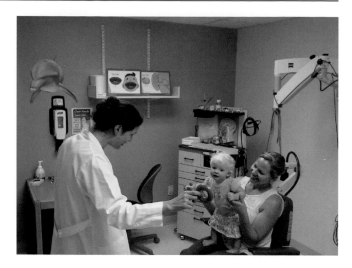

Fig. 15.1 Evaluation of extraocular movements in an infant.

is responsive at birth and continues to mature over the first few years of life. Caloric testing is possible at 2 months of age but is often poorly tolerated in the pediatric population.[17] The cervical vestibular evoked myogenic potential (cVEMP) test can also be used to evaluate saccular function. Although there are some limitations (infants are unable to maintain muscle contraction with head elevation), cVEMPs have been used in newborns and pediatric patients.[15,18,19] Posturography may be helpful, but it is important to note that the vestibular system is not fully developed until age 12, and therefore pediatric normative data are not available.[15,20]

In general, imaging studies should be reserved for vertiginous children with other neurologic symp-

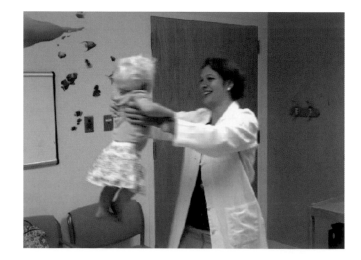

Fig. 15.2 In-office rotatory testing of an infant/child.

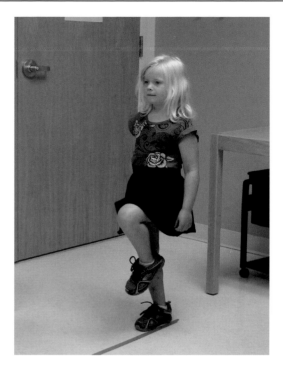

Fig. 15.3 Vestibular testing of the school-age child (BOT-2 exam).

toms, focal neurologic signs, unilateral hearing loss, or severe disease. Imaging studies are costly and frequently require sedation in the pediatric population; therefore, careful consideration is required in each case. Niemensivu et al studied imaging findings in vertiginous children.[21] Out of 23 children with new deviant neurologic findings, 22 children (96%) had associated severe headache or neurologic findings

on exam. They concluded that imaging should not be performed in vertiginous patients without other neurologic findings.[21]

Vestibular Compensation

Patients with congenital vestibular dysfunction may present with minimal symptoms or balance deficits due to central nervous system (CNS) compensation and use of somatosensory visual information.[22] Phenotypic expression may therefore be masked by individual compensatory abilities. Enbom et al evaluated 18 children with congenital or early acquired bilateral vestibular loss. Six of these patients had Usher's syndrome, with two other patients having unspecified hereditary hearing loss. Testing with eyes closed showed no significant difference in body sway velocity until the somatosensory information was perturbed. This study suggested that patients with congenital vestibular anomalies use anticipatory mechanisms in posture and balance to perform similar to controls in most everyday situations.[22]

■ Congenital Vestibular Disorders

Congenital Syndromes

Waardenburg Syndrome

Waardenburg syndrome is inherited in an autosomal dominant pattern and has been linked to six different genes, including *PAX3, MITF, EDN3, EDNRB,*

Table 15.1 Components of the Bruininks-Oseretsky Test of Motor Proficiency, second edition (BOT-2), balance subtest

Task	Maximum Performance	BOT-2 Score
1. Standing on a line (Romberg)		
Eyes open	10 seconds	0–4
Eyes closed	10 seconds	0–4
2. Walking forward on a line (normal gait)	6 steps	0–4
3. Standing on one foot		
Eyes open	10 seconds	0–4
Eyes closed	10 seconds	0–4
4. Walking forward on a line with eyes open (tandem gait)	6 steps	0–4
5. Standing on one foot on balance beam		
Eyes open	10 seconds	0–4
Eyes closed	10 seconds	0–4
6. Heel to toe (tandem Romberg) on balance beam	10 seconds	0–4

SOX10, and *SNAI2.*[23] Incidence of Waardenburg syndrome is estimated to be between 1 in 10,000 and 1 in 20,000.[24] The syndrome is characterized by heterochromia iridis, white forelock, dystopia canthorum (type I), synophrys, hypopigmented areas of the skin, congenital sensorineural hearing loss (SNHL), and hypotrophic nasal alae. There are isolated reports of vestibular anatomic abnormalities, including malformation or absence of the semicircular canals, as well as hypoplasia of the cochlea.[25,26,27] However, a recent review by Kontorinis et al found no abnormalities on the high-resolution computed tomography (CT) scans of 20 patients.[23]

The vestibular findings in Waardenburg syndrome are as variable as the expression of the other phenotypic abnormalities. Black et al found vestibular symptoms to be the most common chief complaint in 22 patients with Waardenburg syndrome.[28] Sixteen patients (73%) had complaints of either disequilibrium or vertigo and 17 patients (77%) had abnormal vestibular function tests. Interestingly, the authors found no differences in vestibular findings based on Waardenburg subtype and noted that vestibular symptoms may be the presenting complaint, even in the absence of hearing loss.[28] Similarly, Marcus et al reported high rates of vestibular dysfunction (21 of 22 subjects) in a study of a family with Waardenburg syndrome.[25]

Branchio-Oto-Renal Syndrome

Branchio-oto-renal (BOR) syndrome is an autosomal dominant disorder of the first and second branchial arches, with causative genes including *EYA1, SIX1,* and *SIX5.* Its prevalence has been reported at 1 in 40,000.[29] BOR syndrome is characterized by hearing loss, malformation of the auricles, preauricular pits, renal anomalies, and branchial cleft fistulas. Hearing loss may be mixed, conductive, or sensorineural. Vestibular findings include unsteadiness in dark environments and delays in ambulation as long as 22 months.[30] Radiographic inner ear malformations are variable. Chen et al looked at temporal bone scans of 12 patients with BOR syndrome and found 11 of 24 ears with enlarged vestibular aqueducts, four enlarged vestibules, and three hypoplastic horizontal semicircular canals.[31] Ceruti et al preformed a review of eight patients in one family and noted abnormal lateral semicircular canals in 14 of 16 ears, and five ears with an enlarged vestibular aqueduct.[32] Despite BOR syndrome's being commonly associated with inner ear malformations, vestibular dysfunction is not well studied in these patients.[31,32,33] There are case reports of hyporeflexia and areflexia on vestibular testing, but no large-scale investigations.[30,34]

Neurofibromatosis Type 2

Neurofibromatosis type 2 (NF2) is an autosomal dominant disorder with a prevalence of 1 in 100,000.[35] It is characterized by multiple nervous system tumors, including bilateral vestibular schwannomas, ocular abnormalities, and skin abnormalities. Although the syndrome is defined by vestibular schwannomas and hearing loss is a common finding, vestibular dysfunction is not commonly a presenting symptom. Choi et al looked at 26 pediatric NF2 patients and found only 20% with vestibular symptoms at the time of diagnosis, presumably due to slow tumor growth.[36] Nunes and MacCollin looked at 12 patients with NF2 and found 25% with abnormal ambulation.[37]

Usher's Syndrome

Usher's syndrome is a rare autosomal recessive syndrome characterized by SNHL, retinitis pigmentosa, and variable presence of vestibular dysfunction.[38,39,40] The prevalence rate is reported to be 3.5 to 6.2 per 100,000.[41,42] Thus far, 11 distinct loci have been discovered related to the syndrome and more overlap is being found between different subtypes.[42] Classically, Usher's syndrome is classified into three main categories based on clinical findings, but genetic advances are allowing for atypical subtypes and further differentiation within the classes.

Type I is characterized by profound deafness, vestibular dysfunction, and early onset of progressive retinitis pigmentosa starting before puberty. Delayed age of ambulation is a frequent finding in this subtype.[39] Vestibular abnormalities of Usher's type IB are described as "vestibulocerebellar ataxia" due to the radiographic finding of cerebellar abnormalities.[43] Although cochlear abnormalities have also been reported, radiographic imaging of the inner ear is typically normal.[26,44] As a result, there is controversy whether the vestibular dysfunction is central or peripheral in origin. Usher's type II is the most common form and is associated with moderate to severe congenital deafness with normal vestibular dysfunction and retinitis pigmentosa beginning in the teenage years.

Type III has variable progressive hearing loss, later onset of retinitis pigmentosa, and variable vestibular dysfunction.[45] Type III is comparatively rare except in Ashkenazi Jewish families.[41] Sadeghi et al studied vestibular function in patients with *USH3* mutation and found 19 of 22 subjects reported walking prior to 18 months. Interestingly, vestibular testing of these adults revealed vestibular hypofunction or areflexia in ten subjects (45%), leading the authors to conclude that some of the patients suffered from a progressive vestibular loss.

Pendred's Syndrome

Pendred's syndrome is an autosomal recessive disorder characterized by profound symmetric SNHL, goiter, and enlarged vestibular aqueduct (**Fig. 15.4**). It is commonly associated with the *SLC26A4* gene.[46] Luxon et al studied vertiginous signs and symptoms and radiographic findings in 33 patients with Pendred's syndrome and profound hearing loss, the vast majority of whom had bilateral dilated vestibular aqueducts.[47] Fifteen of 33 subjects complained of dizziness or vertiginous symptoms. Vestibular testing demonstrated one-third of patients with normal responses, one-third with unilateral vestibular weakness, and one-third with bilateral vestibular deficits. No correlation was found between the degree of hypofunction and either the degree of hearing loss or the presence of an enlarged vestibular aqueduct.[48] In a study of patients with enlarged vestibular aqueducts, Miyagawa et al report on a subset of 15 subjects with Pendred's syndrome,[49] 87% of whom had progressive hearing loss and 80% of whom suffered vertiginous symptoms. Vestibular dysfunction is a common complaint in patients with Pendred's syndrome and should not be overlooked.

Jervell and Lange-Nielsen Syndrome

Jervell and Lange-Nielsen syndrome (JLNS) is a rare autosomal recessive syndrome characterized by prolongation of QT interval, childhood cardiac events, and congenital profound SNHL.[50,51] Incidence has been reported as 1.6 to 6 per 1,000,000.[51] JLNS has been linked to the *KCNQ1* gene, which encodes a potassium ion channel found in epithelial, cardiac, and gastrointestinal tissue, as well as in the inner ear. Winbo and Rydberg evaluated 14 patients with JLNS for vestibular dysfunction.[50] Gross motor developmental delay was reported in 11 out of 12 patients (92%). Postrotary nystagmus test was pathologic in nine patients evaluated, but testing was limited due to fear of provoking a cardiac event.[50] Currently, there are limited data in the literature and more research is needed to better characterize the vestibular dysfunction in JLNS.

X-Linked Deafness with Perilymphatic Gusher

This disorder is classically described as bilateral mixed hearing loss and stapes fixation seen only in the males of a family.[52] Bulbous internal auditory canal and incomplete separation of the bone from the base of the modiolus to the coils of the cochlea have been noted radiographically. *POU3F4* mutations are the underlying cause in 60% of cases.[53] The disorder affects not only males, but also females, who may have moderate hearing loss. Vestibular abnormalities are variable. They may be unilateral or bilateral, and they are not associated with the degree of hearing loss. Although female carriers may demonstrate hearing loss, vestibular deficits have not been described in these patients.[52] Cremars et al published a study of vestibular function in eight males from one family.[54] Responses to caloric stimulation were variable, including normal, unilaterally weak, and bilaterally weak responses. The one consistent finding for all affected males was a shortened decremental time constant of postrotary nystagmus.

CHARGE Association

Vestibular dysfunction is a key feature in CHARGE association and can be demonstrated clinically, radiographically, and on vestibular function testing. CHARGE association is an autosomal dominant disorder named for the combination of clinical features that are frequently associated: *C*oloboma, *H*eart defects, *A*tresia choanae, *R*etarded growth/development, *G*enital hypoplasia, and *E*ar abnormalities. The prevalence is estimated to be 1 in 8,500.[55] Diagnostic criteria have been updated to include cranial nerve dysfunction and hypoplasia of the semicircular canals.[56] CHARGE association is often a result of *CDH7* gene mutations, which have been directly linked to vestibulocochlear defects.[56]

CHARGE is associated with high rates of vestibular developmental abnormalities often detected on imaging and associated reports of balance dysfunc-

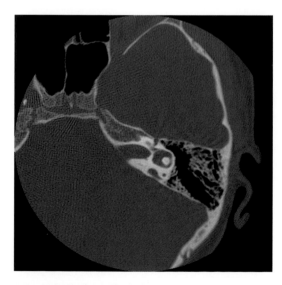

Fig. 15.4 Enlarged vestibular aqueduct.

tion. Radiographic analysis by Morimoto et al of the CT scans of 13 patients with CHARGE association showed all had absence of semicircular canals (**Fig. 15.5**) and 19% had enlarged vestibular aqueducts, and 58% of vestibules were hypoplastic or dysplastic.[57] Similarly, Abadie et al conducted a prospective study of 17 children with CHARGE association and found semicircular canal abnormalities in 94%. In addition to radiographic findings, Abadie et al observed clinically correlated vestibular dysfunction in the patients. They reported milestones were consistently achieved an average of 50% later than normal controls, with 16 of 17 children not walking until after 18 months.[58]

Vestibular testing in patients with CHARGE association is almost uniformly abnormal.[58,59] Murofushi and Graham reported all five CHARGE patients studied demonstrated absent vestibular responses on vestibulo-ocular reflex (VOR) testing and delayed motor development.[59] Deprivation of visual environment led to severe imbalance. Wiener-Vacher et al performed vestibular function tests on seven patients with CHARGE and found universally absent earth-vertical axis rotation (EVAR) responses (consistent with the finding of canal aplasia), with globally normal off-vertical axis rotation (OVAR) responses. They concluded that there was no canal VOR in any patients, but otolith VOR was present and close to normal throughout.[60]

Enlarged Vestibular Aqueduct

Enlarged vestibular aqueduct (EVA) is a sporadic finding in most patients, but it also may be associated with other inner ear malformations or congenital syndromes, such as Pendred's, Waardenburg, distal renal tubular acidosis, X-linked congenital mixed deafness, BOR syndrome, or CHARGE association.[27,61] Its occurrence ranges from 1 to 12% of patients with SNHL.[62] Genetic abnormalities have been linked to several genes. Miyagawa et al studied patients with bilateral enlarged vestibular aqueducts in a Japanese population and discovered *SLC26A4* mutation in 82% and *GJB2* mutations in 8.7%.[49] Their finding of a high prevalence of the *SLC26A4* mutation was consistent with other reported values for eastern Asian populations and is significantly higher than the prevalence in Caucasoid populations.[49]

The diagnosis of EVA is defined by a diameter of greater than 1.5 mm at the midpoint of the postisthmic segment of the aqueduct or greater than 2 mm at the operculum (see **Fig. 15.1**). Characteristically, it is associated with down-sloping SNHL, but normal hearing to profound hearing loss has been reported, as well as a fluctuating, progressive, or sudden pattern of loss.[61,63] Progressive hearing loss is commonly believed to be associated with minor head trauma.

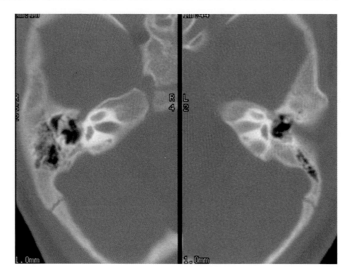

Fig. 15.5 Bilateral vestibular hypoplasia, CHARGE association (axial CT).

Comparatively, vestibular symptoms are less common in EVA than hearing loss and have been reported between 4% and 48%.[27] The exact pathophysiology of vestibular dysfunction in these patients is unknown. The proposed pathologic mechanism is fluctuating transmitted intracranial pressure that affects the otolithic membrane. It is possible that the cochlea is more sensitive to pressure changes than the vestibular system. A second hypothesis is that hyperosmolar fluid refluxes into the cochlear duct, causing vertigo.[64]

Patients with EVA may present with a variety of vestibular complaints. The range extends from minor balance disturbances during observation of rotating objects, to episodic and incapacitating vertigo, or no symptoms at all.[64] There are also reports of Tullio phenomenon. Abnormalities on vestibular testing may range from mild unilateral weakness to bilateral absence of caloric response.[63,64] Children with EVAs may also develop BPPV symptoms.[65] Oh et al presented a 4-year-old girl with EVA who experienced episodes of vertigo 15 to 30 minutes long associated with minor blows to the head.[66] Concern about worsening vestibular function has resulted in some authors recommending avoidance of seemingly innocuous head trauma even in the face of severe to profound hearing loss. Yetiser et al conducted a study of vestibular disturbance in patients with EVA.[63] They noted that 80% of patients had weak bithermal caloric responses, ranging from 22 to 46% and one patient with no response on the affected side. Grimmer and Hedlund examined 21 pediatric patients with EVAs and found vestibular symptoms in 48% of patients, which is equal to the frequency in adults.[64] They found 29% of children presented with episodic vertigo, 10% with motor delay, and 5% with imbalance.

DFNA9

DFNA9 is a subtype of autosomal dominant hearing loss. The disorder includes progressive vestibular dysfunction that accompanies progressive SNHL.[67] Severe bilateral hyporeflexia or unilateral areflexia will eventually develop. The symptoms may manifest as early as the second decade of life. Histologic studies have demonstrated microfibrillar deposits in the membranous labyrinth.

Three affected members from a single family were examined by Verhagen et al.[68] All three patients had ataxic gait, but no nystagmus on clinical examination. Bithermal caloric testing demonstrated bilateral absence of response in two patients and unilateral absence of response in the other. Posturography was abnormal in conditions five and six (vestibular pattern) in all three patients.

Histologic Vestibular Anomalies in Congenital Syndromes

Numerous temporal bone studies have demonstrated congenital malformations of the vestibular system. However, these are without characteristic clinical vestibular features that have been established in the literature. Histopathologic findings in a variety of syndromes are summarized in **Table 15.2**.

Acquired Congenital Disorders

Fetal Alcohol Spectrum Disorder

Fetal alcohol spectrum disorder (FASD) describes a pattern of congenital malformations arising from teratogenic effects of prenatal alcohol exposure. It is characterized by growth retardation, skeletal and internal organ defects, craniofacial abnormalities, ocular abnormalities, and mental impairment. There is some debate about the nature of vestibular dysfunction in this population. Jirikowic et al did a comparison of 10 children with FASD and 10 healthy controls and found poorer sensorimotor performances in children with FASD.[69] However, there was no evaluation of peripheral vestibular function and thus they were unable to determine the root of the abnormality. Church et al studied 22 children with fetal alcohol syndrome and found SNHL in 27 to 29%.[70] VNG and rotatory chair testing were normal in all patients tested; therefore, the investigators concluded there was no evidence of peripheral vestibular dysfunction. The gait ataxia was therefore attributed to cerebellar dysfunction and malformation, which has been previously reported in animal and human studies[70,71]

Table 15.2 Congenital syndromes with histological vestibular anomalies

Alagille syndrome: VA, ASCC, PSCC
Alport's syndrome: E, VA
Anencephaly: V, O, E, VA, PSCC, LSCC
Arnold-Chiari malformation: U, S, E, ASCC, PSCC, LSCC
Atresia auris congenita: V, U, VA, SCC, ASCC, PSCC, LSCC
Branchio-oto-renal syndrome: V, U, VA, ASCC, PSCC, LSCC
Camptomelia: V, U, SCC, ASCC, PSCC
Congenital deafness, keratitis, ichthyosis: S
Congenital heart disease: O, E, SCC, ASCC, PSCC, LSCC
Congenital rubella: S, O
Cornelia de Lange syndrome: SCC, ASCC, VN
DiGeorge syndrome: O, LSCC, VN
Goldenhar's syndrome: O, E, ASCC, PSCC, LSCC
Klippel-Feil syndrome: V, U, S, SCC, ASCC, LSCC, VN
Marfan's syndrome: VA
Möbius's syndrome: V, O, SCC, ASCC
Osler-Weber-Rendu: E, VA
Pierre Robin sequence: U, ASCC, PSCC, LSCC
Potter's syndrome: S, E, LSCC
Scheibe's dysplasia: S
Thalidomide ototoxicity: O, ASCC
Treacher Collins's syndrome: V, U, O, LSCC, VN
Trisomy 13: U, S, E, ASCC, PSCC, LSCC, VN
Trisomy 18: E, ASCC, PSCC, LSCC, VN
Trisomy 21: V, U, E, PSCC
Trisomy 22: E, ASCC, PSCC
Wildervanck syndrome: V, U, S, E, SCC, ASCC

Adapted with permission from Sando I, Orita Y. Vestibular abnormalities in congenital disorders. Ann New York 2001;(412):15–24.

Abbreviations: ASCC, anterior semicircular canal; E, endolymphatic duct/sac; LSCC, lateral semicircular canal; O, oval window; PSCC, posterior semicircular canal; S, saccule; SCC, semicircular canal; U, utricle; V, vestibule; VA, vestibular aqueduct; VN, vestibular nerve.

Cytomegalovirus

Cytomegalovirus (CMV) is the most common congenital infection and can be associated with low birth weight, prematurity, microcephaly, chorioretinitis, petechiae, hepatosplenomegaly, psychomotor retardation, and SNHL.[72,73] Prevalence rates are reported to be between 0.5 and 2.0% of newborns, 90% of whom are asymptomatic at birth.[74] CMV exposure can be confirmed by PCR of the urine or saliva. This test is most valuable within the first few weeks of life. Patients suspected of intrauterine exposure to CMV should have an MRI scan to look for white matter abnormalities.[75] The effects of intrauterine exposure are variable and warrant further discussion.

Although vestibular dysfunction is not commonly viewed as a critical component of congenital CMV infection, it is highly prevalent among the congenital CMV population. Karltorp et al performed a review of 26 patients with congenital CMV and found 88% with vestibular dysfunction. They compared age of ambulation in congenital CMV patients with congenitally deaf controls and found 17 of 23 patients with delayed ambulation in the CMV group, compared with no delays in the deaf controls.[74] Zagolski[76] studied vestibular function and hearing in infants with congenital CMV and compared them to healthy infant controls. VEMP and caloric testing were performed on 66 infants (26 with congenital CMV and 40 healthy controls). Twelve of 52 CMV-infected ears had abnormal VEMP results, compared with none in the control group. Caloric testing was abnormal in 16 of 52 ears in CMV children and in none of the normal children. Interestingly, only eight of 52 ears demonstrated abnormal hearing. Thus, the author concluded that vestibular dysfunction is more common than hearing loss in infants with congenital CMV.

Syphilis

Congenital syphilis is caused by the bacteria *Treponema pallidum,* which can cross the placenta before the fifth month of gestation. The congenital form usually presents in the second to tenth week of life with cutaneous lesions (similar to secondary syphilis) or as the late congenital form that presents in second decade of life. Characteristics include Hutchinson's triad of hearing loss, interstitial keratitis, and notched incisor teeth.

Vestibular dysfunction in syphilis is multifactorial and variable in presentation. Indesteege described vestibular hypofunction presenting later in life.[77] Wilson and Zoller studied seven children with congenital syphilitic otitis and found all had vertigo.[78] In this study, ENG testing revealed both central and peripheral dysfunction in 13 of 14 ears with horizontal canal paresis or absence of responses. They concluded that the vertigo these patients experience has both central and peripheral components.[78] Indesteege and Verstrawte described delayed presentation of congenital syphilis infection later in life with Meniere's symptoms. They evaluated patients presenting with vertiginous episodes in their 50s and 60s with a history of interstitial keratitis and postulated that endolymphatic hydrops explained

the late findings via a luetic infection of the inner ear. It is believed that a mononuclear leukocytic infiltrate causes progressive endarteritis and osteitis leading to fibrosis, endolymphatic hydrops, and degeneration of the membranous labyrinth.[77]

Rubella

Congenital rubella may have a variable presentation, depending on timing and severity, but it is classically described with cataracts, cardiac defects, and SNHL. Nishida et al studied vestibular dysfunction associated with the infection.[79] Caloric and vestibular testing with righting reflex was performed on 80 children with congenital rubella syndrome. They found 38% of patients with vestibular hypofunction, with no correlation between the degree of hearing loss and vestibular dysfunction. Remarkably, roughly half of patients with vestibular hypofunction had normal righting reflexes, suggesting compensatory mechanisms.[79]

■ Peripheral Vestibular Disorders

Meniere's Disease

Meniere's disease is extremely rare in children. The incidence has been reported as 1.5 to 3% of pediatric vertigo patients.[80,81,82,83] The diagnosis is made based on American Academy of Otolaryngology–Head and Neck Surgery (AAO-HNS) diagnostic criteria for Meniere's disease, which can be challenging in this population because young children are often unable to describe and characterize aural symptoms.[84] Case reports of children as young as 4 years old can be found in the literature, but the majority of children present after 10 years of age.[84] Treatment is similar to that for adults, with caffeine and salt restrictions. Diuretics can be added as a second line of therapy if symptoms persist.[83] There have been some case reports of success with pediatric intertympanic injections for refractory cases after failed therapy, but data are limited due to the rarity of the disease in children.[82]

Cochlear Implants

A significant number of congenitally hearing-impaired children (30–70%) have concurrent vestibular dysfunction.[85,86] It is therefore important to understand the potential impact a cochlear implant will have on vestibular function prior to implantation. Jacot et al looked at vestibular function in 89 children before and after implantation and found 71%

of patients with varying postoperative changes and 10% with acquired ipsilateral areflexia. Their study included a wide age range, different surgeons, and different types of implants and no correlation was observed with any of these factors.[86] Eustaquio et al compared balance function in large groups of unilaterally and bilaterally implanted children to nonimplanted hearing-impaired controls and found no clinical differences in scores between the groups.[87] The authors reported the mean of all hearing-impaired groups was below normal and the overall performance was highly variable. The literature postulates that vestibular loss may stem from direct trauma with implantation, leakage of fluids, persistent hyperexcitability though electrode stimulation, or even natural progression of the underlying disorder, but the mechanism is poorly understood.[88,89] Postmortem studies show vestibule fibrosis, collapse of the saccule, and formation of hydrops.[90]

Trauma

Trauma has been cited as the underlying cause of pediatric vertigo in 7 to 30% of cases.[80,91,92,93,94,95] It presents with ataxia, bloody otorrhea, hypoacusis, tinnitus, and hemotympanum. If these symptoms are present, a CT scan should be considered. Vertigo may be caused by tympanic membrane rupture, barotrauma resulting in perilymphatic fistulas, labyrinthine concussion, temporal bone fractures, or a traumatic brain injury. Late complications can include BPPV or endolymphatic hydrops. Vestibular testing may be abnormal, but the incidence has not been widely studied. Choung et al performed rotatory chair testing on four children with traumatic vertigo and found abnormal results in all patients; however, all caloric tests were normal.[95] Trauma is a substantial cause of pediatric vertigo and should not be overlooked.

Infections

Otitis media is another common cause of disequilibrium in children, but the exact incidence is not known. Bower found it to be the most common cause of vertigo in children, but it comprised only 3% of childhood vertigo in the systematic review by Gioacchini.[80,96] Gioacchini attributes this to eardrum abnormalities being exclusion criteria for several of the studies involved and therefore the true prevalence is unknown. Otitis media may cause vestibular dysfunction and motor delays in pediatric patients. Golz et al compared ENG results in children with middle ear effusions with ENG results in healthy controls. They found 58% of children with a middle ear effusion had abnormal ENG findings, compared with 4% of healthy controls. Presumably, the abnormalities were related to the alteration of the caloric effect due to the presence of fluid. Placement of PE tubes resulted in a 96% improvement in ENG findings.[97]

Vestibular neuritis is another potential infectious cause of pediatric vertigo. It typically presents after an upper respiratory viral infection with severe rotatory vertigo, nausea, and vomiting. Caloric testing will characteristically show canal paresis in the acute phase that is expected to slowly recover over years.[98] Infectious causes of vertigo are an important part of the differential diagnosis and should not be ignored.

Benign Paroxysmal Positional Vertigo

Although BPPV commonly occurs in the adult population, it is a rare finding in children. It accounts for approximately 3% of childhood vertigo or dizziness complaints.[99] Presentation is similar to that in adults, with brief recurrent attacks of vertigo and associated rotatory nystagumus. Benign paroxysmal positional vertigo can be distinguished from benign paroxysmal vertigo (BPV) clinically and with bedside exam testing. Children with BPV have a strong family and personal history of migraine and high rates of motion sickness, which is not commonly found in children with BPPV.[100] Diagnosis of BPPV is made with a Dix-Hallpike test, which should be normal in children with BPV.[100] Symptoms can be successfully treated with canal repositioning maneuvers.

Idiopathic Perilymphatic Fistula

The association of perilymphatic fistula and congenital abnormalities was noted by Grundfast and Bluestone[101] in 1978 with the radiographic findings further elucidated by Weissman et al.[102] Associated findings on CT or at surgery were abnormal stapes, abnormal round window, cochlear dysplasia, dysplastic vestibules, and EVAs. The characteristic features of these patients include pressure-induced disequilibrium, positional vertigo, constant disequilibrium, or fluctuating hearing loss. The associated physical findings of Hennebert sign or positional nystagmus are expected. Treatment with conservative measures of head elevation and prevention of Valsalva may be useful.[103] Exploration and closure of the fistula may be required. Beta-transferrin may be useful in confirming the perilymphatic leak.[104] In a recent study of children who have undergone surgical closure of a perilymphatic fistula, 91% of the children with vestibular complaints had symptoms that were improved or stable after surgery.[102]

■ Central Nervous System Disorders

There are many congenital and pediatric CNS disorders that may manifest balance problems. Similar to the peripheral vestibular disorders, some of these are inherited and some are sporadic.

Benign Paroxysmal Vertigo

Benign paroxysmal vertigo (BPV) is the most common cause of pediatric vertigo in several large studies.[2,92,105,106] In one study, the prevalence rate was found to be 2.6% in school children 5 to 15 years old.[3] It is considered part of a spectrum of migrainous disorders. It typically presents in toddlers ages two to three but has been reported in older children and even in adults.[91,95] Benign paroxysmal vertigo is described as recurrent brief attacks of vertigo lasting seconds to minutes and occurring without warning and then resolving spontaneously in otherwise healthy children.[107] It is not associated with headache but is commonly seen in children with a family history of migraines. Vestibular testing findings can be variable. Chang and Young[108] performed caloric and VEMP tests in 20 children with BPV and found abnormal vestibular results in 70% of the patients.[108] Typically, the attacks are self-limited and children will grow out of vertiginous episodes as they get older. However, several studies have shown a high proportion of children with BPV will develop migraines in adulthood.[3,80,109]

Vestibular Migraine

Vestibular migraines are considered part of a spectrum of central vertigo disorders and are twice as common in children with a history of BPV.[3] Depending on the patient population (neurology clinic, primary care clinic, or neuro-otology clinic), vestibular migraines account for 17 to 30% of children with vertigo.[80,91,95,110] They typically are seen in teenagers, have a female predominance, and occur in children with a family history of migraines. Vertigo is described as rotatory in nature and may last 5 minutes to 72 hours. Vertiginous episodes may precede, coincide with, or follow a headache. Associated symptoms include photophobia, phonophobia, nausea, vomiting, aura, and/or fatigue. Vestibular migraines may be accompanied by spontaneous or positional nystagmus but commonly the exam is normal.[111] They are treated with avoidance of triggers (environmental and dietary), and antimigrainous medications can be added if episodes continue.

Somatoform Vertigo

Somatoform vertigo accounts for 4 to 19% of dizzy children.[80,112] It is defined as a psychosomatic disorder associated with psychiatric comorbidities, including anxiety disorder, depression, dissociative disorders, and somatoform disorders.[112] Somatoform vertigo accounts for a relatively small proportion of vertiginous children; however, it is frequently a comorbid condition in children with vestibular migraines. Langhagen et al evaluated 168 pediatric patients referred for vertigo/balance disorders and found that 44% of children with migrainous vertigo also had somatoform vertigo.[112] There is some debate about to what extent the anxiety and comorbid psychiatric conditions stem from vertiginous episodes. Lee et al compared rates of depression and anxiety in vertiginous children to rates in controls with chronic disease. They found 18% of children with vertigo met criteria for depression, compared with none of the controls. Pathologic scores on SCARED (anxiety scale validated in children) were over four times more common in vertiginous children than they were in control children.[113]

Seizures

Vertiginous symptoms have been attributed to the aura preceding a generalized seizure or have been described as an ictal phenomenon.[114] Seizures are associated episodic vertigo lasting minutes.[115] Patients should be evaluated for a family history of seizure disorders, for associated loss of consciousness or changes in sensorium, or for other neurologic findings. Depending on practice setting, 5 to 50% of children with vertigo were found to have vertiginous seizures.[91,105,116,117] Electroencephalography is recommended in all patients with history of altered sensorium.[96]

Friedreich's Ataxia

Friedreich's ataxia is an autosomal recessive neurodegenerative disorder caused by expanded GAA trinucleotide repeats in the frataxin gene. It is characterized by truncal ataxia and dysarthria, with an onset of symptoms in the first or second decades. Patients typically have gait abnormalities on presentation. Progression of the disease from truncal to appendicular deficits generally occurs. Clinical findings including gait abnormalities, dysarthria, axonal sensory neuropathy, bilateral positive Babinski signs, and abnormal eye movements. In addition, electrocardiogram abnormalities, diabetes, pes cavus, and scoliosis may occur. Diagnosis is based on DNA analysis. To date there is neither a cure nor any therapies shown to halt progression of disease.[118]

Arnold-Chiari Malformation

The classification of Arnold-Chiari malformation is based on the degree of herniation of the brainstem and cerebellum through the foramen magnum, with type I Chiari being the most common and accounting for most patients with associated vestibular dysfunction. Radiographically, type I is defined as descent of the cerebellar tonsils more than 5 mm below McRae's line.[119] Patients typically present with a suboccipital headache, but vestibular symptoms are very common. In a study of 627 patients, about half noted instability, 18% reported vertigo, and 15% had nystagmus.[119] Down-beating nystagmus may be noted with type I malformations. MRI can be used to help diagnose and differentiate different types of this condition. Patients show improvement with surgical decompression; therefore, appropriate referrals should be made.[120]

Posterior Fossa Tumors

Posterior fossa tumors are a very rare cause of vertigo in children. They account for less than 1% of all pediatric vertiginous cases.[91] They typically present with equilibrium disturbances and are always associated with neurologic findings or progressive unilateral hearing loss. Magnetic resonance imaging should be obtained in all children with neurologic findings. Most commonly, posterior fossa tumors in children are found to be astrocytomas.[91]

Visually Evoked Dizziness

Motion Sickness

Motion sickness is typically found in school-age children. It is caused by conflicting signals between the vestibular and visual systems. It is thought to arise from a sensory mismatch between vestibular-otolith and vestibular-canal signals.[107] Jahn found that children in this age group were more sensitive to motion sickness than adults, reporting a prevalence of 40% in children 7 to 12 years old.[121] It is postulated that this high prevalence is a result of the maturing vestibular system.[107]

Ophthalmologic Findings

Ocular abnormalities are an important factor in pediatric vertigo and should not be overlooked. They are the cause of vertigo in 5 to 10% of pediatric cases.[91,122] They classically present in younger children (~ 6 years old) and are exacerbated by activities with prolonged attention. Symptoms will be more pronounced after a child has been staring at a television or computer screen for several hours. The vertigo can be described as a sense of rotation or rolling and is often accompanied by a headache. Frequently, symptoms are more pronounced at the end of the day or upon waking. In one study, vestibular testing was borderline abnormal in six of 27 patients, but the testing did not account for the degree of vertigo experienced.[122] Diagnosis can be made with ophthalmologic exam and symptoms can be improved with correction of the visual abnormality.

■ Conclusion

The importance of appropriate family counseling for patients with congenital and pediatric vestibular abnormalities should not be overlooked. A clinician armed with a thorough physiologic understanding of these disorders can provide an explanation of the dizziness symptoms, prognostic information, and appropriate rehabilitative measures. Avoidance of certain physical activities may help to prevent progression of symptoms in some syndromes. Identification of patients with syndromic features or hereditary patterns may be beneficial in investigating other affected organ systems and providing genetic counseling. More work is needed to better define vestibular defects, particularly in cases of nonsyndromic hearing loss, as well as the mechanism of vestibular compensation in these patients.

References

1. O'Reilly RC, Morlet T, Nicholas BD, et al. Prevalence of vestibular and balance disorders in children. Otol Neurotol 2010;31(9):1441–1444

2. Niemensivu R, Pyykkö I, Wiener-Vacher SR, Kentala E. Vertigo and balance problems in children—an epidemiologic study in Finland. Int J Pediatr Otorhinolaryngol 2006;70(2):259–265

3. Abu-Arafeh I, Russell G. Paroxysmal vertigo as a migraine equivalent in children: a population-based study. Cephalalgia 1995;15(1):22–25, discussion 4

4. Anson B, Donaldson J. Surgical anatomy of the temporal bone and ear. 1973. http://scholar.google.com/scholar?hl=en&btnG=Search&q=intitle:Surgical+Anatomy+of+the+Temporal+Bone#0. Accessed May 15, 2015

5. Jackler RK, Luxford WM, House WF. Congenital malformations of the inner ear: a classification based on embryogenesis. Laryngoscope 1987;97(3 Pt 2, Suppl 40): 2–14

6. Richard C, Laroche N, Malaval L, et al. New insight into the bony labyrinth: a microcomputed tomography study. Auris Nasus Larynx 2010;37(2):155–161

7. Jeffery N, Spoor F. Prenatal growth and development of the modern human labyrinth. J Anat 2004; 204(2):71–92

8. Mejdoubi M, Dedouit F, Mokrane FZ, Telmon N. Semicircular canal angulation during fetal life: a computed tomography study of 54 human fetuses. Otol Neurotol 2015;36(4):701–704

9. Donaldson J, Duckert L, Lambert P, Rubel E. Surgical Anatomy of the Temporal Bone. 4th ed. New York, NY: Raven Press; 1992

10. Bast T, Anson B. The Temporal Bone and the Ear. Springfield, IL: Charles C Thomas; 1949

11. Chen EY, Paladin A, Phillips G, et al. Semicircular canal dehiscence in the pediatric population. Int J Pediatr Otorhinolaryngol 2009;73(2):321–327

12. Russo JE, Crowson MG, DeAngelo EJ, Belden CJ, Saunders JE. Posterior semicircular canal dehiscence: CT prevalence and clinical symptoms. Otol Neurotol 2014;35(2):310–314

13. Pyle GM. Embryological development and large vestibular aqueduct syndrome. Laryngoscope 2000; 110(11):1837–1842

14. Kaga K, Sakurai H, Ogawa Y, Mizuatani T, Toriyama M. Morphological changes of vestibular ganglion cells in human fetuses and in pediatric patients. Int J Pediatr Otorhinolaryngol 2001;60(1):11–20

15. Young Y-H. Assessment of functional development of the otolithic system in growing children: a review. Int J Pediatr Otorhinolaryngol 2015;79(4):435–442

16. Foyt D, Slattery WH. Assessment of vestibular dysfunction. In: Lalwani A, Grundfast K, eds. Pediatric Otology and Neurotology. Philadelphia, PA: Lippincott-Raven; 1998

17. Weissman BM, DiScenna AO, Leigh RJ. Maturation of the vestibulo-ocular reflex in normal infants during the first 2 months of life. Neurology 1989;39(4):534–538

18. Chen C-N, Wang S-J, Wang C-T, Hsieh W-S, Young Y-H. Vestibular evoked myogenic potentials in newborns. Audiol Neurootol 2007;12(1):59–63

19. Fife TD, Tusa RJ, Furman JM, et al. Assessment: vestibular testing techniques in adults and children: report of the Therapeutics and Technology Assessment Subcommittee of the American Academy of Neurology. Neurology 2000;55(10):1431–1441

20. Hsu Y-S, Kuan C-C, Young Y-H. Assessing the development of balance function in children using stabilometry. Int J Pediatr Otorhinolaryngol 2009;73(5):737–740

21. Niemensivu R, Pyykkö I, Valanne L, Kentala E. Value of imaging studies in vertiginous children. Int J Pediatr Otorhinolaryngol 2006;70(9):1639–1644

22. Enbom H, Magnusson M, Pyykkö I. Postural compensation in children with congenital or early acquired bilateral vestibular loss. Ann Otol Rhinol Laryngol 1991;100(6):472–478

23. Kontorinis G, Goetz F, Lanfermann H, Luytenski S, Giesemann AM. Inner ear anatomy in Waardenburg syndrome: radiological assessment and comparison with normative data. Int J Pediatr Otorhinolaryngol 2014;78(8):1320–1326

24. Newton VE. Clinical features of the Waardenburg syndromes. Adv Otorhinolaryngol 2002;61:201–208

25. Marcus RE. Vestibular function and additional findings in Waardenburg's syndrome. Acta Otolaryngol 1968;(Suppl 229):229, 1–30

26. Sando I, Orita Y, Miura M, Balaban CD. Vestibular abnormalities in congenital disorders. Ann N Y Acad Sci 2001;942:15–24

27. Santos S, Sgambatti L, Bueno A, Albi G, Suárez A, Domínguez MJ. [Enlarged vestibular aqueduct syndrome. A review of 55 paediatric patients]. Acta Otorrinolaringol Esp 2010;61(5):338–344

28. Black FO, Pesznecker SC, Allen K, Gianna C. A vestibular phenotype for Waardenburg syndrome? Otol Neurotol 2001;22(2):188–194

29. Morisada N, Nozu K, Iijima K. Branchio-oto-renal syndrome: comprehensive review based on nationwide surveillance in Japan. Pediatr Int 2014;56(3):309–314

30. Stinckens C, Standaert L, Casselman JW, et al. The presence of a widened vestibular aqueduct and progressive sensorineural hearing loss in the branchio-oto-renal syndrome. A family study. Int J Pediatr Otorhinolaryngol 2001;59(3):163–172

31. Chen A, Francis M, Ni L, et al. Phenotypic manifestations of branchio-oto-renal syndrome. Am J Med Genet 1995;58(4):365–370

32. Ceruti S, Stinckens C, Cremers CWRJ, Casselman JW. Temporal bone anomalies in the branchio-oto-renal syndrome: detailed computed tomographic and magnetic resonance imaging findings. Otol Neurotol 2002;23(2):200–207

33. Noguchi Y, Ito T, Nishio A, Honda K, Kitamura K. Audiovestibular findings in a branchio-oto syndrome patient with a SIX1 mutation. Acta Otolaryngol 2011;131(4):413–418

34. Kemperman MH, Stinckens C, Kumar S, Huygen PL, Joosten FB, Cremers CW. Progressive fluctuant hearing loss, enlarged vestibular aqueduct, and cochlear hypoplasia in branchio-oto-renal syndrome. Otol Neurotol 2001;22(5):637–643

35. Ruggieri M, Iannetti P, Polizzi A, et al. Earliest clinical manifestations and natural history of neurofibromatosis type 2 (NF2) in childhood: a study of 24 patients. Neuropediatrics 2005;36(1):21–34

36. Choi JW, Lee JY, Phi JH, et al. Clinical course of vestibular schwannoma in pediatric neurofibromatosis type 2. J Neurosurg Pediatr 2014;13(6):650–657

37. Nunes F, MacCollin M. Neurofibromatosis 2 in the pediatric population. J Child Neurol 2003;18(10):718–724

38. Kimberling WJ, Möller CG, Davenport SL, et al. Usher syndrome: clinical findings and gene localization studies. Laryngoscope 1989;99(1):66–72

39. Möller CG, Kimberling WJ, Davenport SL, et al. Usher syndrome: an otoneurologic study. Laryngoscope 1989;99(1):73–79

40. Matthews TW, Poliquin J, Mount J, MacFie D. Is there genetic heterogeneity in Usher's syndrome? J Otolaryngol 1987;16(2):61–66

41. Cohen M, Bitner-Glindzicz M, Luxon L. The changing face of Usher syndrome: clinical implications. Int J Audiol 2007;46(2):82–93

42. Yan D, Liu XZ. Genetics and pathological mechanisms of Usher syndrome. J Hum Genet 2010;55(6):327–335

43. Sun JC, van Alphen AM, Wagenaar M, et al. Origin of vestibular dysfunction in Usher syndrome type 1B. Neurobiol Dis 2001;8(1):69–77

44. Jatana KR, Thomas D, Weber L, Mets MB, Silverman JB, Young NM. Usher syndrome: characteristics and outcomes of pediatric cochlear implant recipients. Otol Neurotol 2013;34(3):484–489

45. Sadeghi M, Cohn ES, Kimberling WJ, Tranebjaerg L, Möller C. Audiological and vestibular features in affected subjects with USH3: a genotype/phenotype correlation. Int J Audiol 2005;44(5):307–316

46. Stinckens C, Huygen PL, Joosten FB, Van Camp G, Otten B, Cremers CW. Fluctuant, progressive hearing loss associated with Ménière like vertigo in three patients with the Pendred syndrome. Int J Pediatr Otorhinolaryngol 2001;61(3):207–215

47. Phelps PD, Coffey RA, Trembath RC, et al. Radiological malformations of the ear in Pendred syndrome. Clin Radiol 1998;53(4):268–273

48. Luxon LM, Cohen M, Coffey RA, et al. Neuro-otological findings in Pendred syndrome. Int J Audiol 2003;42(2):82–88

49. Miyagawa M, Nishio S-Y, Usami S; Deafness Gene Study Consortium. Mutation spectrum and genotype-phenotype correlation of hearing loss patients caused by SLC26A4 mutations in the Japanese: a large cohort study. J Hum Genet 2014;59(5):262–268

50. Winbo A, Rydberg A. Vestibular dysfunction is a clinical feature of the Jervell and Lange-Nielsen Syndrome. Scand Cardiovasc J 2015;49(1):7–13

51. Yanmei F, Yaqin W, Haibo S, et al. Cochlear implantation in patients with Jervell and Lange-Nielsen syndrome, and a review of literature. Int J Pediatr Otorhinolaryngol 2008;72(11):1723–1729

52. Nance WE, Setleff R, McLeod A, Sweeney A, Cooper C, McConnell F. X-linked mixed deafness with congenital fixation of the stapedial footplate and perilymphatic gusher. Birth Defects Orig Artic Ser 1971;07(4):64–69

53. Cremers CW, Snik AF, Huygen PL, Joosten FB, Cremers FP. X-linked mixed deafness syndrome with congenital fixation of the stapedial footplate and perilymphatic gusher (DFN3). Adv Otorhinolaryngol 2002;61:161–167

54. Cremers CW, Hombergen GC, Scaf JJ, Huygen PL, Volkers WS, Pinckers AJ. X-linked progressive mixed deafness with perilymphatic gusher during stapes surgery. Arch Otolaryngol 1985;111(4):249–254

55. Issekutz KA, Graham JM Jr, Prasad C, Smith IM, Blake KD. An epidemiological analysis of CHARGE syndrome: preliminary results from a Canadian study. Am J Med Genet A 2005;133A(3):309–317

56. Sanlaville D, Verloes A. CHARGE syndrome: an update. Eur J Hum Genet 2007;15(4):389–399

57. Morimoto AK, Wiggins RH III, Hudgins PA, et al. Absent semicircular canals in CHARGE syndrome: radiologic spectrum of findings. AJNR Am J Neuroradiol 2006;27(8):1663–1671

58. Abadie V, Wiener-Vacher S, Morisseau-Durand MP, et al. Vestibular anomalies in CHARGE syndrome: investigations on and consequences for postural development. Eur J Pediatr 2000;159(8):569–574

59. Murofushi T, Ouvrier RA, Parker GD, Graham RI, da Silva M, Halmagyi GM. Vestibular abnormalities in CHARGE association. Ann Otol Rhinol Laryngol 1997;106(2):129–134

60. Wiener-Vacher SR, Amanou L, Denise P, Narcy P, Manach Y. Vestibular function in children with the CHARGE association. Arch Otolaryngol Head Neck Surg 1999;125(3):342–347

61. González-García JA, Ibáñez A, Ramírez-Camacho R, Rodríguez A, García-Berrocal JR, Trinidad A. Enlarged vestibular aqueduct: Looking for genotypic-phenotypic correlations. Eur Arch Otorhinolaryngol 2006;263(11):971–976

62. Madden C, Halsted M, Benton C, Greinwald J, Choo D. Enlarged vestibular aqueduct syndrome in the pediatric population. Otol Neurotol 2003;24(4):625–632

63. Yetiser S, Kertmen M, Özkaptan Y. Vestibular disturbance in patients with large vestibular aqueduct syndrome (LVAS). Acta Otolaryngol 1999;119(6):641–646

64. Grimmer JF, Hedlund G. Vestibular symptoms in children with enlarged vestibular aqueduct anomaly. Int J Pediatr Otorhinolaryngol 2007;71(2):275–282

65. Song J-J, Hong SK, Kim JS, Koo J-W. Enlarged vestibular aqueduct may precipitate benign paroxysmal positional vertigo in children. Acta Otolaryngol 2012;132(January, Suppl 1):S109–S117

66. Oh AK, Ishiyama A, Baloh RW. Vertigo and the enlarged vestibular aqueduct syndrome. J Neurol 2001;248(11):971–974

67. Khetarpal U. DFNA9 is a progressive audiovestibular dysfunction with a microfibrillar deposit in the inner ear. Laryngoscope 2000;110(8):1379–1384

68. Verhagen WI, Bom SJ, Fransen E, et al. Hereditary cochleovestibular dysfunction due to a COCH gene mutation (DFNA9): a follow-up study of a family. Clin Otolaryngol Allied Sci 2001;26(6):477–483

69. Jirikowic TL, McCoy SW, Lubetzky-Vilnai A, et al. Sensory control of balance: a comparison of children with fetal alcohol spectrum disorders to children with typical development. J Popul Ther Clin Pharmacol 2013;20(3):e212–e228

70. Church MW, Eldis F, Blakley BW, Bawle EV. Hearing, language, speech, vestibular, and dentofacial disorders in fetal alcohol syndrome. Alcohol Clin Exp Res 1997;21(2):227–237

71. Sowell ER, Jernigan TL, Mattson SN, Riley EP, Sobel DF, Jones KL. Abnormal development of the cerebellar vermis in children prenatally exposed to alcohol: size reduction in lobules I–V. Alcohol Clin Exp Res 1996;20(1):31–34

72. Huygen PL, Admiraal RJ. Audiovestibular sequelae of congenital cytomegalovirus infection in 3 children presumably representing 3 symptomatically different types of delayed endolymphatic hydrops. Int J Pediatr Otorhinolaryngol 1996;35(2):143–154

73. Pappas DG. Hearing impairments and vestibular abnormalities among children with subclinical cytomegalovirus. Ann Otol Rhinol Laryngol 1983;92(6 Pt 1):552–557

74. Karltorp E, Löfkvist U, Lewensohn-Fuchs I, et al. Impaired balance and neurodevelopmental disabilities among children with congenital cytomegalovirus infection. Acta Paediatr 2014;103(11):1165–1173

75. Lanari M, Capretti MG, Lazzarotto T, et al. Neuroimaging in CMV congenital infected neonates: how and when. Early Hum Dev 2012;88(Suppl 2):S3–S5

76. Zagólski O. Vestibular-evoked myogenic potentials and caloric stimulation in infants with congenital cytomegalovirus infection. J Laryngol Otol 2008;122(6):574–579

77. Indesteege F, Verstraete WL. Menière's disease as a late manifestation of congenital syphilis. Acta Otorhinolaryngol Belg 1989;43(4):327–333

78. Wilson WR, Zoller M. Electronystagmography in congenital and acquired syphilitic otitis. Ann Otol Rhinol Laryngol 1981;90(1 Pt 1):21–24

79. Nishida Y, Ueda K, Fung KC. Congenital rubella syndrome: function of equilibrium of 80 cases with deafness. Laryngoscope 1983;93(7):938–940

80. Gioacchini FM, Alicandri-Ciufelli M, Kaleci S, Magliulo G, Re M. Prevalence and diagnosis of vestibular disorders in children: a review. Int J Pediatr Otorhinolaryngol 2014;78(5):718–724

81. Choung YH, Park K, Kim CH, Kim HJ, Kim K. Rare cases of Ménière's disease in children. J Laryngol Otol 2006;120(4):343–352

82. Akagi H, Yuen K, Maeda Y, et al. Ménière's disease in childhood. Int J Pediatr Otorhinolaryngol 2001;61(3):259–264

83. Rodgers GK, Telischi FF. Meniere's disease in children. Otolaryngol Clin North Am 1997;30(6):1101–1104

84. Brantberg K, Duan M, Falahat B. Ménière's disease in children aged 4-7 years. Acta Otolaryngol 2012;132(5):505–509

85. Kaga K, Shinjo Y, Jin Y, Takegoshi H. Vestibular failure in children with congenital deafness. Int J Audiol 2008;47(9):590–599

86. Jacot E, Van Den Abbeele T, Debre HR, Wiener-Vacher SR. Vestibular impairments pre- and post-cochlear implant in children. Int J Pediatr Otorhinolaryngol 2009;73(2):209–217

87. Eustaquio ME, Berryhill W, Wolfe JA, Saunders JE. Balance in children with bilateral cochlear implants. Otol Neurotol 2011;32(3):424–427

88. Licameli G, Zhou G, Kenna MA. Disturbance of vestibular function attributable to cochlear implantation in children. Laryngoscope 2009;119(4):740–745

89. Thierry B, Blanchard M, Leboulanger N, et al. Cochlear implantation and vestibular function in children. Int J Pediatr Otorhinolaryngol 2015;79(2):101–104

90. Handzel O, Burgess BJ, Nadol JB Jr. Histopathology of the peripheral vestibular system after cochlear implantation in the human. Otol Neurotol 2006;27(1):57–64

91. Wiener-Vacher SR. Vestibular disorders in children. Int J Audiol 2008;47(9):578–583

92. D'Agostino R, Tarantino V, Melagrana A, Taborelli G. Otoneurologic evaluation of child vertigo. Int J Pediatr Otorhinolaryngol 1997;40(2-3):133–139

93. Casselbrant ML, Mandel EM. Balance disorders in children. Neurol Clin 2005;23(3):807–829, vii

94. O'Reilly R, Grindle C, Zwicky EF, Morlet T. Development of the vestibular system and balance function: differential diagnosis in the pediatric population. Otolaryngol Clin North Am 2011;44(2):251–271, vii

95. Choung Y-H, Park K, Moon S-K, Kim C-H, Ryu SJ. Various causes and clinical characteristics in vertigo in children with normal eardrums. Int J Pediatr Otorhinolaryngol 2003;67(8):889–894

96. Bower CM, Cotton RT. The spectrum of vertigo in children. Arch Otolaryngol Head Neck Surg 1995;121(8):911–915

97. Golz A, Netzer A, Angel-Yeger B, Westerman ST, Gilbert LM, Joachims HZ. Effects of middle ear effusion on the vestibular system in children. Otolaryngol Head Neck Surg 1998;119(6):695–699

98. Taborelli G, Melagrana A, D'Agostino R, Tarantino V, Calveo MG, Calevo. Vestibular neuronitis in children: study of medium and long term follow-up. Int J Pediatr Otorhinolaryngol 2000;54(2-3):117–121

99. Saka N, Imai T, Seo T, et al. Analysis of benign paroxysmal positional nystagmus in children. Int J Pediatr Otorhinolaryngol 2013;77(2):233–236

100. Marcelli V, Piazza F, Pisani F, Marciano E. Neuro-otological features of benign paroxysmal vertigo and benign paroxysmal positioning vertigo in children: a follow-up study. Brain Dev 2006;28(2):80–84

101. Grundfast KM, Bluestone CD. Sudden or fluctuating hearing loss and vertigo in children due to perilymph fistula. Ann Otol Rhinol Laryngol 1978;87(6 Pt 1):761–771

102. Weissman JL, Weber PC, Bluestone CD. Congenital perilymphatic fistula: computed tomography appearance of middle ear and inner ear anomalies. Otolaryngol Head Neck Surg 1994;111(3 Pt 1):243–249

103. Weber PC, Bluestone CD, Perez B. Outcome of hearing and vertigo after surgery for congenital perilymphatic fistula in children. Am J Otolaryngol 2003; 24(3):138–142

104. Weber PC, Kelly RH, Bluestone CD, Bassiouny M. b2-transferrin confirms perilymphatic fistula in children. Otolaryngol Head Neck Surg 1994;110(4):381–386

105. Batu ED, Anlar B, Topçu M, Turanlı G, Aysun S. Vertigo in childhood: a retrospective series of 100 children. Eur J Paediatr Neurol 2015;19(2):226–232

106. McCaslin DL, Jacobson GP, Gruenwald JM. The predominant forms of vertigo in children and their associated findings on balance function testing. Otolaryngol Clin North Am 2011;44(2):291–307, vii

107. Jahn K, Langhagen T, Heinen F. Vertigo and dizziness in children. Curr Opin Neurol 2015;28(1):78–82

108. Chang C-H, Young Y-H. Caloric and vestibular evoked myogenic potential tests in evaluating children with benign paroxysmal vertigo. Int J Pediatr Otorhinolaryngol 2007;71(3):495–499

109. Batuecas-Caletrío A, Martín-Sánchez V, Cordero-Civantos C, et al. Is benign paroxysmal vertigo of childhood a migraine precursor? Eur J Paediatr Neurol 2013;17(4):397–400

110. Tusa RJ, Saada AA Jr, Niparko JK. Dizziness in childhood. J Child Neurol 1994;9(3):261–274

111. Lempert T. Vestibular migraine. Semin Neurol 2013; 33(3):212–218

112. Langhagen T, Schroeder AS, Rettinger N, Borggraefe I, Jahn K. Migraine-related vertigo and somatoform vertigo frequently occur in children and are often associated. Neuropediatrics 2013;44(1):55–58

113. Lee CH, Lee SB, Kim YJ, Kong WK, Kim HM. Utility of psychological screening for the diagnosis of pediatric episodic vertigo. Otol Neurotol 2014;35(10):e324–e330

114. MacGregor DL. Vertigo. Pediatr Rev 2002;23(1):10–16

115. Weiss AH, Phillips JO. Congenital and compensated vestibular dysfunction in childhood: an overlooked entity. J Child Neurol 2006;21(7):572–579

116. Eviatar L, Eviatar A. Vertigo in children: differential diagnosis and treatment. Pediatrics 1977;59(6):833–838

117. Erbek SH, Erbek SS, Yilmaz I, et al. Vertigo in childhood: a clinical experience. Int J Pediatr Otorhinolaryngol 2006;70(9):1547–1554

118. Abrahão A, Pedroso JL, Braga-Neto P, Bor-Seng-Shu E, de Carvalho Aguiar P, Barsottini OGP. Milestones in Friedreich ataxia: more than a century and still learning. Neurogenetics 2015;16(3):151–160

119. Guerra Jiménez G, Mazón Gutiérrez Á, Marco de Lucas E, Valle San Román N, Martín Laez R, Morales Angulo C. Audio-vestibular signs and symptoms in Chiari malformation type I. Case series and literature review. Acta Otorrinolaringol Esp 2015;66(1):28–35

120. Aitken LA, Lindan CE, Sidney S, et al. Chiari type I malformation in a pediatric population. Pediatr Neurol 2009;40(6):449–454

121. Jahn K. Vertigo and balance in children—diagnostic approach and insights from imaging. Eur J Paediatr Neurol 2011;15(4):289–294

122. Anoh-Tanon MJ, Bremond-Gignac D, Wiener-Vacher SR. Vertigo is an underestimated symptom of ocular disorders: dizzy children do not always need MRI. Pediatr Neurol 2000;23(1):49–53

16 Migraines As a Source of Vestibular Disorders: Diagnosis and Management

Ana H. Kim and Michele M. Gandolfi

◼ Introduction

Migraine and vertigo are two common neurologic complaints in the general population. The prevalence of migraine has been shown to be elevated among patients with dizziness, and in particular among patients with unclassified recurrent vertigo.[1,2,3] Conversely, significantly more patients with migraine reported vertigo compared with patients with tension headache, namely 27% versus 8%.[4,5] Vertigo was also more common in migraine patients than in headache-free controls in two case-control studies.[6,7] Migraine and vestibular symptoms co-occur more than three times more often than by chance alone. As migraine has a lifetime prevalence of 14% and vestibular vertigo of 7%, the absolute chance consensus is expected to occur in 1% of the population, but was actually found in 3.2% in a large, population-based study.[8,9]

Various terms have been used to describe the recurring vestibular symptoms in migraine when an alternative diagnosis has been ruled out. These include migraine-associated dizziness, migraine-related vestibulopathy, migrainous vertigo, and vestibular migraine. These terms imply a link between migraine and the vestibular symptoms based on epidemiology.[5,6] Migraine associated with vertigo/dizziness, with the principal feature being the symptom of vertigo, is referred to as vestibular migraine (VM). The presentation of VM varies from spontaneous and positional vertigo, head motion vertigo/dizziness, and ataxia of variable duration, ranging from seconds to days. Most episodes have no sequential relationship with the headache, which patients experience as a separate episode. VM is considered to be the second most common cause of vertigo and the most common cause of spontaneous episodic vertigo.[10]

Recently, the Bárány Society, which represents the international community of physicians committed to vestibular research, mandated a classification group to develop diagnostic criteria for VM.

Their classification, developed in conjunction with the Migraine Classification Committee of the International Headache Society, resulted in a joint document defining VM and probable VM.[11] The criteria are included in the third edition of the *International Classification of Headache Disorders* (ICHD-3), where they appear in the appendix of new disorders that need further research for validation (**Table 16.1**). In addition, the classification of VM is part of the evolving Classification of Vestibular Disorders of the Bárány Society. The new ICHD-3 includes only VM, while the Bárány classification also contains probable VM (**Table 16.2**).

◼ Clinical Presentation

Migraine is divided into two major subtypes, migraine without aura and migraine with aura. Migraines without aura are recurrent headaches manifesting as attacks lasting 4 to 72 hours. Typical characteristics of the headache are unilateral location, pulsating quality, moderate or severe intensity, aggravation by routine physical activity, and association with nausea and/or photophobia and phonophobia. Migraine with aura is the occurrence of an aura or a perceptual disturbance before the headache begins. It often manifests as the perception of a strange light, an unpleasant smell, or confusing thoughts or experiences. Auras vary by individual; some people experience smells, lights, or hallucinations.[12] Less well-known ocular symptoms include disturbances where the eyes roll back in the head due to photosensitivity-like symptoms. A sufferer of this type of aura may experience tearfulness of the eyes and uncontrollable sensations of light, followed by reduced symptoms after ~ 20 minutes. The diagnosis of a migraine-related condition is based on a transient sign or symptom in the absence of conventional visual aura or prodrome. The headache may or may not be present.

Table 16.1   Diagnostic criteria for vestibular migraine (ICHD-3)

A.   At least five episodes fulfilling criteria C and D

B.   A current or past history of migraine without aura or migraine with aura

C.   Vestibular symptoms of moderate or severe intensity, lasting between 5 minutes and 72 hours

D.   At least 50% of episodes are associated with at least one of the following three migrainous features:
1. headache with at least two of the following four characteristics: a) unilateral location, b) pulsating quality, c) moderate or severe intensity, d) aggravation by routine physical activity
2. photophobia and phonophobia
3. visual aura

E.   Not better accounted for by another ICHD-3 diagnosis or by another vestibular disorder

From Headache Classification Committee of the International Headache Society (HIS). Data from *The International Classification of Headache Disorders*, 3rd ed.

Table 16.2   Diagnostic criteria for vestibular migraine and probable vestibular migraine

A.   At least five episodes with vestibular symptoms[a] of moderate or severe intensity,[b] lasting 5 minutes to 72 hours[c]

B.   Current or previous history of migraine with or without aura according to the International Classification of Headache Disorders (ICHD)[d]

C.   One or more migraine features with at least 50% of the vestibular episodes[e]:
• Headache with at least two of the following characteristics: one-sided location, pulsating quality, moderate or severe pain intensity, aggravation by routine physical activity
• Photophobia and phonophobia[f]
• Visual aura[g]

D.   Not better accounted for by another vestibular or ICHD diagnosis[h]

Probable vestibular migraine

A.   At least five episodes with vestibular symptoms[a] of moderate or severe intensity[b], lasting 5 minutes to 72 hours[c]

B.   Only one of criteria B and C for vestibular migraine is fulfilled (migraine history or migraine features during the episode)

C.   Not better accounted for by another vestibular or ICHD diagnosis[h]

[a] Vestibular symptoms, as defined by the Bárány Society's Classification of Vestibular Symptoms and qualifying for a diagnosis of vestibular migraine, include:
• Spontaneous vertigo including:
– Internal vertigo, a false sensation of self-motion
– External vertigo, a false sensation that the visual surround is spinning or flowing
• Positional vertigo, occurring after a change of head position
• Visually induced vertigo, triggered by a complex or large moving visual stimulus
• Head motion-induced vertigo, occurring during head motion
• Head motion-induced dizziness with nausea. Dizziness is characterized by a sensation of disturbed spatial orientation. Other forms of dizziness are currently not included in the classification of vestibular migraine.
[b] Vestibular symptoms are rated "moderate" when they interfere with, but do not prohibit, daily activities, and "severe" if daily activities cannot be continued.
[c] Duration of episodes is highly variable: About 30% of patients have episodes lasting minutes, 30% have attacks for hours, and another 30% have attacks lasting several days. The remaining 10% have attacks lasting seconds only, which tend to occur repeatedly during head motion, visual stimulation, or after changes of head position. In these patients, episode duration is defined as the total period during which short attacks recur. At the other end of the spectrum, there are patients who may take 4 weeks to fully recover from an episode. However, the core episode rarely exceeds 72 hours.
[d] Migraine categories 1.1 and 1.2 of the ICDH-2.
[e] One symptom is sufficient during a single episode. Different symptoms may occur during different episodes. Associated symptoms may occur before, during, or after the vestibular symptoms.
[f] Phonophobia is defined as sound-induced discomfort. It is a transient and bilateral phenomenon that must be differentiated from recruitment, which is often unilateral and persistent. Recruitment leads to an enhanced perception and often distortion of loud sounds in an ear with decreased hearing.
[g] Visual auras are characterized by bright scintillating lights or zigzag lines, often with a scotoma that interferes with reading. Visual auras typically expand over 5 to 20 minutes and last for less than 60 minutes. They are often, but not always, restricted to one hemifield. Other types of migraine aura, for example, somatosensory or dysphasic auras, are not included as diagnostic criteria because their phenomenology is less specific and most patients also have visual auras.
[h] History and physical examinations do not suggest another vestibular disorder or such a disorder is considered, but ruled out by appropriate investigations, or such disorder is present as a comorbid or independent condition, but episodes can be clearly differentiated. Migraine attacks may be induced by vestibular stimulation. Therefore, the differential diagnosis should include other vestibular disorders complicated by superimposed migraine attacks.

Patients with VM typically report spontaneous or positional vertigo. Some experience a sequence of spontaneous vertigo that transforms into positional vertigo after several hours or days.[13] This positional vertigo is distinct from benign paroxysmal positional vertigo (BPPV) with regard to duration of individual attacks (often as long as the head position is maintained in VM versus seconds only in BPPV), duration of symptomatic episodes (minutes to days in VM versus weeks in BPPV), and nystagmus findings. Altogether, 40 to 70% of patients experience positional vertigo in the course of the disease, but not necessarily with every attack.[14] A frequent additional symptom is head motion intolerance, i.e., imbalance, illusory motion, and nausea aggravated or provoked by head movements.[9,15] Visually induced vertigo, that is vertigo provoked by moving visual scenes, such as traffic or movies, can be another prominent feature of VM.[16] Nausea and imbalance are frequent, but nonspecific, accompaniments of acute VM.

Benign paroxysmal vertigo of childhood is an early manifestation of VM that is recognized by the ICHD-3. It is characterized by brief attacks of vertigo or disequilibrium, anxiety, and often nystagmus or vomiting, recurring for months or years in otherwise healthy young children.[17] Many of these children later develop migraines, often years after vertigo attacks have ceased. A family history of migraine in first-degree relatives is increased twofold in these children compared with controls. In a population-based study, the prevalence of recurrent vertigo probably related to migraine was estimated at 2.8% in children between 6 and 12 years old.[18]

VM often misses not only the duration criterion for an aura as defined by the ICHD-3, but also the temporal relationship to migraine headaches: vertigo can lead to headache (as would be typical for an aura), may begin with headache, or may appear late in the headache phase. Many patients experience attacks both with and without headache,[19] or attenuated headache with their vertigo as compared with their usual migraine.[15] In some patients, vertigo and headache never occur together.[19,20] Along with the vertigo, patients may experience photophobia, phonophobia, osmophobia, and visual or other auras. These phenomena are of diagnostic importance because they may represent the only apparent connection of vertigo and migraine. Patients need to be asked specifically about these migraine symptoms because they often do not volunteer them. A dizziness diary can be useful for prospective recording of associated features.

■ Pathophysiology

The pathogenesis of isolated vertigo in migraine likely shares a mechanism similar to other transient events observed in migraine, such as tinnitus, hyperacusis, hemiplegia, visual aura, torticollis, and headache. Current theories focus on disturbances in serotonergic and noradrenergic neurons of the brainstem due to an inherited voltage-gated calcium channelopathy. A primary neuronal initiation begins a cascade of neurochemical processes, culminating in a spreading wave of cortical neuronal depolarization and regional oligemia.[21] The transient vestibular events of migraine could be explained by the same focal brain dysfunction that also causes migraine-associated hemiplegia, visual aura, torticollis, and headache. However, other than discovery that a regional hyperpolarization of neurons exists in the cortical areas of the regions responsible for visual aura, the precise physiology of neurologic events in migraine remains obscure.[22] The current pathophysiologic model of VM is based on the overlap in CNS pathways responsible for pain, equilibrium, and a sense of well-being, and modulators mediated largely by norepinephrine and serotonin.[23]

The development of diagnostic criteria for migrainous vertigo was an important step in bringing together diagnostic standards for a condition like VM, which lacks any biomarkers. The term *vestibular migraine* has been convincingly advocated as a condition that stresses particular vestibular manifestations of migraine and therefore best avoids confusion with nonvestibular dizziness associated with migraine.[24]

■ Clinical Evaluation

Traditionally, patients with recurrent vertigo associated with migraine are seen in consultation by neurologists. Otolaryngologists and internists are now becoming more familiar with this condition. In patients with vertigo and migraine, clinicians must determine whether they have vertigo that is caused by migraine or rather dizziness/vertigo of an unrelated cause, which may occur by chance in a migraine patient. Of note, VM accounted for only a third of migraine patients with a history of vertigo, which indicates the need for a thorough neurotologic work-up for exclusion of other diagnoses.[25] The clinical evaluation of migraine as a source of vestibulopathy is often a time-consuming task, because the associated vestibular symptoms are so often varied. Histories taken without careful consideration of associated symptoms often focus on the intensity of vertigo and the accompanying emotional and systemic symptoms, ignoring minor neurologic symptoms. Details concerning the episodes of vertigo are most critical, with careful scrutiny given to how random or provoked the episodes are, the precise duration of episodes, the exact episode frequency, and the temporal relationship of the episodes to other symptoms. Recording these details early in the course of the illness, even when the importance is not immediately obvious, may be critical later when symptoms of accompanying conditions can obscure details of past symptoms.

Episodic vertigo is commonly accompanied by the unpleasant vegetative symptoms of motion sickness. A history of childhood motion sickness is important because it often defines the severity of these symptoms in vestibular disorders. Vestibular symptoms in migraine include an altered visuospatial awareness, an ill-defined sense of dizziness or giddiness, lightheadedness, near-fainting sensation, ataxia or disequilibrium, or an illusion of motion. The vague description of these vestibular symptoms opens up the differential diagnosis to include transient cerebral ischemia, epilepsy, presyncope, and panic disorder. Complicating differentiation, some patients have features of both migraine and Meniere's disease. Auditory symptoms are rare compared with vestibular symptoms but nevertheless there is evidence that hearing loss and tinnitus do occur.[26] Hamed et al, on the other hand, found only minor changes of no significance in persons with migraine.[27] Tinnitus is common in migraine.

Many of the dietary and environmental triggers for migraineurs are the same as those for patients with nonmigrainous vestibular dysfunction (**Table 16.3**). Hormonal fluctuations, foods, and weather changes (barometric pressure variations) often exacerbate both conditions. If patients are examined acutely when vertiginous, there is usually minimal or no spontaneous nystagmus. This provides a differential feature from peripheral vestibular syndromes. When nystagmus is present, it is often directed vertically (e.g., up-beating or down-beating). Vertically directed spontaneous nystagmus is unusual in other contexts, providing another differential point.

■ Testing

There is no "test" for VM that by itself is specific and diagnostic. VM is diagnosed from the clinical pattern and by excluding alternatives. Neuroimaging studies, although rarely diagnostic, are helpful to rule out obscure pathologic entities.[28,29] A combination of audiologic and vestibular function tests is typically employed. These include positional testing with video-oculography, oculomotor and vestibulo-ocular reflex assessments with gaze stability and/or dynamic visual acuity testing, horizontal canal testing with video electronystagmography (VNG) with calorics, audiogram, and vestibular evoked myogenic potential (VEMP).

Nystagmus observed can have peripheral, central, or mixed features.[30] Vestibular test abnormalities usually cited in migraine patients include shorter vestibulo-ocular reflex (VOR) time constants, higher VOR gain, larger VOR bias, and more caloric asymmetry.[22,31] Audiometric testing in VM typically reveals no changes in function other than occasional hyperacusis, which usually is temporary and resolves shortly after the migraine event ends. However, there are also some reports of transient cochlear symptoms, usually a transient, mild, nonprogressive, low-frequency hearing loss.[27] There is no useful genetic test for ruling in or ruling out competing diagnoses.

Rather than seeking a specific test for migraine, consider narrowing the differential diagnosis of vestibular disorders causing episodic dizziness, with a careful process of inclusion or exclusion differentiating the clinical features of an otogenic source from neurogenic, cervicogenic, cardiogenic, or psychogenic sources. This is particularly important in chronic cases, where more than one source may be involved.

Table 16.3 Food triggers

Foods	Examples
Aged or ripened cheeses	Cheddar, Gruyère, Emmenthaler, Stilton, Brie, Gouda, Romano, Parmesan, feta, Bleu, Camembert
Monosodium glutamate (MSG)	East Asian foods often have large amounts of MSG
Smoked, cured, or processed meats	Bacon, sausage, ham, salami, pepperoni, pickled herring, bologna, chicken livers, hot dogs
Alcohol	Especially red wine, port, sherry, Scotch, gin, bourbon
Chocolate, cocoa	
Nuts, peanut butter	
Caffeine	Excessive tea, coffee, cola drinks
Certain fruits	Figs, avocados, raisins, red plums, passion fruit, papaya, banana, citrus fruit

Data from Tusa RJ. Diagnosis and management of neuro-otologic disorders due to migraine. In: Herdman SJ, ed. Philadelphia, PA: F.A. Davis Co., 1994.

■ Treatment

Pharmacologic Treatment

Pharmacologic treatment of migraine can be divided into two types: symptomatic and prophylactic. Symptomatic treatment of migraine vestibulopathy differs from migraine headache in two important ways. First, the headache phase is rarely the focus of symptom management. Second, the severe autonomic symptoms prevent the bioavailability of oral agents. Triptan medications used to abort migraine headache have yet to show promise in symptomatic treatment of vertigo associated with migraine.[32] This is anticipated by the effect of triptans at vascular serotonergic receptors ($5\text{-HT}_{1b\text{-}1d}$) only during the headache phase, not the aura phase, because of their activity in the trigeminal system and inhibition of dural vasodilation. They are contraindicated in the symptomatic treatment of basilar migraine.[33]

Successful symptomatic management of the vertigo and the accompanying autonomic symptoms in migraine vestibulopathy does not differ from symptomatic management of episodic vertigo.[34] Several different vestibular suppressant medications are available with variability in their degree of sedation[35]:

- Meclizine 12.5–50 mg po every 6 hours
- Dimenhydrinate 50 mg po every 4–6 hours, 100 mg prn every 12 hours
- *Diphenhydramine 25–50 mg every 4–6 hours
- Lorazepam 0.5–1.0 mg sublingually every 4 hours
- *Lorazepam 0.5–2 mg IM/IV every 6–8 hours
- *Diazepam 2–10 mg po/IV/IM every 6–8 hours
- Droperidol 2.5–5 mg IV/IM every 3–4 hours
- Promethazine 12.5–25 mg po/pr/IV/IM every 4–6 hours
- Prochlorperazine 5–10 mg po/pr/IV/IM every 6–8 hours
- Scopolamine patch 0.5 mg per 24 hours every 3 days
- * (An asterisk denotes off-label usage, not FDA approved. po = by mouth; pr = per rectum; prn = pro re nata, when necessary; IV = intravenously; IM = intramuscularly)

The nonbenzodiazepine medications useful in treating episodic vertigo include meclizine, dimenhydrinate, and diphenhydramine. They often are given chronically yet have no proven prophylactic benefit in migraine. Scopolamine is a potent parenteral vestibular suppressant, yet it is a slow-acting agent more effective for motion sickness than for vertigo. Its chronic use (more than 9 days) and withdrawal often produce significant neurologic symptoms. The off-label use of benzodiazepines has been the mainstay of treatment for episodic vertigo, yet their chronic daily usage is complicated by uncertain pharmacokinetics, exacerbation of migraine headache, abuse potential, and significant neurologic risks of withdrawal. The parenteral administration of benzodiazepines is appropriate in the emergency department or hospital setting for the acute reduction in vertigo intensity. Sublingual lorazepam to reduce the intensity of the vertigo attack, leading to less provocation of the autonomic and emotional effects, has also proved useful, although no evidence-based confirmation of its efficacy exists.

Migraine occurring more than once a week or persisting more than 24 hours may benefit from migraine prophylaxis. There is no clinical evidence to suggest a preferential efficacy of one medication or class over another in the treatment of migraine. The first medication chosen should be a result of collaboration between doctor and patient. A return visit to assess efficacy requires waiting ~ 2 months after reaching therapeutic dosage. For appropriate treatment of migraine, the American Academy of Neurology (AAN) has published treatment guidelines, dividing prophylactic medications into various groups, defined by evidence of proven efficacy.[33] Because these medications are drawn from a diverse group of agents released for other indications, patients often become confused. It is important for the doctor to discuss this prior to beginning therapy, as the patient's confusion can polarize the therapeutic relationship. Fortunately, the diversity of effective migraine prophylactic medications usually does not require trials of medications without proven efficacy. These agents include antihypertensives, antidepressants, and neuroleptics (**Fig. 16.1**).

All of these medications require titration from a low, nontherapeutic dosage to therapeutic dosage. The dose is advanced slowly over a course of weeks to months. This allows for considerable accommodation to side effects but delays expected outcomes. Patience is required, as often side effects are a poor predictor of eventual outcome. Weight changes and psychiatric, cardiopulmonary, and other side effects complicate compliance and treatment outcome. Each drug has different side effects. A trial should not be considered adequate until a therapeutic dose is reached and maintained for a minimum of 2 to 3 months.[36] Once stabilized, effective treatment requires at least 6 months of continued administration before consideration is made to taper off the medication. Withdrawal from these agents too early can produce relapse. Evidence confirming the efficacy of migraine prophylaxis in migraine vestibulopathy is complicated by the lack of standardized diagnostic criteria. However, several case series have been reported, usually with medications that are not AAN group 1 agents. These studies find 33 to 92% improvement using β-blockers, calcium channel blockers, tricyclic antidepressants, acetazolamide, and clonazepam.

There are certain caveats to treatment of VM. Chronic daily headache or head pain suggests the

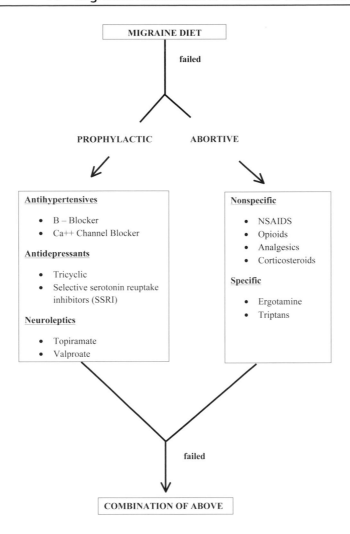

Fig. 16.1   Migraine treatment flowsheet.

patient will do best to address the headache control first. These patients will require a headache clinic approach to management of their head pain before any promise of a response to migraine prophylaxis for their vestibular complaints. In refractory cases, it is important to reconsider disorders that masquerade as migraine. These include the early stages of Meniere's disease, superior semicircular canal dehiscence syndrome, and a myriad of sporadic and familial neurodegenerative disorders.

Nonpharmacologic Treatment

Successful nonpharmacologic treatment requires a careful history focused on an attempt to identify why a change in the frequency of migraine phenomena has occurred. Changes in lifestyle, sleep, stress, perimenopause/hormonal changes, and diet are often easily identified as the source. Assuming exacerbating factors for migraine cannot be identified, migraine

prophylaxis should be discussed individually with each patient to set realistic goals of modulation through medication. For those with sleep disturbances resulting in sleep deprivation and symptoms of excessive daytime somnolence, strategies should focus on reestablishing restorative sleep cycles. For those in whom anxiety is an issue and reassurance is unsuccessful, behavioral techniques and/or antianxiety medications should be considered. Suggestions to avoid activities or places where the patient feels most vulnerable can reinforce atypical panic disorder.

Physical therapy for VM often fails because standard treatment is intended to facilitate dysfunctional vestibular pathways. When vestibular rehabilitation fails in cases of peripheral vestibulopathy, it is often due to a combination with VM. Once migraine control has been established, a reassessment for vestibular physical therapy afterward is helpful. Often the physical therapist can best approach such patients with techniques to restore confidence in postural stability and mobility, and reverse harmful avoidant behaviors.

Questions

Q1: The following are all diagnostic criteria for vestibular migraine except:

A. At least five episodes with vestibular symptoms of moderate or severe intensity each lasting 5 minutes to 72 hours.

B. Current or previous history of migraine with or without aura according to the International Classification of Headache Disorders (ICHD).

C. One or more migraine features with at least 75% of the vestibular episodes. Headache with at least two of the following characteristics: one-sided location, pulsating quality, moderate or severe pain intensity, or aggravation by routine physical activity, photophobia, phonophobia, and visual aura.

D. Not better accounted for by another vestibular or ICHD diagnosis.

Q2: Vestibular test abnormalities usually cited in migraine patients include which of following?

A. Longer vestibulo-ocular reflex (VOR) time constants.

B. Higher VOR gain.

C. Smaller VOR bias.

D. Less caloric asymmetry.

Q3: Studies found a 92% improvement in migraine prophylaxes using all of the following except:

A. β-blockers

B. Calcium channel blockers

C. Benzodiazepams

D. Tricyclic antidepressants

Q4: The following nonbenzodiazepine medications are useful in treating episodic vertigo except:

A. Meclizine

B. Dimenhydrinate

C. Diphenhydramine

D. Triptans

Q5: Effective nonpharmacologic treatment of migraine vestibulopathy includes:

A. Lifestyle modifications, herbal remedies, mind-body relaxation techniques, physical therapy, and psychotherapy.

B. High-salt diet, abstaining from exercise, and avoiding social situations.

C. High-stress environment, seeking situations that provoke symptoms of vertigo and migraine, high amounts of caffeine.

References

1. Neuhauser H, Leopold M, von Brevern M, Arnold G, Lempert T. The interrelations of migraine, vertigo, and migrainous vertigo. Neurology 2001;56(4):436–441

2. Lee H, Sohn SI, Jung DK, et al. Migraine and isolated recurrent vertigo of unknown cause. Neurol Res 2002;24(7):663–665

3. Cha YH, Lee H, Santell LS, Baloh RW. Association of benign recurrent vertigo and migraine in 208 patients. Cephalalgia 2009;29(5):550–555

4. Kayan A, Hood JD. Neuro-otological manifestations of migraine. Brain 1984;107(Pt 4):1123–1142

5. Akdal G, Baykan B, Ertaş M, et al. Population-based study of vestibular symptoms in migraineurs. Acta Otolaryngol 2015;135(5):435–439

6. Kuritzky A, Ziegler DK, Hassanein R. Vertigo, motion sickness and migraine. Headache 1981;21(5):227–231

7. Vuković V, Plavec D, Galinović I, Lovrencić-Huzjan A, Budisić M, Demarin V. Prevalence of vertigo, dizziness, and migrainous vertigo in patients with migraine. Headache 2007;47(10):1427–1435

8. Jensen R, Stovner LJ. Epidemiology and comorbidity of headache. Lancet Neurol 2008;7(4):354–361

9. Neuhauser HK, von Brevern M, Radtke A, et al. Epidemiology of vestibular vertigo: a neurotologic survey of the general population. Neurology 2005;65(6):898–904

10. Bisdorff A. Migraine and dizziness. Curr Opin Neurol 2014;27(1):105–110

11. Lempert T, Olesen J, Furman J, et al. Vestibular migraine: diagnostic criteria. J Vestib Res 2012;22(4):167–172

12. Gupta SN, Gupta VS, Borad N. Spectrum of migraine variants and beyond: the individual syndromes in children. Brain Devel 2015, June 13

13. Roceanu A, Antochi F, Bajenaru O. Chronic migraine—new treatment options. Maedica (Buchar) 2014;9(4):401–404

14. von Brevern M, Radtke A, Clarke AH, Lempert T. Migrainous vertigo presenting as episodic positional vertigo. Neurology 2004;62(3):469–472

15. Furman JM, Marcus DA, Balaban CD. Migrainous vertigo: development of a pathogenetic model and structured diagnostic interview. Curr Opin Neurol 2003;16(1):5–13

16. Waterston J. Chronic migrainous vertigo. J Clin Neurosci 2004;11(4):384–388

17. Krams B, Echenne B, Leydet J, Rivier F, Roubertie A. Benign paroxysmal vertigo of childhood: long-term outcome. Cephalalgia 2011;31(4):439–443

18. Abu-Arafeh I, Russell G. Paroxysmal vertigo as a migraine equivalent in children: a population-based study. Cephalalgia 1995;15(1):22–25, discussion 4

19. Cutrer FM, Baloh RW. Migraine-associated dizziness. Headache 1992;32(6):300–304

20. Lempert T, Neuhauser H. Epidemiology of vertigo, migraine and vestibular migraine. J Neurol 2009; 256(3):333–338

21. Goadsby PJ, Lipton RB, Ferrari MD. Migraine—current understanding and treatment. N Engl J Med 2002;346(4):257–270

22. Wray SH, Mijović-Prelec D, Kosslyn SM. Visual processing in migraineurs. Brain 1995;118(Pt 1):25–35

23. Furman JM, Balaban CD. Vestibular migraine. Ann N Y Acad Sci 2015;1343:90–96

24. Brandt T, Strupp M. Migraine and vertigo: classification, clinical features, and special treatment considerations. Headache Currents 2006;3:12–19

25. Neuhauser HK, Radtke A, von Brevern M, et al. Migrainous vertigo: prevalence and impact on quality of life. Neurology 2006;67(6):1028–1033

26. Battista RA. Audiometric findings of patients with migraine-associated dizziness. Otol Neurotol 2004;25(6):987–992

27. Hamed SA, Youssef AH, Elattar AM. Assessment of cochlear and auditory pathways in patients with migraine. Am J Otolaryngol 2012;33(4):385–394

28. Gizzi M, Riley E, Molinari S. The diagnostic value of imaging the patient with dizziness. A Bayesian approach. Arch Neurol 1996;53(12):1299–1304

29. MacDonald CB, Melhem ER. An approach to imaging the dizzy patient. J Neuroimaging 1997;7(3):180–186

30. von Brevern M, Zeise D, Neuhauser H, Clarke AH, Lempert T. Acute migrainous vertigo: clinical and oculographic findings. Brain 2005;128(Pt 2):365–374

31. Baloh RW. Neurotology of migraine. Headache 1997;37(10):615–621

32. Neuhauser H, Radtke A, von Brevern M, Lempert T. Zolmitriptan for treatment of migrainous vertigo: a pilot randomized placebo-controlled trial. Neurology 2003;60(5):882–883

33. Silberstein SD. Practice parameter: evidence-based guidelines for migraine headache (an evidence-based review): report of the Quality Standards Subcommittee of the American Academy of Neurology. Neurology 2000;55(6):754–762

34. Bisdorff AR. Management of vestibular migraine. Ther Adv Neurol Disord 2011;4(3):183–191

35. Oas JC. Episodic vertigo. In: Rakel RE, Bope ET, eds. Conn's Current Therapy. Philadelphia, PA: WB Saunders; 2002

36. Tfelt-Hansen PC. Evidence-based guideline update: pharmacologic treatment for episodic migraine prevention in adults: report of the Quality Standards subcommittee of the American Academy of Neurology and the American Headache Society. Neurology 2013;80(9):869–870

Answers	
A1:	C
A2:	B
A3:	C
A4:	D
A5:	A

17 Rare Causes of Unilateral Peripheral Vestibulopathy

Alan G. Micco

■ Introduction

Peripheral vestibulopathy indicates an injury or change in the vestibular function of the inner ear. The typical presentation is the onset of vertigo, which is one of the most common neurologic complaints. Although the patient will usually give a clear history of vertigo, the absence of such complaint does not rule out a peripheral vestibulopathy. Other symptoms may include lightheadedness, imbalance, or syncope. It is important to carefully evaluate patients with these latter complaints so that a true peripheral vestibular disorder is not missed.

■ Applied Vestibular Physiology

The vestibular system works like a push–pull pairing between each ear. There is an equal and opposite effect that is created with head movement that stimulates the vestibulo-ocular reflex (VOR). When this process is disturbed, eye movements are not coordinated, which can lead to the clinical finding of nystagmus and a patient complaint of vertigo. In essence, when there is an unequal and opposite coordination of the eye, the brain will think the head is moving when it is not.[1] The fast phase of the nystagmus will move in the direction of the stronger (normal ear) signal. Another way to think of it is that the eyes will slowly drift toward the weak side and the normal side will create the fast-phase compensatory motion. Therefore, the fast phase of the nystagmus is usually in the direction of the normal ear.

■ Etiology

Vertigo symptoms with different disorders will vary in intensity and duration. A careful history is critical to develop a diagnosis. Commonly recognized causes of peripheral vertigo, such as Meniere's disease, viral labyrinthitis/neuronitis, benign paroxysmal positional vertigo (BPPV), and perilymphatic fistula, are covered in other chapters. In this chapter, we discuss rare causes of peripheral vestibulopathy, including bacterial, traumatic, iatrogenic, and neoplastic causes. Presenting signs and symptoms, as well as clinical findings, are reviewed. Finally, work-up and treatment are covered. Ototoxicity is the usual cause of bilateral vestibulopathy, and that is covered at the end of the chapter.

■ Types and Treatment of Peripheral Vestibulopathy due to Rare Causes

Bacterial Infections

Infectious etiologies of peripheral vestibulopathy are usually viral in origin. The usual viruses considered are cytomegalovirus (CMV), mumps (i.e., paramyxovirus), and rubella (i.e., togavirus). Although rare, labyrinthitis can be caused by bacterial sources. Bacteria can enter the inner ear and cause a suppurative labyrinthitis, leading to vestibular damage. The bacteria can reach the inner ear through the round window, a fistula created by a neoplasm, or via the cerebrospinal fluid (CSF) space, internal auditory canal (IAC), or cochlear/vestibular aqueduct, as they do in meningitis. Neoplasms include cholesteatoma, glomus tumors, and metastatic disease. Histopathology usually shows an acute inflammatory response of neutrophils that eventually leads to destruction of the membranous labyrinth. Eventually, there is macrophage infiltration leading to formation of a granuloma and permanent scarring.[2,3] This may eventually lead to osteoblast formation and subsequent bone formation, as we see in meningitis. Obviously, the damage causes hearing loss, as well as a peripheral vestibulopathy. In the case of meningitis, the symptoms could be bilateral.

Appropriate antimicrobial coverage is necessary. Patients will have acute symptoms, with hearing loss and violent vertigo. They will usually be febrile. Appropriate antibiotics with broad-spectrum coverage should be used. Typically, the bacterial agent is similar to the ones that cause otitis media. Antibiotics that can travel across the blood–brain barrier are recommended because the perilymph space is, in essence, an extension of the CSF space. If there is a neoplasm, it will obviously need surgical management and creation of a barrier in the area of the fistula. This is discussed later in this chapter.

Another bacterial cause of vertigo is Lyme disease, which should be considered if the patient lives in an endemic area or has a history of a visit to such an area. Appropriate antibiotic therapy, such as doxycycline, should be used. Serum titers are followed for recovery.[4]

Tertiary syphilis can lead to a lymphocytic infiltrate of the temporal bone that can be damaging to the membranous labyrinth, leading to the formation of endolymphatic hydrops. In fact, presenting symptoms can be very similar to Meniere's disease.[5] Diagnosis requires a suspicion as well as a history of syphilis. The tertiary infection may develop years after the initial primary infection. Tertiary syphilis reaches its peak in the fifth or sixth decade of life.[6] There may be an associated fluctuating hearing loss. Clinically, there may be a finding of Tullio phenomenon secondary to the intralabyrinthine scarring.[7] A rapid plasma reagin (RPR) test and a fluorescent treponemal antibody test are usually positive. The sensitivity of the fluorescent treponemal antibody absorbed (FTA-ABS) is usually higher for tertiary syphilis. Ultimately, a cerebrospinal fluid Venereal Disease Research Laboratory (VDRL) test will be positive. Spirochetes may also be seen under dark-field exam of the CSF.[8] Treatment consists of crystalline penicillin G, 2 million to 4 million units IV every 4 hours for 10 days. Prednisone is added if not contraindicated.[9]

Trauma

The most common form of posttraumatic vertigo is BPPV. Also, endolymphatic hydrops can occur as a result of trauma. (These topics are covered in other chapters.) A temporal bone fracture with or without associated hemorrhage can lead to direct injury or concussion to the inner ear or vestibular nerve itself. Meniere's disease has also been seen to occur after trauma.[10,11] Other traumas without fracture, including airbag trauma, can induce vertigo.[11,12]

As expected, there is a higher incidence of injury to the vestibular system with transverse fractures.[13,14] Typically, patients will have severe rotatory vertigo and may also have associated hearing loss. Testing should include electronystagmography (ENG), which will likely show reduced caloric function on that side. Expectant treatment with antivertigo medication, such as meclizine or lorazepam, and antinausea medication, such as promethazine or prochlorperazine, is the usual initial therapy.[15] Usually the problem is self-limiting; however, vestibular rehabilitation may hasten recovery.[16]

Barotrauma refers to injury sustained from a failure to equalize the pressure of an air-containing space with that of the surrounding environment. The most common examples of barotrauma occur in air travel and scuba diving.[17,18] Barotrauma can also affect several different areas of the body, including the face and lungs. Barotrauma is caused by a difference in pressure between the external environment and the internal parts of the ear. Fluids do not compress under pressures experienced during diving or flying. Therefore, a fluid-containing space does not alter its volume under these pressure changes. However, the air-containing spaces of the ear do compress, resulting in damage to the ear if the pressure cannot be equalized.

Symptoms of barotrauma include fullness of the ear, ear pain, hearing loss, dizziness, tinnitus, and hemorrhage from the ear. The main concern with barotrauma is that the associated sensorineural hearing loss may be permanent. The other concern is that there is associated vertigo. This usually happens around the onset of the trauma. The vertigo is usually self-limiting but may be prolonged. Treatment can include decongestants; however, if there are signs of sudden hearing loss and vertigo, a course of steroids should be started.[19]

Perilymphatic fistula can also develop as a result of direct trauma or barotrauma. Leakage of perilymph can occur around the oval or round window. With severe blunt or penetrating trauma, there can be an obvious stapes dislocation leading to the fistula formation. The patient will complain of vertigo symptoms with head position change or Valsalva. Also, changes in pressure, such as in airplanes or elevators, can cause symptoms. Fistula testing can be conducted by pressurizing the canal with a pneumatic otoscope. Electronystagmography or electrocochleography testing may or may not show any positive findings.[20]

Initially, conservative treatment is recommended if there is no associated hearing loss. This includes activity restriction, bed rest with head elevated, and laxatives. If there is associated hearing loss, it is recommended that exploration be done relatively quickly to maximize the potential for hearing return. Also, if conservative therapy for the vertigo symptoms fails, then exploratory surgery with packing off of the round and/or oval window may be indicated.[21,22,23] The surgery is performed under local or general anesthetic. The surgical procedure for perilymphatic fistula repair is covered in a separate chapter. There is some debate whether the windows should be plugged if no obvious leak is seen. The biggest possible side effect is a conductive hearing loss from scarring in the area of the oval window. If the history and/or exam are suspicious for a fistula, the windows should be packed off even if nothing is seen during Valsalva.

Another type of vertigo, called alternovertigo, can occur when the pressure between the two middle ear spaces is different, which stimulates the vestibular (balance) end-organs asymmetrically, thus resulting in vertigo. This can be elicited by forcefully equalizing the middle ear pressure with a Politzer maneuver. This causes an unequal inflation of the middle ear space.[24,25]

Cervical vertigo is another condition that can result from trauma. This is a condition where vertigo or dizziness accompanies a neck injury.[26] Cervical vertigo should be considered when there is a related whiplash injury. The usual symptom is dizziness or vertigo that is associated with neck movement. There are usually no hearing symptoms, but there may be otalgia.

There are two thoughts about the causes of cervical vertigo. One thought is that there is vascular compression of the vertebral arteries in the neck. Chronic arthritis, previous surgery, and chiropractic manipulation can increase the incidence of symptoms after an accident. The other thought is that there is abnormal sensory input from neck proprioceptors.

To diagnose cervical vertigo, other entities need to be ruled out, especially BPPV, since the symptoms are very similar. As stated earlier, there should be no hearing symptoms or findings, but there may be otalgia, as part of the ear is supplied by sensory afferents from the high cervical nerve roots.

If cervical vertigo still seems likely after excluding reasonable alternatives, confirmatory tests should be ordered. Magnetic resonance angiography (MRA) and vertebral Doppler procedures are rarely abnormal and sometimes are used as a screening procedure to decide whether vertebral angiography is necessary. A magnetic resonance imaging (MRI) scan of the neck and flexion-extension X-ray films of the neck should be obtained. If warranted, angiography of the vertebral arteries should be undertaken. Treatments must include neck physiotherapy, but labyrinthine suppressants can be used when necessary.[27]

Epileptic vertigo and dizziness are usually characterized by a brief episode of vertigo. Patients typically experience vertigo lasting less than 30 seconds; however, some patients experience episodes lasting much longer. The source is thought to be in the temporal lobe. Symptoms can range from mild unsteadiness to rotatory vertigo. The condition usually affects younger patients with a family history of seizure disorder. This entity can present similar to BPPV. Careful history and exam are necessary. Electroencephalography usually shows temporal anomalies. Seizure treatment usually helps in the control of the episodes.[28]

Chiari malformations can also cause brief vertigo that can also be confused with BPPV. A Chiari malformation causes herniation of the cerebellar tonsils through the foramen magnum. The clinical suspicion has to be high to consider imaging the patient.[29]

It is important to keep in mind that ear pathologies that primarily cause hearing loss can also lead to vestibular symptoms. One of the more common pathologies is otosclerosis. A majority of patients with otosclerosis show abnormalities of the ocular VEMP, which likely result from involvement of the saccule.[30]

Iatrogenic Causes

Whenever otologic surgery is performed, there is always a risk of iatrogenic injury to the vestibular system. Although iatrogenic injury occurs less than 1% of the time, it has to be disclosed to the patient as a risk. The more common injuries include inadvertent drilling into the labyrinth or traumatic disruption of the ossicles. Also, a perilymphatic fistula can be created, especially after stapedectomy or ossiculoplasty.[31] If an injury is noted during the course of surgery, it should be packed off with soft tissue. This can include fat or fascia. Typically, if there is a full entry into the lateral canal, there is complete loss of hearing and balance functioning in that ear. Although the hearing is unlikely to recover in this situation, the vertigo and balance issues usually resolve. Whether there is recovery of the function or not, it is well known that roughly 90% of patients with a vestibular injury will recover and function normally. Fortunately, the brain is able to compensate and function on less than full caloric function. As in trauma patients, vestibular rehabilitation may hasten recovery. Usually, the patient will get back to normal in ~ 3 months.

Neoplasms

Any neoplasm that erodes the labyrinth can lead to vertigo. In fact, vertigo could be the sole presenting complaint from a patient with a tumor. Cholesteatomas are known to erode into the inner ear. Typically, the cholesteatoma erodes into the labyrinth at the level of the lateral semicircular canal.[32] Preoperative CT scans can help alert the surgeon to this potential complication. Care must be taken when removing the tumor. If the matrix is removed, it should be done under irrigation to prevent rapid decompression of the inner ear, which leads to permanent damage. The fenestration then needs to be covered with soft tissue. Obviously, if matrix is left on the fenestration to preserve inner ear function, a canal-wall-down mastoidectomy has to be performed.

Although not common, an acoustic neuroma can lead to symptoms of vertigo. It has been well documented that most patients with acoustic neuroma have decreased caloric function on the affected side. Other tumors that can erode into the labyrinth include glomus tumors, cerebellopontine angle tumors, cholesterol granulomas, and metastatic disease.[33] The patient must be informed preoperatively of the possibility of not only hearing loss but also vertigo. If attempts are made to preserve hearing and balance, care should be taken when removing tumor from the labyrinth.

Autoimmune Disorders

Vertigo can be associated with various autoimmune or collagen vascular diseases.[34] Patients with connective tissue disorders, such as scleroderma, rheumatoid arthritis, and lupus erythematosus, may have vertigo symptoms. Inflammatory conditions can lead to fluctuating hearing loss, as well as to vertigo. These disorders are typically treated with steroids. A response is indicative of these types of problems. If prolonged therapy is necessary, oral chemotherapeutic agents, such as cyclophosphamide or methotrexate, may be more beneficial than long-term steroid use.

Cogan's syndrome is defined as nonsyphilitic interstitial keratitis and bilateral audiovestibular deficits. There is generally a brief episode of inflammatory eye disease followed by bilateral audiovestibular symptoms. The symptoms typically deteriorate progressively within days. Whereas the erythrocyte sedimentation rate, white blood cell count, and C-reactive protein tests may be abnormal, and there can be an associated thrombocytosis or anemia, none of these findings is a reliable indicator of the disease. A slit-lamp examination is essential. Recent work has suggested that high-resolution MRI and antibodies to inner ear antigens may be helpful for diagnosis. The presentation can mimic that of Meniere's disease.[35]

Ototoxicity

Ototoxicity is a well-recognized entity. Many drugs can cause damage to the inner ear. Although this chapter focuses on vestibular toxicity, these drugs can also lead to hearing loss. There are several classes of drugs that are well recognized as ototoxic. These include, but are not limited to, salicylates, nonsteroidal anti-inflammatory drugs, aminoglycosides, loop diuretics, and platinum-based chemotherapeutic agents.

Ototoxic drugs usually lead to the formation of free radicals, usually as a result of an oxidation-reduction reaction. Prevention of the formation of these radicals with antioxidants or chelators has been shown to prevent the ototoxic damage.[36]

Salicylates and nonsteroidal anti-inflammatory drugs typically have cochlear effects, leading to tinnitus and hearing loss. Quinine has similar effects to salicylates; however, there is a known vestibular toxicity from quinine. It is known to induce transient positional abnormalities on ENG testing.

Loop diuretics, such as furosemide and ethacrynic acid, are known to be primarily cochleotoxic. These drugs inhibit the Na-K ATPase of the stria vascularis. This leads to reduction of the endocochlear potential. Platinum-based chemotherapeutic agents are typically cochleotoxic. Their major effect is on the outer hair cells in the cochlea. Although there has been notation of their vestibulotoxicity, there has been no clear or consistent evidence of this.

By far, the most common vestibulotoxic medicines are the aminoglycoside antibiotics. There is a continuum of aminoglycosides, starting with streptomycin and gentamicin, which are primarily vestibulotoxic, to neomycin and kanamycin, which are primarily cochleotoxic. With all aminoglycosides, however, cochlear and vestibular toxicity can occur.

Aminoglycosides are normally cleared by the kidney, so renal function has to be monitored.[37] Serum peak and trough levels are also closely monitored. It should be kept in mind, however, that aminoglycosides could remain in the cells of the inner ear for up to 6 months. Therefore, the duration of the therapy also has to be taken into consideration to prevent ototoxicity. Usually, systemic application leads to bilateral vestibulopathy. As soon as a patient begins to complain of otologic symptoms, the therapy should be stopped.

The typical finding in these patients is bilateral caloric deficits. Even more important, the rotatory chair test result will be abnormal. Typically, there is an increase in the phase and decrease in the gain on the chair test. The patients usually end up with oscillopsia, requiring extensive physical therapy and perhaps a wheelchair.

Unilateral vestibulopathy is commonly seen with intratympanic administration of the aminoglycoside. Although this is an expected outcome when the drug is used for vestibular ablation, one has to be careful when using aminoglycoside drops in the ear. Drops containing aminoglycosides are not recommended if the tympanic membrane is perforated or the status of the membrane is unknown. Ototopicals have been shown to cause vestibular damage as well as hearing loss when used inappropriately.[38,39,40,41] For this reason, ophthalmic preparations that contain either gentamicin or tobramycin as well as otologic preparations that contain neomycin are not recommended for use in the ear, especially if the tympanic membrane is not intact.[41,42,43,44] As with systemic usage of aminoglycoside, as soon as a patient begins to complain of otologic symptoms, the therapy should be stopped.

There is a genetic predisposition in certain patients who have been found to be more susceptible to aminoglycoside ototoxicity.[45] Because it affects only a portion of the population, routine screening is not efficacious.

■ Conclusion

The entities covered in this chapter are causes of vertigo that should be considered when the patient does not fall into the usual diagnoses. Although the chapter is not exhaustive, these causes are not uncommonly seen and should be easily recognized. As with any illness, a thorough history and complete exam are paramount. Ancillary testing is ordered based on the findings. A high degree of suspicion is usually necessary as well. Timely diagnosis of most of these problems will be beneficial in the ultimate outcome for the patient.

References

1. Zee DS, Leigh RJ. Disorders of eye movements. Neurol Clin 1983;1(4):909–928

2. Cureoglu S, Schachern PA, Rinaldo A, Tsuprun V, Ferlito A, Paparella MM. Round window membrane and labyrinthine pathological changes: an overview. Acta Otolaryngol 2005;125(1):9–15

3. Harris JP, Heydt J, Keithley EM, Chen MC. Immunopathology of the inner ear: an update. Ann N Y Acad Sci 1997;830:166–178

4. Goldfarb D, Sataloff RT. Lyme disease: a review for the otolaryngologist. Ear Nose Throat J 1994; 73(11):824–829

5. Pulec JL. Meniere's disease of syphilitic etiology. Ear Nose Throat J 1997;76(8):508–510, 512, 514 passim

6. Steckelberg JM, McDonald TJ. Otologic involvement in late syphilis. Laryngoscope 1984;94(6):753–757

7. Pillsbury HC III, Postma DS. The Tullio phenomenon, fistula test, and Hennebert's sign: clinical significance. Otolaryngol Clin North Am 1983;16(1):205–207

8. Ruckenstein MJ, Prasthoffer A, Bigelow DC, Von Feldt JM, Kolasinski SL. Immunologic and serologic testing in patients with Ménière's disease. Otol Neurotol 2002;23(4):517–520, discussion 520–521

9. Gleich LL, Linstrom CJ, Kimmelman CP. Otosyphilis: a diagnostic and therapeutic dilemma. Laryngoscope 1992;102(11):1255–1259

10. Shea JJ Jr, Ge X, Orchik DJ. Traumatic endolymphatic hydrops. Am J Otol 1995;16(2):235–240

11. Fitzgerald DC. Head trauma: hearing loss and dizziness. J Trauma 1996;40(3):488–496

12. Ferber-Viart C, Postec F, Duclaux R, Dubreuil C. Perilymphatic fistula following airbag trauma. Laryngoscope 1998;108(8 Pt 1):1255–1257

13. Wennmo C, Svensson C. Temporal bone fractures. Vestibular and other related ear sequele. Acta Otolaryngol Suppl 1989;468:379–383

14. Fredrickson JM, Griffith AW, Lindsay JR. Transverse fracture of the temporal bone, a clinical and histopathological study. Arch Otolaryngol 1963;78:770–784

15. Friedman JM. Post-traumatic vertigo. Med Health R I 2004;87(10):296–300

16. Dieterich M, Pöllmann W, Pfaffenrath V. Cervicogenic headache: electronystagmography, perception of verticality and posturography in patients before and after C2-blockade. Cephalalgia 1993;13(4):285–288

17. Farmer JC Jr. Diving injuries to the inner ear. Ann Otol Rhinol Laryngol Suppl 1977;86(1 Pt 3, Suppl 36):1–20

18. Fee GA. Traumatic perilymphatic fistulas. Arch Otolaryngol 1968;88(5):477–480

19. Parris C, Frenkiel S. Effects and management of barometric change on cavities in the head and neck. J Otolaryngol 1995;24(1):46–50

20. Campbell KC, Savage MM, Harker LA. Electrocochleography in the presence and absence of perilymphatic fistula. Ann Otol Rhinol Laryngol 1992;101(5):403–407

21. Black FO, Pesznecker S, Norton T, et al. Surgical management of perilymphatic fistulas: a Portland experience. Am J Otol 1992;13(3):254–262

22. Fitzgerald DC. Persistent dizziness following head trauma and perilymphatic fistula. Arch Phys Med Rehabil 1995;76(11):1017–1020

23. Glasscock ME III, Hart MJ, Rosdeutscher JD, Bhansali SA. Traumatic perilymphatic fistula: how long can symptoms persist? A follow-up report. Am J Otol 1992;13(4):333–338

24. Uzun C, Yagiz R, Tas A, et al. Alternobaric vertigo in sport SCUBA divers and the risk factors. J Laryngol Otol 2003;117(11):854–860

25. Tjernström O. Further studies on alternobaric vertigo. Posture and passive equilibration of middle ear pressure. Acta Otolaryngol 1974;78(3-4):221–231

26. Jongkees LB. Cervical vertigo. Laryngoscope 1969; 79(8):1473–1484

27. Bracher ES, Almeida CI, Almeida RR, Duprat AC, Bracher CB. A combined approach for the treatment of cervical vertigo. J Manipulative Physiol Ther 2000;23(2):96–100

28. Tarnutzer AA, Lee SH, Robinson KA, Kaplan PW, Newman-Toker DE. Clinical and electrographic findings in epileptic vertigo and dizziness: a systematic review. Neurology 2015;84(15):1595–1604

29. Unal M, Bagdatoglu C. Arnold-Chiari type I malformation presenting as benign paroxysmal positional vertigo in an adult patient. J Laryngol Otol 2007;121(3):296–298

30. Lin KY, Young YH. Role of ocular VEMP test in assessing the occurrence of vertigo in otosclerosis patients. Clin Neurophysiol 2015;126(1):187–193

31. Caparosa RJ, Shamblin JD, Junker CW. Stapedectomy—fistula repair. Laryngoscope 1977;87(8):1373–1377

32. Kobayashi T, Sakurai T, Okitsu T, et al. Labyrinthine fistulae caused by cholesteatoma. Improved bone conduction by treatment. Am J Otol 1989;10(1):5–10

33. Thompson LD, Bouffard JP, Sandberg GD, Mena H. Primary ear and temporal bone meningiomas: a clinicopathologic study of 36 cases with a review of the literature. Mod Pathol 2003;16(3):236–245

34. Barrs DM. Neurotologic issues. Semin Neurol 2003; 23(3):315–324

35. Baumann A, Helbling A, Oertle S, Häusler R, Vibert D. Cogan's syndrome: clinical evolution of deafness and vertigo in three patients. Eur Arch Otorhinolaryngol 2005;262(1):45–49

36. Rybak LP, Ramkumar V. Ototoxicity. Kidney Int 2007; 72(8):931–935

37. Saunders JE. Vestibulotoxicity: a risk of home aminoglycoside therapy. J Okla State Med Assoc 2005; 98(12):596–600

38. Rauch SD. Vestibular histopathology of the human temporal bone. What can we learn? Ann N Y Acad Sci 2001;942:25–33

39. Lundy LB, Graham MD. Ototoxicity and ototopical medications: a survey of otolaryngologists. Am J Otol 1993;14(2):141–146

40. Zappia JJ, Altschuler RA. Evaluation of the effect of ototopical neomycin on spiral ganglion cell density in the guinea pig. Hear Res 1989;40(1-2):29–37

41. Roland PS, Rybak L, Hannley M, et al. Animal ototoxicity of topical antibiotics and the relevance to clinical treatment of human subjects. Otolaryngol Head Neck Surg 2004;130(3, Suppl):S57–S78

42. Haynes DS. Topical antibiotics: strategies for avoiding ototoxicity. Ear Nose Throat J 2004;83(1, Suppl):12–14

43. Daniel SJ, Kozak FK, Fabian MC, et al; Expert round table of pediatric and general otolaryngologists, pediatricians, and family physicians. Guidelines for the treatment of tympanostomy tube otorrhea. J Otolaryngol 2005;34(Suppl 2):S60–S63

44. Matz G, Rybak L, Roland PS, et al. Ototoxicity of ototopical antibiotic drops in humans. Otolaryngol Head Neck Surg 2004;130(3, Suppl):S79–S82

45. Fischel-Ghodsian N. Genetic factors in aminoglycoside toxicity. Pharmacogenomics 2005;6(1):27–36

18 Central Vertigo and Disequilibrium

Peter C. Weber and Samuel C. Levine

■ Introduction

Vertigo or disequilibrium associated with central lesions or as a symptom of known diagnoses is well established and easy to ascertain, control, or manage. The real dilemmas occur when the vertigo is acute and ascribed to a peripheral etiology rather than a life-threatening central bleed/stroke. However, the money spent in evaluating every patient with an acute vertiginous attack is staggering. This chapter assesses various methods of differentiating the central from the peripheral in a cost-effective manner so that not every acute vertiginous attack receives an MRI, vascular studies, cardiac tests, laboratory analysis, and hospital admission.

Because peripheral causes of vertigo are so much more common and can be determined with some degree of certainty with bedside tests and laboratory analysis, they should be considered first if the patient exhibits no other overt central neurologic pathology/symptoms. Thus, physicians need to understand the complexities of these conditions and be well versed in the head thrust test, vestibulo-ocular reflex (VOR), nystagmus, and benign paroxysmal positional vertigo (BPPV).[1,2]

In the classic paper by Fisher,[3] written almost 50 years ago, the notion that acute vertigo could have a central cause was described. Since then, other papers have demonstrated the severity of some of the consequences, such as death. With the advent of MRI, we now know that smaller central bleeds can be the root cause of an acute vertiginous attack. The problem is whether the acute vertigo is really due to the pathology on the scan, since the age of the lesion is typically not able to be determined.

■ Diagnostic Evaluation of the Acute Vertiginous Attack

This section predicates that the patient has no focal neurologic signs/symptoms that would negate a peripheral cause. In those cases where the patient does exhibit these signs/symptoms (such as dysarthria, unilateral weakness or numbness, disorientation), diffusion-weighted MRI (MRI-DWI) with and without contrast is indicated. History is also extremely important. Whether the episode is a constant one lasting days to weeks to months versus multiple small spells of vertigo associated with movements that then subside when not moving is important. Thus, history as well as bedside evaluation is extremely useful in pinpointing a peripheral versus central cause.

The examination should include testing for dysmetria and truncal ataxia, both key central pathology findings. However, it is eye movement, nystagmus, that can be very revealing of central or peripheral etiologies. Some of the more common central findings include bidirectional nystagmus, gaze-evoked nystagmus in the vertical or horizontal plane, inability to suppress the vertical ocular reflex (VOR), rebound nystagmus, and abnormal saccades or smooth pursuit testing. It is the smooth pursuit and positional testing that prove to be the more difficult.

Bedside testing of smooth pursuit is performed with the patient following the examiner's finger or a high-contrast focal point, such as a penlight, which the examiner moves back and forth. This test does require adequate vision and therefore it may be difficult in some elderly patients, especially those with cataracts. Normal patients can easily track the moving source in a fluid motion, while central lesions induce a jerky path of following, often termed a *saccadic pursuit pattern*. In addition, testing for suppression of the VOR can be done by having the patient extend his arm out and hold up his thumb. While the patient fixates on the thumb, the chair is rotated back and forth. The slow visual tracking system should be able to suppress the VOR, and if it cannot, then a central pathology is indicated. Abnormal smooth pursuits can be associated with any central pathology but in patients with acute vertigo, the most common etiology is a midline cerebellar lesion.

The only time that abnormal smooth pursuit is found with a peripheral etiology is in acute labyrinthitis, when the patient has high-velocity nystagmus.

In this case, the smooth pursuit may be abnormal in the direction of the fast phase.

Positional testing can also reveal central pathology. In BPPV, the typical nystagmus is in the horizontal-rotary direction and is fatiguable. Central findings typically include nonfatiguable nystagmus, the vertical or downbeating nystagmus (although superior canal otoliths can cause a downbeat nystagmus), and inability to cure the problem with typical bedside maneuvers. The most common central lesions in these instances involve the cerebellum's flocculonodular lobe and include Chiari malformation, tumor, or a cerebellar degenerative process.

Recent papers suggest a new test may be important in places like the emergency department for assessing central versus peripheral pathology in acute vertigo.[4,5,6,7] The test is known as HINTS, and it is a battery of three tests of oculomotor physiology performed at the bedside. HINTS stands for *h*ead *i*mpulse test, *n*ystagmus, *t*est of *s*kew. It is relatively simple to perform. The horizontal head impulse test (h-HIT) described by Halmagyi and Curthoys in 1988 is utilized to assess the VOR; the findings are abnormal in peripheral disease but typically normal with a central etiology. In assessing nystagmus, one identifies central etiologies if the nystagmus fails to suppress with visual fixation or there is a direction-changing gaze component. In skew deviations, typically the eye is tilted vertically and the head is tilted. From HINTS came the INFARCT acronym (impulse normal, fast phase alternating, refixation on cover test). Presence of any one of three eye findings (bilaterally normal h-HIT, direction-changing gaze-evoked nystagmus, or skew deviation) means an infarct is highly likely. In one study of 101 patients, the sensitivity was 100% and the specificity 96%. In fact, HINTS was more sensitive than initial MRI-DWI for stroke identification in the acute setting.[4]

■ Specific Central Vertigo and Disequilibrium Pathologies

Transient Ischemic Attacks (TIAs)

Transient ischemic attacks are some of the more difficult etiologies to assess without imaging. Typically, TIAs are recurrent, but the patient is typically recovered by the time he/she gets medical attention. The vertigo is usually the most noticeable symptom, or the only one, and thus masks other central symptoms that may lead one to a central etiology more quickly. Typically, the spells are brief (minutes) and have recently begun (in the past few months). The most common vessel involved is the vertebral basilar artery. The clinician must determine if vertigo occurs with head extension only, which could be due to spinal compression of the artery. If hearing loss also occurs, rather than Meniere's disease, the pathology could involve the anterior inferior communicating artery.

Stroke

It is important to be able to differentiate stroke and acute peripheral neuronitis. Aside from other focal neurologic complaints, the onset of vertigo is typically different in the two conditions. In acute neuronitis, although the vertigo starts suddenly, as in a stroke, the intensity typically builds over a couple of hours, while in a stroke the vertigo is most intense immediately. The bedside head thrust test is important here. If the patient has a positive head thrust test without other focal neurologic findings, it is almost certain the lesion is peripheral. This is true for brainstem strokes as well. Cerebellar infarctions may have isolated vertigo but abnormal gaze-evoked nystagmus and ambulation difficulties are common. Cerebellar infarcts should never produce an abnormal head impulse test, since the VOR remains intact.[7]

Individuals at risk for stroke, but with acute vertigo as the only sign and with a normal MRI, may have a posterior circulatory stroke of the labyrinthine artery only, effectively mimicking acute neuronitis. Contrast-enhanced MRI may help in the diagnosis, because it is thought that a viral etiology may demonstrate a bright nerve or labyrinth.

Patients may demonstrate multiple small-vessel disease on brain MRI with multiple hyperintensities. These patients typically give a history of imbalance as well as small cognitive impairments. They tend to complain of dizziness and not vertigo. Typically, this is in the form of lightheadedness that is worse when they are upright, thus leading to the imbalance.

Cerebellar Degeneration

The causes of cerebellar degeneration include chronic alcoholism, autoimmune cerebellar disease, multisystem atrophy, and the most prevalent causes, hereditary conditions. Numerous genes/loci have been identified (SCA1–27, OMIM) and the hereditary disorders usually present with a gradual onset and progression of ataxia/disequilibrium, oculomotor abnormalities, cognitive impairment, Parkinsonism, and myoclonus.[8] However, early on, findings are usually just mild disequilibrium, abnormal smooth pursuit, and fixation suppression of the VOR. Interestingly, the SCA6 lesion seems to be associated more often with episodic vertigo that responds more to acetazolamide than to hydrochlorathiazide/triamterene.

Demyelinating Lesions

Multiple sclerosis (MS) is commonly associated with vertigo at some point during the disease process. However, vertigo may be the initial complaint in ~ 5% of patients.[9,10] Typically, plaque causing episodic vertigo alone may be located at the root entry zone of cranial nerve VIII, while it may be in other locations if other symptoms are experienced. Technically, the diagnosis is made if a minimum of two distinct clinical episodes occur with two separate lesions. With only one plaque and one episode, a lumbar puncture may be useful to analyze the CSF. For acute episodes, steroids are extremely useful. Newer medications have been developed that are taken on a long-term basis to help limit or retard the spread of disease.

Central Tumors

The most common tumors are acoustic neuromas and meningiomas in the cerebellopontine angle region. The associated vertigo may be acute, typically brought on by sudden pressure on, or inflammation of, the nerve. More commonly, the patient notices disequilibrium that he/she cannot explain and that occurs gradually over time as the tumor infiltrates or compresses the vestibular nerve. True CNS tumors, such as cerebellar lesions, present with positional vertigo, disequilibrium, and headaches. Brainstem lesions typically cause positional vertigo that has down-beat nystagmus and is nonfatigable, as well as headaches. Some tumors produce hydrocephalus, which can cause ataxia. All of the tumors are readily identified on MRI, with and without contrast. Finally, bleeding by some tumors into the subarachnoid space can cause a superficial siderosis leading to auditory vestibular complaints.[11,12]

Episodic Ataxia

Episodic ataxia may arise by one of two pathways—a potassium channel mutation (EA1) or a calcium channel mutation (EA2)—although six types have now been described. The typical manifestation is recurrent episodes of ataxia (imbalance) but patients may also exhibit recurrent vertigo attacks.[13] However, the real complaint is typically not spinning but rather being uncoordinated. In EA2, patients may have a spontaneous nystagmus during episodes, over time developing impaired smooth pursuit, truncal ataxia, and even positional nystagmus. Acetazolamide may be used during episodes to help control them, with significant effect.

Migraine

Migraine, by definition, is a paroxysmal, multifactorial, multigenetic, neurovascular disorder. Although migraine is best known for the headaches it produces, migraine-associated vertigo does not need to be associated with a headache, analogous to optic migraines. Benign vertigo of childhood is now thought to be a precursor to migraines. A patient's history may demonstrate other family members with migraines, motion intolerance/sickness with car or carnival rides, or loss of hearing in one ear. Meniere's symptoms are typical of migraines and migraines are now believed to be the most common cause of Meniere's disease. Other associations include BPPV in young patients, drop attacks, vestibular paresis, and hearing loss. Clearly, there are measurable peripheral deficits and this occurs with migraine, possibly vasospasm, is still not entirely clear.[14]

Treatment is both acute and preventative.[15] Acutely, the vertiginous attack can be treated with promethazine (Phenergan), which has both antiemetic and antivertiginous effects. Promethazine is much more effective than meclizine or Zofran. Ativan or valium may also be useful. Immetrix is very useful for the acute headaches of migraine and possibly for the acute peripheral spells as well. The real key is prevention, and just like in Meniere's disease, the side effects of the two most common medications, Tegretol and Effexor, must be balanced by how often the episodes occur and how intense they are for the individual patient. To determine if the medication is effective, a trial of 6 to 8 weeks at therapeutic doses is needed. Dietary control and elimination of other triggers may also prove useful in the prevention of attacks.

Panic Attacks

Panic attacks are typically episodic, with dizziness/vertigo, but may also include palpitations, sweating, shortness of breath, choking, trembling, nausea, fear of losing control or dying, paresthesias, chills, hot flashes, and derealization or depersonalization. Indeed, for panic attacks to be diagnosed, the patient needs to experience at least four of these symptoms during an attack and needs to have multiple attacks.[16] In addition, one of the attacks must be due to persistent concern about additional attacks or a significant change in behavior due to the attacks. Panic attacks are a medical condition caused by hypersensitivity of the parts of the brain that control fear and autonomic nervous system responses. The disorder is believed to be familial and is treated or controlled with medications, cognitive-behavior therapy, or both.

■ Conclusion

Central causes of vertigo are very real, and the ability to ascertain a central etiology in the acute phase is a necessity in providing appropriate patient care. The new HINTS test, along with the future development of the Quantitative HIT and the "eye ECG," could well give us that.[17]

References

1. Halmagyi GM, Curthoys IS. Clinical testing of otolith function. Ann N Y Acad Sci 1999;871:195–204

2. Aw ST, Todd MJ, Aw GE, McGarvie LA, Halmagyi GM. Benign positional nystagmus: a study of its three-dimensional spatio-temporal characteristics. Neurology 2005;64(11):1897–1905

3. Fisher CM. Vertigo in cerebrovascular disease. Arch Otolaryngol 1967;85(5):529–534

4. Kattah JC, Talkad AV, Wang DZ, Hsieh YH, Newman-Toker DE. HINTS to diagnose stroke in the acute vestibular syndrome: three-step bedside oculomotor examination more sensitive than early MRI diffusion-weighted imaging. Stroke 2009;40(11):3504–3510

5. Handschu R, Poppe R, Rauss J, Neundörfer B, Erbguth F. Emergency calls in acute stroke. Stroke 2003; 34(4):1005–1009

6. Kattah JC, Gujrati M. Familial positional downbeat nystagmus and cerebellar ataxia: clinical and pathologic findings. Ann N Y Acad Sci 2005;1039:540–543

7. von Campe G, Regli F, Bogousslavsky J. Heralding manifestations of basilar artery occlusion with lethal or severe stroke. J Neurol Neurosurg Psychiatry 2003;74(12):1621–1626

8. Takahashi H, Ishikawa K, Tsutsumi T, et al. A clinical and genetic study in a large cohort of patients with spinocerebellar ataxia type 6. J Hum Genet 2004;49(5):256–264

9. Pula JH, Newman-Toker DE, Kattah JC. Multiple sclerosis as a cause of the acute vestibular syndrome. J Neurol 2013;260(6):1649–1654

10. Marrie RA, Cutter GR, Tyry T. Substantial burden of dizziness in multiple sclerosis. Mult Scler Relat Disord 2013;2(1):21–28

11. Miwa T, Minoda R, Matsuyoshi H. Vestibular function in superficial siderosis. BMC Ear Nose Throat Disord 2013;13:5

12. Sydlowski SA, Cevette MJ, Shallop J. Superficial siderosis of the central nervous system: phenotype and implications for audiology and otology. Otol Neurotol 2011;32(6):900–908

13. Nachbauer W, Nocker M, Karner E, et al. Episodic ataxia type 2: phenotype characteristics of a novel CACNA1A mutation and review of the literature. J Neurol 2014;261(5):983–991

14. Seemungal B, Kaski D, Lopez-Escamez JA. Early diagnosis and management of acute vertigo from vestibular migraine and Meniere's disease. Neurol Clin 2015;33:551–564

15. Neuhauser H, Radtke A, von Brevern M, Lempert T. Zolmitriptan for treatment of migrainous vertigo: a pilot randomized placebo-controlled trial. Neurology 2003;60(5):882–883

16. Teggi R, Caldirola D, Colombo B, et al. Dizziness, migrainous vertigo and psychiatric disorders. J Laryngol Otol 2010;124(3):285–290

17. Newman-Toker DE, Curthoys IS, Halmagyi GM. Diagnosing stroke in the acute vertigo: The HINTS family of eye movement tests and the future of the "Eye ECG". Semin Neurol 2015;35(5):506–521

19 Medications Used in Treating Acute and Chronic Vertigo and Various Vestibular Disorders

Candice Colby and Tina C. Huang

■ Introduction

The vestibular system is critical for perception of one's position in space. It is composed of three building blocks interacting in complex order: the labyrinth within the inner ear, the visual system, and the somatosensory system. If a mismatch occurs between any of these three systems, the brain may perceive a sensation of dizziness or vertigo. Vertigo is the sensation of motion without true motion, and is typically a spinning sensation. True rotatory vertigo is secondary to lesions or dysfunction within the vestibular system. When prescribing medication to relieve dizziness, it is critical to attempt to define what type of dizziness the patient is experiencing, and therefore which of the three systems may be malfunctioning. This chapter focuses on medication used to treat vertigo and other various vestibular disorders.

The goals of pharmacotherapy for vertigo include eliminating the vertigo, enhancing vestibular compensation, and decreasing the neurovegetative and psychoaffective symptoms that often accompany vertigo and that may limit the patient's ability to compensate. The neurovegetative symptoms, such as nausea, vomiting, and prostration, are often more bothersome to the patient than the vertigo itself. Many patients also experience anxiety that may be quite disabling and can limit activity required for compensation. Although the immediate goal is to reduce the vertigo, several medications that reduce vertigo may also reduce the brain's ability to compensate for the reduction in vestibular function, and therefore may be indicated only for a short time. Sensory feedback is essential for adaptation to occur and treatment must balance immediate relief of symptoms with long-term correction. Therefore, treatment for vertigo commonly combines therapies aimed at both the vertigo itself and the secondary symptoms. **Fig. 19.1** shows a schematic of the relationship between the causes and symptoms of vertigo.

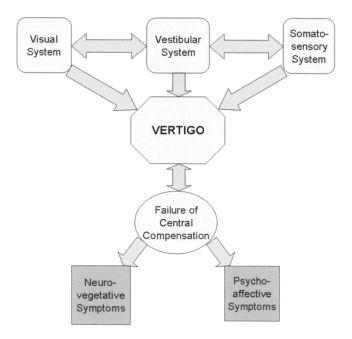

Fig. 19.1 Interaction between the visual, vestibular, and somatosensory systems leading to vertigo and the failure of compensation leading to adjunctive symptoms.

Currently, medical treatment of vertigo is primarily treatment of symptoms. If the vertigo is secondary to a defined etiology, such as infection or vascular insufficiency, the underlying cause must be treated in addition to treating the vertigo itself. If a specific vestibular disorder causing episodic dizziness is suspected, such as Meniere's disease, particular medications may be given to help prevent future attacks and to treat symptoms as they arise. Lastly, several medications also cause vertigo either due to direct peripheral ototoxic effects or due to effects on the central vestibular pathways. Although the effects may be temporary, multiple medications can cause irreversible damage to the vestibular system.

◼ Neuropharmacology of Pathways in the Vestibular System Involved in Vertigo

The medial vestibular nucleus contains histamine, glutamate, and muscarinic acetylcholine receptors.[1] Glutamate is the primary excitatory neurotransmitter at the vestibular hair cell-vestibular nerve synapse and the vestibular nerve-vestibular nucleus synapse and may work through N-methyl-D-aspartate (NMDA) receptors.[2,3] M_2 acetylcholine muscarinic receptors involved in vertigo are found in the pons and medulla and in the vestibular nuclei complex.[2] The efferent nerves to the vestibular neuroepithelium contain cholinergic receptors.[2,4] Gamma-aminobutyric acid (GABA) is one of the inhibitory neurotransmitters in the connection of the vestibular system to the oculomotor neurons. Histamine is found throughout the central vestibular system. A high density of H_1 receptors has been found within the medical vestibular nuclei.[1] Both H_1 and H_2 histamine receptors affect the vestibular response.[5] Norepinephrine modulates the reaction to vestibular stimuli centrally, and dopamine also modulates the vestibular system centrally.

The area postrema, located within the brainstem, contains the chemoreceptor trigger zone. Stimulation of this area causes vomiting. This response is reduced by blockade of the dopaminergic receptors.[3] Signaling from the gastrointestinal tract to the brain to induce vomiting is via serotonin, and serotonin blockers ($5HT_3$) block this response. Medications may act on one or multiple neurotransmitter pathways. The complexity of the interactions can make defining the exact location of action difficult.

◼ Medications for Treatment of Acute Vertigo

The treatment of acute vertigo consists mainly of controlling the associated symptoms of nausea and vomiting, and allowing the patient to perform the activities of daily living. One must ensure that life-threatening and more serious causes have been ruled out, and the etiology and further recommended treatment may be determined once the patient's symptoms have improved.

Antihistamines

Antihistamines are the most common agents used in the treatment of acute vertigo, and multiple medications from this class have shown efficacy: diphenhydramine, dimenhydrinate, cyclizine, meclizine, promethazine, cinnarizine, and astemizole. The most commonly prescribed is meclizine, due to its side effect profile. These drugs are thought to work centrally but it is difficult to pinpoint their exact mechanism, as many of these drugs have multiple sites of action. Many of the antihistamines listed also have anticholinergic activity. The most effective antihistamines are unfortunately those with the most anticholinergic properties as well,[4] causing the side effects of sedation and dry mouth.[3] These drugs are administered orally, with a duration of action between 4 and 12 hours.

Interestingly, although antihistamines are effective against vertigo, histamine itself has also been used as a treatment for vertigo. It has primarily been used to treat vertigo thought to be of vascular origin. Histamine is administered intravenously, subcutaneously, or sublingually. It increases capillary and venous volume and is a regulator of the microcirculation.[4] Betahistine, an analogue of L-histidine, is a partial H_1 postsynaptic agonist and an H_3 presynaptic antagonist[3,5] that can be taken orally and has largely replaced histamine in use. It increases inner ear blood flow and may have central effects as well. Adverse effects include headache and nausea, and it is contraindicated in patients with a history of gastroduodenal ulcer or pheochromocytoma. It has been shown to be effective for patients with Meniere's disease, both in the treatment of acute vertigo and in preventing the attacks.[6]

Anticholinergics

Anticholinergics are some of the oldest agents used to control vertigo. This class includes atropine, homatropine, and the more commonly used scopolamine (hyoscine). These drugs are nonselective and block all muscarinic receptor subtypes, both centrally and peripherally. Only anticholinergics that cross the blood–brain barrier are effective in reducing vertigo.[3] Effects after oral administration last ~ 4 hours; however, scopolamine has been developed into a transdermal patch for prolonged administration with a decreased side-effect profile and lasts ~ 4 days. In addition to improving symptoms of dizziness, the central blockade of muscarinic receptors also causes some undesired effects, such as sedation, memory problems, and confusion, particularly in the elderly. Side effects from peripheral parasympathetic blockade include mydriasis, cycloplegia, dry mouth, constipation, and urinary retention. Closed-angle glaucoma and prostatic hypertrophy are contraindications to their use.

Benzodiazepines

Benzodiazepines are GABA receptor potentiators and are often used for severe acute vertigo. Intravenous administration can be effective in preventing attacks of vertigo, and the area of action may be at the lateral vestibular nucleus.[4] Low doses of oral benzodiazepines may be effective both for treatment during an acute attack and in preventing attacks. The anxiolytic property is often useful in reducing the anxiety that often accompanies vertigo.[3] Etizolam, a benzodiazepine currently not available in the United States, has been shown in one recent study to help patients with BPPV return to daily life more rapidly and comfortably after a canalith-repositioning maneuver,[7] and it may help patients undergo treatment. Typically, diazepam is the agent of choice due to its length of action. However, in addition to being potentially addictive, diazepam can prolong compensation and recovery time if given during an acute vestibular crisis. Other adverse effects include sedation, memory impairment, and an increased risk of falls. Although benzodiazepines are efficacious, some physicians recommend benzodiazepines not be used for treatment of chronic vertigo because of their lack of selectivity for the vestibular system and their addictive potential.[2]

Calcium Channel Blockers

Calcium channel blockers have been proven effective in the treatment of acute vertigo, as well as in the prevention of vestibular migraine. Recent randomized-controlled trials from Europe and India have shown efficacy for both cinnarizine and flunarizine alone or in combination with an antihistamine.[8,9,10] Cinnarizine and flunarizine have been used primarily in Europe for the treatment of acute vertigo. These drugs have not been approved by the U.S. Food and Drug Administration (FDA), and are therefore not available for use in the United States. Cinnarizine is an antagonist of histamine, norepinephrine, nicotine, and angiotensin, as well as a calcium channel blocker. Flunarizine is its derivative and is a potent H_1 blocker with antidopaminergic properties. Neither has anticholinergic properties. Although their mechanism is not completely known, they are vestibular suppressants and likely work by blocking the entry of extracellular calcium into cells, including endothelial cells causing vasodilation. Both are administered orally. Flunarizine has a long half-life, and steady-state concentrations are not reached until 2 months. Adverse effects include sedation, weight gain, extrapyramidal reactions, and depression,[11] all of which are worsened with prolonged administration or in the elderly. Therefore, these drugs should not be used for more than a month, particularly in the elderly population.[3]

Corticosteroids

Steroids have long been advocated for the treatment of acute vertigo, although the evidence often is equivocal. In addition to treatment for autoimmune inner ear disease, steroids are used to treat early vestibular neuritis or Meniere's attacks.[2,12,13] Glucocorticoid receptors have been found in cochlear and vestibular tissue, leading researchers to speculate that steroids themselves may influence inner ear function.[14] A Cochrane review from early 2011 on the use of steroids for the treatment of vestibular neuritis found insufficient evidence from these trials to support the administration of corticosteroids to patients with idiopathic acute vestibular dysfunction.[15] However, a subsequent study from later that year found glucocorticoids administered within 3 days after onset of vestibular neuronitis improve long-term recovery of vestibular function and reduce length of hospital stay.[16] Several studies using intratympanic corticosteroid administration have also been performed, with varying results.[14]

Antidopaminergics

Other adjunctive medications to reduce the neurovegetative symptoms associated with vertigo include antidopaminergic drugs, such as phenothiazine derivatives, butyrophenones, and benzamides.[3] Some antihistamines, such as promethazine, are also dopamine antagonists, and several of the antidopaminergic medications also possess anticholinergic properties, which may contribute to vestibular suppression. Even the agents that do not cross the blood–brain barrier are effective antiemetics because the area postrema is permeable. They can be administered orally, rectally, or by injection, and their duration of action ranges from 4 to 12 hours. Adverse effects include orthostatic hypotension, somnolence, Parkinsonism, tardive dyskinesia, acute dystonia, endocrine abnormalities, and all of the anticholinergic adverse effects. Neuroleptic malignant syndrome, characterized by rigidity, mental status changes, autonomic changes, and hyperthermia, can also occur, although it is extremely rare.[13]

■ Medications for the Treatment of Vascular Insufficiency

Vascular insufficiency may be a cause of acute vertigo. Cerebrovascular accidents can present with vertigo but typically present with other focal signs or symptoms associated with the vertigo. Treatment of a stroke should be directed at the underlying cause. The blood supply to the inner ear (anterior vestibular artery, common cochlear artery) is supplied by end arteries and has no collateral circulation. Hypertension, diabetes, hyperlipidemia, or any other systemic disease that disrupts the microcirculation can cause vascular compromise. Vascular agents have previously been used in an attempt to reperfuse the vestibular system and decrease vertigo symptoms, but studies have been inconsistent as to their efficacy.[4] Agents include carbon dioxide, papaverine, buphenine, naftidrofuryl, and thymoxamine. Vasodilators may not be effective, because they work systemically, rather than locally on the vessels of the inner ear.

■ Medications for the Treatment of Autoimmune Inner Ear Disease

Autoimmune inner ear disease typically presents with hearing loss (in addition to vertigo) that may be unilateral or bilateral. If the patient has a known autoimmune disease, treatment should be instituted for that diagnosis, and steroids should also be initiated. If the patient has no known history of an autoimmune disorder and one is suspected based on presentation, laboratory investigation can confirm the diagnosis and specific treatment can begin, typically in addition to high-dose steroids if they are tolerated by the patient.

■ Other Medications

Several medications are used to treat vertigo either off label or with no clinical studies proving their efficacy. Acetylleucine is mainly used in France. Anxiolytics other than the benzodiazepines can be used to treat vertigo or the associated anxiety.[13] *Ginkgo biloba*, piribedil, and ondansetron have all been reported to be effective; however, no controlled clinical trials have proven efficacy.[3]

■ Medications for Treatment of Chronic Vertigo

Although medication may play a role in control of chronic vertigo, vestibular rehabilitation is the mainstay of treatment. Adaptation can occur only if the brain senses a mismatch between the vestibular, ocular, and somatosensory pathways, and it cannot occur if there continues to be fluctuations in those pathways. Several studies have shown improvements in function for patients who underwent vestibular rehabilitation.[13] Medication may be used as an adjunct to vestibular exercises.

Meniere's Disease

Meniere's disease may cause both acute and chronic vertigo. Treatment for acute attacks of vertigo is similar to treatment for any peripheral cause of acute vertigo. Chronic therapy is aimed at reducing the amount of fluid within the endolymphatic space, thus preventing endolymphatic hydrops. Medical management with salt restriction and use of salt-wasting diuretics is the mainstay of treatment in the United States.

Diuretics

Table 19.1 lists the classes of diuretics and examples of medications within each class. Any class of diuretic may be used, although loop diuretics should be used with caution, as they can be ototoxic. Combination medications containing potassium-sparing agents are the most commonly used, such as hydrochlorothiazide-triamterene.

Acetazolamide

Acetazolamide may reduce the vertigo in Meniere's disease by two mechanisms. First, it acts as a diuretic, thereby decreasing fluid volume. Second, it is a carbonic anhydrase inhibitor. Carbonic anhydrase catalyzes the hydration of carbon dioxide and the dehydration of carbonic acid and is found throughout the body, including the inner ear.[4] Inhibition of carbonic anhydrase may have direct effects on the physiology of the inner ear. However, there have been conflicting reports regarding the effectiveness of acetazolamide in the treatment of Meniere's disease, including incidences of tinnitus and vertigo in patients placed on the medication.

Acetazolamide can also be used to treat episodic ataxia type 2, which is a disorder defined by recurrent attacks of ataxia provoked by stress or exer-

Table 19.1   Classes of diuretics

Class	Example
Loop	Furosemide Bumetanide Ethacrynic acid
Thiazide and thiazidelike	Hydrochlorothiazide Chlorthalidone Metolazone Indapamide
Potassium-sparing	Triamterene Amiloride Spironolactone

cise that can last several hours to days. During the attack-free interval, a central oculomotor dysfunction, mainly downbeat nystagmus, is seen in nearly all patients. Episodic ataxia type 2 is an autosomal dominant hereditary disorder with mutations of the calcium channel gene.[17]

Betahistine

Betahistine is also used in the treatment of acute and chronic Meniere's disease, more often in Europe than the United States. It is thought to improve the microcirculation of the inner ear by acting on the precapillary sphincters of the stria vascularis, and therefore likely reduces the production and increases the absorption of endolymph.[17] A recent meta-analysis showed therapeutic benefit of betahistine on vertiginous symptoms in treatment of the disease[6] and the frequency of the attacks.[17]

Nimodipine

Nimodipine is a voltage-sensitive calcium channel blocker that is FDA approved for reduction of the severity of neurologic deficits resulting from vasospasm in subarachnoid hemorrhage patients and is being used off label as prophylactic treatment for both vestibular migraine and Meniere's disease. In a 2012 study, nimodipine showed an effect on the control of vertigo attacks, tinnitus annoyance, and sensorineural hearing loss when used in combination with betahistine.[18] Calcium channels have been described in the peripheral auditory systems of different species, and it has been shown that they primarily mediate neurotransmitter release from hair cells[19] and increase the latency of the action potential in a reversible manner.[20] The mobility of the outer hair cells in the organ of Corti is inhibited by the presence of nimodipine, suggesting a protective role against abnormal mechanical stimulation due to the hydropic pressure on the cochlear structures.[18]

Vestibular Migraine

Vestibular migraine is now recognized as a common cause of spontaneous episodic vertigo. An attack can consist of any combination of vertigo, ataxia, and oculomotor dysfunction, with or without head pressure, pain, nausea, or vomiting. The duration of the attack can vary from minutes to several days. Many authors have recommended first-line treatment of vestibular migraine with a β-blocker, such as propranolol or metoproplol, or tricyclic antidepressants. Topiramate is an alternative medication for prophy-

lactic treatment of vestibular migraine if the other medications are not tolerated.[17]

Chronic Subjective Dizziness (or Persistent Postural Perceptual Dizziness or Phobic Postural Vertigo)

Chronic subjective dizziness is another syndrome characterized by a persistent or fluctuating sense of unsteadiness or postural imbalance, with or without recurrent spells of vertigo. The patients' symptoms are often worsened by visually complex stimuli, such as checkerboard floors, fluorescent lights, or tall shelving in stores. The patients typically have normal vestibular testing. The condition often begins after a major stressor or a physical illness or after a true vestibular disorder, such as vestibular neuritis. Patients then develop phobic behavior and avoidance. Treatment is aimed at self-controlled desensitization within the context of behavioral therapy by repeated exposure, and if no improvement is seen within a few months, concomitant medical treatment is recommended. The first-line therapy is a selective serotonin reuptake inhibitor, such as paroxetine.[17]

Vestibular Paroxysmia

Vestibular paroxysmia is characterized by attacks of rotatory or to-and-fro vertigo that last seconds and can occur up to 30 times a day. The suspected pathophysiologic mechanism is a neurovascular cross-compression of the eighth nerve near the brainstem that leads to local demyelination.[17] Antiepileptic sodium channel blockers, such as carbamazepine and oxcarbamazepine, have shown effect, and successful treatment with these medications can be used to support the diagnosis.

Chronic Vertigo with Nystagmus

Baclofen

Baclofen is used to treat the acquired form of periodic alternating nystagmus. The nystagmus in this disorder often beats horizontally and changes its direction every 60 to 180 seconds. Patients report that their oscillopsia is less when they turn their head in the direction of the quick phase of the nystagmus.[17] This is a central vestibular disorder typically secondary to posterior fossa lesions, which may be caused by instability within central vestibular connections.[1] Baclofen is thought to reduce nystagmus by potentiating inhibition within the central vestibular pathways. It has not been shown to be effective in other central vestibular disorders.

4-Aminopyridine (Dalfampridine or Fampridine)

4-Aminopyridine is a potassium channel blocker. Dalfampridine, the sustained-release form of 4-aminopyridine, has shown a decrease in the slow-phase velocity and improved visual acuity in patients with downbeat nystagmus.[21] Downbeat nystagmus may be caused by impaired function of cerebellar Purkinje cells, and patients report oscillopsia, blurred vision, and reduced visual acuity, as well as gait or stance difficulties. The most common reported side effects of 4-aminopyridine are abdominal discomfort and dizziness.[21]

4-Aminopyridine can also be used to treat episodic ataxia type 2 (described previously) as well as upbeat nystagmus. Upbeat nystagmus is a rare oculomotor disorder in which oscillopsia is due to retinal slip of the visual scene and postural instability. It can be evoked by lesions in the brainstem or cerebellum, or in conditions like multiple sclerosis, ischemia, tumors, Wernicke's encephalopathy, cerebellar degeneration, and dysfunction due to intoxication. This condition is not permanent in most patients and spontaneously resolves within weeks.[17]

Intractable Peripheral Vertigo

Gentamicin

The mainstay of treatment for patients with intractable peripheral vertigo due to any cause who have been unresponsive to other forms of medical therapy is ablation of the peripheral vestibular system. Although a surgical labyrinthectomy is the gold standard for ablation of the peripheral vestibular end-organs, chemical labyrinthectomy using aminoglycoside antibiotics, particularly gentamicin, has shown great promise as a more noninvasive form of therapy.[4] Though gentamicin is not selectively vestibulotoxic, it is more vestibulotoxic than cochleotoxic.[22] Early forms of therapy involved administering intravenous injections to ablate the vestibular system; however, this often led to bilateral dysfunction and hearing loss. Current therapy uses local administration, either through direct intratympanic injection or via gentamicin drops administered after placement of a pressure equalization tube.[23] This eliminates the systemic effects of the medication and although a risk of hearing loss exists, reducing the dosage and prolonging the schedule of drug administration have minimized it. Multiple studies have shown that intratympanic delivery of gentamicin is effective and relatively safe.[23] The ototoxic effects of aminoglycoside antibiotics are discussed in detail in the next section of this chapter.

■ Ototoxic Medications: Medications That Can Cause Vertigo

Aminoglycosides

The ototoxic nature of the aminoglycoside antibiotics has been known since their introduction in the 1950s. Although the antibiotics have different levels of vestibulotoxicity versus cochleotoxicity, all toxicity depends on the serum concentration of the drug and the duration of treatment. Because the aminoglycosides are excreted by the kidney, impaired renal function will increase serum concentrations. This is compounded by the fact that the aminoglycosides are also nephrotoxic. In addition, clearance of aminoglycosides within the inner ear has been shown to be slower than their elimination from plasma or cerebrospinal fluid.[22] Within the vestibular neuroepithelium, the crista ampullaris of the semicircular canals is the most sensitive. The saccule is the least sensitive, and the utricle is midway between the two. The type I hair cells are more sensitive than the type II hair cells. The antibiotic binds to the cell membranes and disrupts calcium uptake by the cell,[4,22] and this cell damage is permanent. A genetic susceptibility to toxicity has been shown in patients with the *A1555G* mitochondrial RNA mutation, as well as those with other mitochondrial abnormalities.

Loop Diuretics

Furosemide, ethacrynic acid, and bumetanide are loop diuretics that are known to be ototoxic.[4] Their diuretic mechanism of action is to block the reabsorption of sodium and chloride in the ascending loop of Henle. High doses and impaired renal function are risk factors for ototoxicity, although their mechanism of toxicity is unknown. Typically, cochlear function is impaired, but vestibular function can be affected as well and this impairment may be temporary or permanent. It is important to note that the combination of a loop diuretic with an aminoglycoside antibiotic increases the overall ototoxicity of both drugs. Other risk factors for developing toxicity from any ototoxic drug include the previous use of an ototoxic agent, exposure to multiple ototoxic agents, duration of treatment longer than 14 days, multiple courses of ototoxic agents, and advanced age.[24]

■ Drugs Causing Central Vestibular Symptoms

A central vestibular syndrome has been reported with several medications,[3] and symptoms include ataxia, disequilibrium, and gaze-paretic nystagmus. Antiepileptics, tricyclic antidepressants, anxiolytics, opiates, neuroleptics, alcohol, and other recreational drugs, such as phencyclidine, that depress the central nervous system (CNS) have been implicated. Medications in the hydantoin family, toluene, and chemotherapeutic agents have been known to cause irreversible cerebellar damage as well.

■ Less Common Medications

Table 19.2 lists other medications that can cause vertigo. It is by no means a comprehensive list, as almost any medication can potentially cause a sensation of vertigo and/or disequilibrium. In addition, several drugs can cause orthostatic hypotension, which patients often report as dizziness, including antihypertensives, antiadrenergic agents, vasodilators (nitroglycerine), and anti-Parkinsonism medications (levodopa and dopamine agonists). Sedative medications and antidiabetic medications causing hypoglycemia can also bring on a sensation of dizziness or lightheadedness. Even withdrawal after the chronic use of vestibular suppressants can cause dizziness.[13]

Table 19.2 Medications that can cause vertigo

Class	Example
Aminoglycoside antibiotics	Amikacin
	Dibekacin
	Dihydrostreptomycin
	Gentamicin
	Kanamycin
	Lividomycin
	Neomycin
	Netilmicin
	Sisomicin
	Tobramycin
Other antibiotics	Chloramphenicol
	Clindamycin
	Erythromycin
	Isoniazid
	Lincomycin
	Minocycline
	Polymyxin B
	Ristocetin
	Vancomycin
	Viomycin
Antimalarials	Carbon sulfide
	Chloroquine
	Mefloquine
	Quinine
	Toluene
Loop diuretics	Bumetanide
	Ethacrynic acid
	Furosemide
	Piretanide
Nonsteroidal anti-inflammatories	Aspirin
	Indomethacin
	Salicylates
Antiarrhythmics	Amiodarone
	Quinidine

Class	Example
Anticonvulsants	Barbiturates
	Carbamazepine
	Phenytoin
Antidepressants	Amitriptyline
	Imipramine
Hypnotics/tranquilizers	Chlordiazepoxide
	Flurazepam
	Meprobamate
	Triazolam
Muscle relaxants	Cyclobenzaprine
	Methocarbamol
	Orphenadrine
Cytotoxic agents	Carboplatin
	Chlormethine
	Cisplatin
	Floxuridine
	Fluorouracil
	Gold
	Methchlorethamine
	Methotrexate
	Nitrogen mustard
	Procarbazine
	Vinblastine
Chemicals	Aniline dyes
	Arsenic
	Ethyl alcohol
	Lead
	Manganese
	Mercury
	Mineral oils
	Povidone iodine scrub solution
	Propylene glycol
	Styrene
	Tin
	Trichloroethylene

■ Conclusion

The ideal medication for the treatment of vertigo has yet to be found. A plethora of choices exists for symptomatic improvement, with few drugs established as preventative medication. Many medications are vestibular suppressants, which will reduce the asymmetry between the two vestibular systems and reduce the symptoms, but also often decreases the vestibular compensation by reducing the sensory feedback of the asymmetric signal. Unfortunately, the practitioner must often force the patient to feel worse through the compensation period before the symptoms will begin to improve. An underlying cause for the vertigo must also be sought and treatment initiated for the primary disease.

References

1. Zee DS. Perspectives on the pharmacotherapy of vertigo. Arch Otolaryngol 1985;111(9):609–612
2. Darlington CL, Smith PF. Drug treatment for vertigo and dizziness. N Z Med J 1998;111(1073):332–334
3. Rascol O, Hain TC, Brefel C, Benazet M, Clanet M, Montastruc JL. Antivertigo medications and drug-induced vertigo. A pharmacological review. Drugs 1995; 50(5):777–791
4. Norris CH. Drugs affecting the inner ear. A review of their clinical efficacy, mechanisms of action, toxicity, and place in therapy. Drugs 1988;36(6):754–772
5. Timmerman H. Pharmacotherapy of vertigo: any news to be expected? Acta Otolaryngol Suppl 1994; 513:28–32
6. Nauta JJ. Meta-analysis of clinical studies with betahistine in Ménière's disease and vestibular vertigo. Eur Arch Otorhinolaryngol 2014;271(5):887–897
7. Jung HJ, Koo JW, Kim CS, Kim JS, Song JJ. Anxiolytics reduce residual dizziness after successful canalith repositioning maneuvers in benign paroxysmal positional vertigo. Acta Otolaryngol 2012;132(3):277–284
8. Lepcha A, Amalanathan S, Augustine AM, Tyagi AK, Balraj A. Flunarizine in the prophylaxis of migrainous vertigo: a randomized controlled trial. Eur Arch Otorhinolaryngol 2014;271(11):2931–2936
9. Hahn A, Novotný M, Shotekov PM, Cirek Z, Bognar-Steinberg I, Baumann W. Comparison of cinnarizine/dimenhydrinate fixed combination with the respective monotherapies for vertigo of various origins: a randomized, double-blind, active-controlled, multicentre study. Clin Drug Investig 2011;31(6):371–383
10. Scholtz AW, Schwarz M, Baumann W, Kleinfeldt D, Scholtz HJ. Treatment of vertigo due to acute unilateral vestibular loss with a fixed combination of cinnarizine and dimenhydrinate: a double-blind, randomized, parallel-group clinical study. Clin Ther 2004;26(6):866–877
11. Taghdiri F, Togha M, Razeghi Jahromi S, Refaeian F. Cinnarizine for the prophylaxis of migraine associated vertigo: a retrospective study. Springerplus 2014;3:231
12. Goebel JA. Management options for acute versus chronic vertigo. Otolaryngol Clin North Am 2000;33(3):483–493
13. Tusa RJ. Dizziness. Med Clin North Am 2003;87(3): 609–641, vii
14. Barrs DM. Intratympanic corticosteroids for Meniere's disease and vertigo. Otolaryngol Clin North Am 2004;37(5):955–972, v
15. Fishman JM, Burgess C, Waddell A. Corticosteroids for the treatment of idiopathic acute vestibular dysfunction (vestibular neuritis). Cochrane Database Syst Rev 2011;(5):CD008607
16. Karlberg ML, Magnusson M. Treatment of acute vestibular neuronitis with glucocorticoids. Otol Neurotol 2011;32(7):1140–1143
17. Huppert D, Strupp M, Mückter H, Brandt T. Which medication do I need to manage dizzy patients? Acta Otolaryngol 2011;131(3):228–241
18. Monzani D, Barillari MR, Alicandri Ciufelli M, et al. Effect of a fixed combination of nimodipine and betahistine versus betahistine as monotherapy in the long-term treatment of Ménière's disease: a 10-year experience. Acta Otorhinolaryngol Ital 2012;32(6):393–403
19. Sueta T, Zhang SY, Sellick PM, Patuzzi R, Robertson D. Effects of a calcium channel blocker on spontaneous neural noise and gross action potential waveforms in the guinea pig cochlea. Hear Res 2004;188(1-2):117–125
20. Chen L, Sun W, Salvi RJ. Effects of nimodipine, an L-type calcium channel antagonist, on the chicken's cochlear potentials. Hear Res 2006;221(1-2):82–90
21. Claassen J, Feil K, Bardins S, et al. Dalfampridine in patients with downbeat nystagmus—an observational study. J Neurol 2013;260(8):1992–1996
22. Nakashima T, Teranishi M, Hibi T, Kobayashi M, Umemura M. Vestibular and cochlear toxicity of aminoglycosides—a review. Acta Otolaryngol 2000; 120(8):904–911
23. Carey J. Intratympanic gentamicin for the treatment of Meniere's disease and other forms of peripheral vertigo. Otolaryngol Clin North Am 2004;37(5):1075–1090
24. Vasquez R, Mattucci KF. A proposed protocol for monitoring ototoxicity in patients who take cochleo- or vestibulotoxic drugs. Ear Nose Throat J 2003; 82(3):181–184

20 Vestibular Rehabilitation

Bryan D. Hujsak

Introduction

Vestibular rehabilitation is a highly specialized form of neurologic rehabilitation using activities and movement that challenge an individual's ability to maintain gaze stability, balance, and sensory organization. The net result is integration of the altered vestibular state with other sensory cues to develop a new internal construct of the physical self and its orientation to the surrounding environment. Vestibular disorders cover a broad spectrum of diseases and conditions that affect the vestibular apparatus, its connection to the central nervous system, and the subsequent regions of integration. Common symptoms associated with these disorders include vertigo, dizziness, disorientation, nausea, oscillopsia, and disequilibrium. These disorders are classified not only by the disease or condition but by the location of the lesion, in an attempt to develop an accurate prognosis for recovery. As the vestibular system is not readily visible by direct physical examination, proper assessment of the system requires the careful assessment of many of the associated reflexes. These findings, combined with results of performance-based tasks, standardized balance tests, and symptom patterns within the subjective report, are critical to developing an effective treatment plan. The intent of this chapter is to give the clinician a detailed contextual framework to use in the approach to patients with vestibular disorders.

Classification Schema

Vestibular disorders can be broadly defined as either stable or unstable lesions. Stable lesions are typically the result of a one-time insult to the system, such as vestibular neuritis or labyrinthitis. Episodic disorders that have been ameliorated through medical or surgical management can also be classified as stable. Examples include patients with Meniere's disease who have responded to a low-sodium diet and diuresis, ablative therapy through intratympanic gentamicin injection, vestibular nerve sectioning, or labyrinthectomy. Unstable lesions are those that continue to cause episodic bouts of vertigo, dizziness, and disequilibrium, potentially resulting in further degradation of the vestibular system. Examples include unmanaged Meniere's disease, vestibular migraine, endolymphatic hydrops, and vestibular autoimmune disorders. Although a customized rehabilitation program for patients with Meniere's disease will have little effect on the episodes associated with unstable lesions, patients may benefit from the secondary hypofunction that develops as the disorder progresses. Residual weakness that results in symptoms of instability, chronic dizziness, and decreased function has been shown to benefit from vestibular rehabilitation.[1] Vestibular migraine can also be classified as an unstable lesion due to its episodic and unpredictable nature. Although rehabilitation techniques will not prevent migraine episodes directly, there is evidence that they can significantly reduce symptoms and improve quality of life.[2,3,4,5,6,7,8] Optimal outcomes are obtained when unstable lesions are stabilized through medical and surgical intervention.

Vestibular disorders can be further classified as unilateral or bilateral, incomplete or complete, symmetric or asymmetric, and peripheral, central, or mixed. Peripheral disorders include any pathology that affects the vestibular end-organs or the vestibular portion of the eighth cranial nerve. An example of a unilateral peripheral dysfunction is vestibular neuritis. Widely studied, patients with peripheral disorders generally compensate within a few weeks if no other limiting factors are present. In patients whose symptoms persist, there is compelling evidence that they improve greatly with a customized rehabilitation program.[9,10,11,12,13,14,15]

Bilateral peripheral dysfunctions can be seen with ototoxicity from intravenous aminoglycoside administration and with Meniere's disease. Any of the bilateral peripheral disorders can cause partial or complete loss of function. In the case of complete bilateral loss, patients will experience profound instability, poor gaze stability,[16] and be at a higher risk for falls.[17,18,19] Rehabilitation in this population focuses on sensory substitution, facilitating optimization of visual and sensory cues to compensate for the lack of vestibular information. Patient education and functional strategies are an integral part of the program. There is some evidence that patients do improve with a customized program,[20] but it is asserted that expectations for complete recovery should be guarded.[17,18,19]

Central disorders include any pathology that affects the vestibular nuclei and their myriad connections throughout the brainstem, cerebellum, thalamus, and cortical centers. Recent work with patients recovering from concussion has demonstrated benefit from customized vestibular rehabilitation,[20,21,22,23,24,25,26,27] as postconcussion dizziness has been a negative predictor of outcome.[28,29] In the case of cerebral vascular accident, dizziness and instability arising from posterior circulation insult were significantly improved following therapeutic modalities, including vestibular rehabilitation techniques,[30,31] but progress is expected to be slower than in patients with peripheral disorders.[32] Demyelination at the nerve-root entry zone of cranial nerve VIII occurs in multiple sclerosis and can be classified as a mixed peripheral-central disorder. Other mixed disorders include vestibular schwannomas compromising the cerebellopontine angle, and acquired brain injury with labyrinthine concussion as a sequela.

Classification of vestibular disorders in these categories can assist in prognosis and may determine the most appropriate rehabilitation approach. A combination of vestibular function testing, the bedside clinical exam, performance-based balance measures, and patient reporting will aid in determining the type of vestibular dysfunction that is present.

■ Disablement Model

The currently accepted model in rehabilitation is the International Classification of Function, Disability, and Health (ICF) developed by the World Health Organization (WHO). This multidirectional interaction model takes into account how the pathologic condition causes impairments in body structure and function and its subsequent impact on an individual's activity level and participation in activities of daily living. The ICF model is the first to formally acknowledge the influence of personal and environmental factors. The significance of the ICF model lies in its broadened view of how the disease process impacts a person's ability to function in society.[33] In addition to trying to mitigate the impairments related to the vestibular pathology, all practitioners participating in the care of these individuals need to be mindful of the personal and environmental factors that either help or hinder in the patient's recovery.

■ Subjective Questionnaires

No two patients are alike, of course. Even individuals with the same diagnosis will have completely different experiences, time to recovery, and perception of disability. The experience of dizziness and disequilibrium is often difficult for the patient to articulate, much less quantify. To measure the subjective experience and quantify change over time, there are several questionnaires designed specifically for patients with vestibular dysfunction or that have been later validated for this population. Some of the more common questionnaires are listed in **Table 20.1**.

■ Objective Testing

Not every patient will arrive for their first therapy session having undergone a complete battery of vestibular function tests, imaging studies, and a complete medical work-up. The number of locales that permit direct access to therapy is growing, and it is incumbent on the treating clinician not only to thoroughly examine the vestibular system (see Chapters 1 and 2 of this book), but also to recognize other red flags that give cause for additional medical assessment. Therefore, it is recommended that every exam include a modified systems review that encompasses the patient's musculoskeletal system, cardiopulmonary system, and neuromuscular system. A medication review is warranted, because new medications or changes in dosages may contribute to the patient's symptoms.

Even if the patient has had a complete medical work-up with all possible testing, it is critical that the systems review and bedside examination be repeated, for three reasons. First, there may have been a lapse in time since the patient has seen the referring physician, during which the patient's medical status has changed. Second, the patient may have experienced additional episodes that have resulted in further insult to the system. As the signs and symptoms pattern has changed, the current working diagnosis may have to be revisited. What was once thought to be a stable process may have been only the first episode in an unstable pathologic process. Finally, the rehabilitation examination of the patient goes beyond diagnosis and prognosis. It is prescriptive. Deficits detected on examination will determine what activities and exercises are used to best facilitate compensation.

Table 20.1 Subjective questionnaires

Questionnaire	Description	Psychometrics
DHI: Dizziness Handicap Inventory	DHI is a 25-question survey assessing the physical, emotional, and functional impact of symptoms.	Internal consistency (α = 0.89) and reliability (r = 0.97)[34]
ABC: Activities-specific Balance Confidence Scale	ABC is a 16-question rating scale that rates confidence in balance from 0 to 100%.	Internal consistency (α = 0.95) and reliability (ICC for individual items = 0.67–0.92)[35]
VADL: Vestibular Disorders Activities of Daily Living Scale	VADL has 28 items assessing functional tasks, ambulation activities, and instrumental activities.	Internal consistency (α = 0.90) and reliability (r = 0.87)[36,37]
VAP: Vestibular Activities and Participation	VAP is a 34-item scale assessing walking and instrumental tasks scored on a 5-point scale. Results for activities and participation level are correlated with the ICF*.	Test–retest (ICC = 0.95) and agreement per item (k = 0.41–0.80)[38]
SVQ: Situational Vertigo Questionnaire	Developed to assess visual vertigo symptoms in environments of sensory conflict between motion sensitivity and visual motion sensitivity.[39]	Not reported.
PANAS: Positive and Negative Affective Scale	Patients rate relevance of positive and negative words on a scale of 0–5. Scoring low on the positive scale may indicate depression. Scoring high on the negative scale may indicate anxiety.[40]	Internal consistency (positive items α = 0.88; negative items α = 0.87) and reliability (r = 0.76–0.92)[40]

*ICF, International Classification of Function, Disability, and Health (ICF).

■ Functional Outcomes Measures

In addition to the clinical exam, the therapist has several functional outcome measures that have been validated for the vestibular population. The advantage of these measures are that they tend to be independent of the exercises that the patient performs daily, and therefore measure performance progress, and not simply practice effect. In addition, some of the outcome measures have predictive validity with respect to falls.

Dynamic Gait Index (DGI)

The DGI is an 8-item instrument that assesses the ability to walk with head turns, changes of speed, and negotiation of obstacles. The score for each item ranges from 0 to 3, where 0 is severe impairment and 3 is normal. The highest possible score is 24.[41] The ability of the DGI to classify older adults at risk for falls, with scores of < 19/24, has been reported to have a sensitivity of 59% and a specificity of 64%.[42] Optimal identification of individuals over 60 with balance dysfunction was obtained at a score cutoff point of 22 (sensitivity = 82%, specificity = 88%). The cutoff score for those under 60 was 23 (sensitivity = 96%, specificity = 94%).[43]

Functional Gait Assessment (FGA)

The FGA is a modification of the DGI that was developed to improve the reliability of the DGI and to reduce the ceiling effect seen with the DGI in patients with vestibular disorders.[44,45] The FGA is a 10-item clinical gait test during which subjects are asked to perform the following gait activities: walk at normal speeds, at fast and slow speeds, with vertical and horizontal head turns, with eyes closed, over obstacles, in tandem, backward, and while negotiating stairs. The FGA is scored on a 4-level (0–3) ordinal scale ranging from 0 to 30, with lower scores indicating greater impairment. The interrater reliability of the FGA in individuals with vestibular disorders was reported as r = 0.86, and the intrarater reliability as r = 0.74. In community-dwelling individuals, the FGA has excellent interrater reliability (ICC = 0.93).[46]

Modified Clinical Test of Sensory Integration and Balance (mCTSIB)

The Clinical Test of Sensory Integration and Balance (CTSIB) closely mirrors the sensory organization test (SOT) component of computerized dynamic posturography (CDP) by evaluating the visual, somatosensory, and vestibular components of balance.[47] The modified version (mCTSIB) does not use the visual conflict components and tests balance under four conditions: eyes open on firm surface, eyes closed on firm surface, eyes open on foam, and eyes closed on foam (**Fig. 20.1**).[48] Scores on mCTSIB have a moderate correlation with the SOT. This correlation is greater when the feet are positioned together than when they are slightly apart.[49] One of the major benefits to this test is that it requires only a stopwatch and a piece of foam.

Balance Error Scoring System (BESS) Test

The BESS test has been used in several studies for measuring balance deficits connected with sport-related concussion.[50,51] The test utilizes a combination of static balance positions with variations in base of support and surface. Patients are scored by the amount of errors observed in each position. Higher scores represent poorer balance performance. Iverson et al[52] provided preliminary normative reference values stratified by age groups for the BESS in community-dwelling adults. Psychometric analysis indicated test–retest reliability improved when male (0.92) and female (0.91) participants were evaluated independently.[53]

Four Square Step Test (FSST)

Originally developed to assess risk for falls in community-dwelling older adults,[54] the FSST has been validated in patients with vestibular disorders.[55] Patients are timed as they step clockwise and counterclockwise over four canes arranged in a cross pattern. The FSST has good reliability (ICC = 0.93) and a fall risk cut-off score of 12 seconds (sensitivity = 80%, specificity = 92%).[56]

■ Concepts of Recovery

There are many terms in the literature used to define recovery following vestibular insult. Terms like *compensation, adaptation, habituation,* and *substitution* are used often as distinct entities in the recovery process and in the development of treatment strategies. Compensation can be defined as the functional recovery of the patient, in which the patient has returned to the premorbid activity level with a minimum of symptoms. Adaptation is considered to be a restoration of prior responses at the neurologic level. Habituation is the diminution of a given symptom response by a controlled repeated presentation

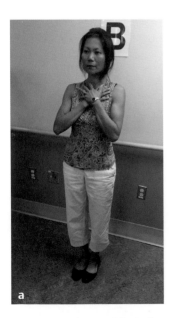 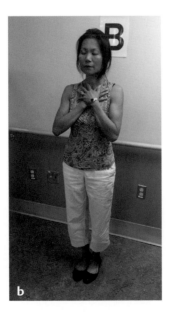 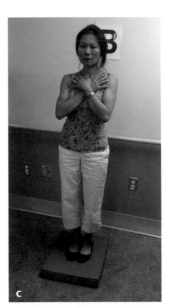 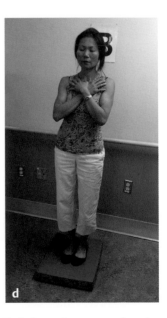

Fig. 20.1 The Modified Clinical Test of Sensory Integration and Balance (mCTSIB). The patient's static balance is measured under four conditions: **(a)** Condition 1, Romberg eyes open on a firm surface; **(b)** Condition 2, Romberg eyes closed on a firm surface; **(c)** Condition 3, Romberg eyes open on a compliant surface; and **(d)** Condition 4, Romberg eyes closed on a compliant surface. Assumptions about functional balance under varying sensory cues can be ascertained by comparing scores between conditions. Poorer scores on Condition 2 than on Condition 1 are thought to indicate deficient balance performance with somatosensory cues. Increased difficulty on Condition 3 compared with Condition 1 is indicative of difficulties in using vision to maintain balance. Abnormalities in Condition 4 compared with Condition 3 indicate of deficiency in utilizing vestibular cues in maintaining static balance.

of a stimulus. Substitution is the utilization of alternate sensations or responses to maintain orientation or perform a given task. Although it does not completely compensate for the vestibular loss, substitution can allow for improved function. Historically, the concepts of recovery have been presented in a hierarchical manner, with substitution at the lowest level, adaptation at its pinnacle, and habituation in between. The reality is that all types of recovery have a role in returning the patient to their prior level of function (**Fig. 20.2**).

Patients are also known to *decompensate* during times of profound physical or emotional stress and will experience a return of their symptoms in the absence of new pathology.

In early recovery, there is a tonic rebalancing of the vestibular system that occurs not only at the processing level, but at the cellular level as well. For example, loss of one labyrinth results in changes of both the ipsilesional and contralesional vestibular nuclei. Their interaction results in changes of both the tonic and phasic type I and type II neurons.[56] At the cellular level, animal studies have revealed changes in neural proteins and the proportion of irregular and regular afferents in Scarpa's ganglion after unilateral labyrinthectomy.[57] As a result of these and other changes, there is progressive resolution of the static oculomotor and postural deficits over the initial weeks following the vestibular insult. Dynamic compensation follows static stabilization. But unlike the tonic changes observed with the vestibular nuclei, compensation from dynamic deficits is a result of a multitude of sensory and oculomotor substitutions.[58,59,60,61] Because of the extensive neural processing of vestibular information, there are many opportunities for the system to adapt to, habituate to, and substitute for decreased vestibular input. The role of treatment is to provide these opportunities.

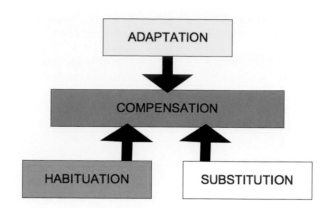

Fig. 20.2 Recovery Interaction Model: compensation from vestibular insult is a combination of habituation, substitution, and adaptation. The net result is improved system performance and functional recovery.

to be based on the deficiencies in gaze stability, balance, and sensory organization determined on evaluation, and should be at a level that the patient can perform with small errors and only mild to moderate symptoms. Although there is always an element of habituation inherent in most exercises, the emphasis should be on skill re-acquisition for balance, orientation, and gaze stability. In improving motor control, training effects with task acquisition is most robust when presented in an incremental fashion.[62,63] Especially in the case of chronic dizziness, positive experience with movement needs to be facilitated, as avoidance behavior is high in this population.

Dynamic Gaze Stability

One of the major areas of treatment in vestibular rehabilitation is restoring dynamic gaze stability. This ability to maintain clarity and stability of an image while the head is in motion is primarily mediated by the vestibulo-ocular reflex (VOR) and is supplemented by the cervical ocular reflex (COR). The visual system also contributes via smooth pursuit, saccades, and optokinetic nystagmus. Following injury to the vestibular system, impairments in the VOR are readily observed. Patients will primarily experience dizziness with head motion, but may also complain of visual blurring. In the case of bilateral vestibular loss, they may experience oscillopsia, or a bouncing of their visual world, especially during gait.

Multiple animal and human studies have explored the process of adaptation and recovery of an impaired VOR. Many of the early studies used passive, sinusoidal, low-frequency rotation to measure adaptive changes. Newer research has studied

■ Treatment

The goal of treatment for patients with vestibular dysfunction is to restore function while minimizing, if not eliminating, symptoms. The approaches to treatment can be divided into two distinct camps: mechanical treatment and performance-based treatment. Mechanical treatment encompasses the various approaches and maneuvers in the management of benign paroxysmal positional vertigo (see Chapter 9). Here, we discuss the performance-based treatment options available to the clinician in facilitating dynamic vestibular compensation.

Customized home exercise programs are crucial to a successful outcome. As with any skill acquisition, frequent purposeful practice is the key to improving the performance of the system. The exercises need responses to active and passive head movement at higher frequencies and has yielded greater understanding of how little VOR adaptation occurs following vestibular insult. Instead, we see that the brain is able to substitute rapid saccades during head movement.[64] Known as covert saccades,[65] they are undetectable to the viewer and the clinician, requiring specialized equipment to be observed. Covert saccades are much different from the overt saccade observed during bedside head impulse testing, as they occur while the head is in motion, not after.[66,67]

Activities prescribed to restore functional dynamic gaze stability are active, not passive. Dynamic visual acuity improves more readily with self-generated head motions over unpredictable head movement.[68,69] Patients with a unilateral or bilateral vestibular hypofunction demonstrate improved dynamic gaze stability if they are able to predict timing, direction, and amplitude of head motion.[70,71,72,73,74,75] The head movements used in therapy are patient generated while fixating on a stationary or moving target. Described as X1 and X2 viewing, respectively, the exercises should have a simple target and should allow the patient to discern if visual acuity and stability are maintained. In X1 viewing, the patient fixates on a discrete target while oscillating their head through a 30° arc in the yaw and pitch planes. This results in eye movement velocity equal to the velocity of the head, or a *gain* of 1 (the mathematical ratio of eye movement to head movement). With X2 viewing, the target, held by the patient, is moved opposite the head. The net result is eye velocity twice the speed of the head velocity, or a gain of 2. The controlled variable in the activity is speed of head movement. The patient is instructed to slow the rate of head rotation should the visual image become distorted or unstable. Often, initially training at slower speeds will result in habituation to any dizziness generated by the head motion.[76]

As speed increases, *retinal slip* will occur. Retinal slip describes the difference between eye velocity and the target velocity. A 2° retinal slip is considered the optimal error signal responsible for improvements in dynamic gaze stability.[77,78] With complete bilateral vestibular loss, the COR is optimized via the same paradigm, but it is limited to head frequencies of up to 1 Hz.[79,80] In combination with contributions from the visual system, oscillopsia is minimized and dynamic gaze stability is restored.[81,82]

Static and Dynamic Balance

Addressing deficits in postural stability is an important component of a rehabilitation program. Modalities range from simple static and dynamic exercises that the patient performs independently to sophisticated virtual reality systems. The overall goal is to decrease the degree of postural sway during quiet stance and gait. Multiple reflexes are associated with postural control. Specific to the vestibular system, the medial and lateral vestibulospinal reflex (VSR) and vestibulocolic reflex (VCR) play a critical role in maintenance of balance following displacement relative to the gravity axis, as well as postural changes associated with active head yaw, pitch, and roll. These reflexes, combined with contributions from lower-extremity proprioceptive input, cervical spinal proprioceptive input, and visual cues, comprise the afferent information used in the body's balance reactions. In addition, integrating this information in the thalamus and vestibular cortex creates an internal construct of our position in space, and our relationship to the surrounding environment. Following unilateral insult, there is a postural shift toward the affected side.[83] Termed *lateralpulsion*, this static deviation tends to decrease and diminish in the initial weeks.[84]

To facilitate balance and orientation skill reacquisition, static and dynamic balance activities are employed. Static balance activities include the patient's attempting to maintain their equilibrium using a progressively narrowed base of support. The patient can be challenged to perform the exercises with the eyes closed, reducing the visual dependence that often accompanies vestibular deficits. Introducing altered proprioceptive information (i.e., foam cushioning, rocker board) further challenges the patient's equilibrium. Dynamic equilibrium compensation with this population involves gait activities. Progressively narrowing a patient's base of support and incorporating head motion during gait facilitates improvement in patient performance in the areas where the VSR is deficient. As with dynamic gaze stability training, it is important to titrate the intensity of the exercise. Regaining balance is a skill acquisition and therefore the patient should not be challenged beyond what provides an incremental training effect.

Sensory Organization

It is common for patients with vestibular dysfunction to rely on their visual system to maintain orientation.[85,86,87] Although this is effective in visually static environments, problems can arise when the patient encounters dynamic visual environments. Patients will complain of dizziness provoked in grocery store aisles, walking through crowds, negotiating theaters, or riding in elevators or on escalators.[88] The incongruity between the sensory systems in these environments results in sensory conflict and a dizziness of disorientation known as *visual vertigo*. Various treatment modalities, including full-field visual movement,[39] virtual reality,[89,90,91] and off-the-shelf gaming consoles[92,93,94] have shown promising results in this area. Low-tech approaches, such as balancing with eyes closed on a soft surface, or visually following a ball tossed from hand to hand, can also assist in improving orientation in visually challenging environments.

Barriers to Recovery

One of the major challenges in care of patients with chronic vestibulopathy is determining why they have not recovered spontaneously. Often, associated comorbidities either impair movement or decrease motivation for movement. Orthopedic issues, especially in the lower extremities, can have a negative impact on recovery. The psychological impact of disability can also negatively affect recovery.[95] Some conditions, such as peripheral lower extremity neuropathy or visual perceptual disorders, result in erroneous afferent information that, in combination with the altered vestibular state, only deepens the disorientation that the patient experiences. Visual perceptual dysfunction and its impact on recovery are briefly discussed next.

Visual Perceptual Dysfunction

Although the vestibular system and somatosensory system provide discrete information about body position in space and segmental orientation, it is the visual system that is the primary orientation sense. It is our most far-reaching sense, and 90% of all sensory information processing by the brain is dedicated to the visual system. The role of vision has been demonstrated in equilibrium. Visual inputs improve responses to linear acceleration[96] and righting reflexes.[97] When visual motion is withheld from subjects, delays in recovery of equilibrium have been observed.[98,99,100,101]

Since adaptation of the VOR relies on responses to the discrete error signal of retinal slip no greater than 2°, any errors inherent to the visual system will confound this process. Animal studies indicate that visual stimulation is required for VOR adaptation. Animals with lesions restricted to dark environments[59] or who underwent bilateral occipital lobectomy did not recover.[102,103] VOR adaptation was also lost following occipital lobectomy.[59] Independent of the vestibular nuclei, VOR function is dependent on cranial nerves III, IV, and VI and their respective nuclei, the flocculus and vermis of the cerebellum, the inferior olive, and the interstitial nucleus of Cajal. Lesions seen in multiple sclerosis, cerebrovascular accidents, or acquired brain injury have resulted in impairments of these structures.

Issues with visual acuity will also impact dynamic gaze stability. Any pathology that impairs the structures of refraction, the retina, or its subsequent central connections will have a negative impact on dynamic gaze stability and postural stability. These include such common conditions as cataracts, glaucoma, age-related macular degeneration, and convergence insufficiency. The use of multifocal lenses can also have a negative impact on gaze stability and balance. Not only do the lenses restrict a patient's visual field, but also patients with instability tend to look down when walking, often looking through the reading portion of the lens. Multifocal lenses can also have a direct impact on VOR gain adaptation[104] and are considered contraindicated in patients with vestibular dysfunction.[105]

In light of the importance of the visual system in adaptation and balance, it is imperative that the treating clinician properly screen each patient for dysfunction. A patient will often minimize, or be unaware of, visual issues, because the brain's ability to compensate for the aberrations is profound (**Fig. 20.3**). Careful assessment of visual acuity, oculomotor control, visual fields, ocular dominance, and convergence should be part of the comprehensive evaluation.

Conclusion

Vestibular rehabilitation is two parts science and one part art. Over the years, a tremendous amount of research has been directed toward the anatomy, physiology, and pathophysiology of this unique system. Because the study of vestibular disorders involves many disciplines, decoding the literature can be quite challenging. The therapist must be able to use this knowledge to assess, treat, and educate patients about their conditions. Often, the therapist is counselor by proxy, and must have a compassionate and empathetic approach, as patients with chronic vestibulopathy commonly present with a high level of anxiety and depression related to their condition. It is the clinician as the artist who not only reassures patients, but also convinces them to commit to a program that can initially increase their degree of symptoms without an immediate sense of benefit. For the patient with chronic vestibulopathy, simply identifying the primary vestibular dysfunction and prescribing the appropriate exercises is often not enough. The clinician needs to try to determine why the individual's natural history has not resulted in compensation. Therefore, the clinician must recognize and attempt to mitigate the comorbidities that slow or halt the process of compensation.

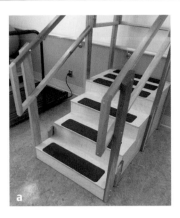 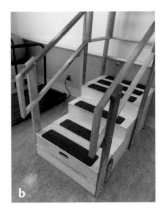 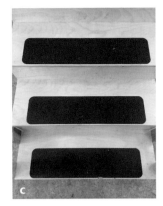 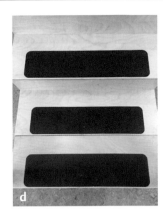

Fig. 20.3 Functional Visual Perception Test. **(a)** The patient is asked to ascend and descend the stairs three times. The patient is distracted with a "balance" test at the top of the stairs: standing with bilateral upper extremity support with eyes closed, the patient is asked to count down aloud from 100 by seven. **(b)** The therapist covertly adds the additional step. The patient is assured that they performed well on the "test" and is asked to descend the stairs. Patients with intact vision will notice the additional step. Those with profound visual problems, especially with depth perception, will not notice the additional step. **(c)** Their visual system is relying on the visual "cue" of the striped pattern on the riser and **(d)** knowledge of prior experience. Failure on this screen indicates the need for further exploration of the patient's vision.

References

1. Clendaniel RA, Tucci DL. Vestibular rehabilitation strategies in Meniere's disease. Otolaryngol Clin North Am 1997;30(6):1145–1158

2. Pavlou M, Bronstein AM, Davies RA. Randomized trial of supervised versus unsupervised optokinetic exercise in persons with peripheral vestibular disorders. Neurorehabil Neural Repair 2013;27(3):208–218

3. Bisdorff AR. Management of vestibular migraine. Ther Adv Neurol Disord 2011;4(3):183–191

4. Baker BJ, Curtis A, Trueblood P, Vangsnes E. Vestibular functioning and migraine: comparing those with and without vertigo to a normal population. J Laryngol Otol 2013;127(12):1169–1176

5. Vitkovic J, Winoto A, Rance G, Dowell R, Paine M. Vestibular rehabilitation outcomes in patients with and without vestibular migraine. J Neurol 2013; 260(12):3039–3048

6. Lin E, Aligene K. Pharmacology of balance and dizziness. NeuroRehabilitation 2013;32(3):529–542

7. Pavlou M, Quinn C, Murray K, Spyridakou C, Faldon M, Bronstein AM. The effect of repeated visual motion stimuli on visual dependence and postural control in normal subjects. Gait Posture 2011;33(1):113–118

8. Gottshall KR, Moore RJ, Hoffer ME. Vestibular rehabilitation for migraine-associated dizziness. Int Tinnitus J 2005;11(1):81–84

9. Shepard NT, Telian SA. Programmatic vestibular rehabilitation. Otolaryngol Head Neck Surg 1995; 112(1):173–182

10. Horak FB, Jones-Rycewicz C, Black FO, Shumway-Cook A. Effects of vestibular rehabilitation on dizziness and imbalance. Otolaryngol Head Neck Surg 1992; 106(2):175–180

11. Gill-Body KM, Krebs DE, Parker SW, Riley PO. Physical therapy management of peripheral vestibular dysfunction: two clinical case reports. Phys Ther 1994; 74(2):129–142

12. Shepard NT, Telian SA, Smith-Wheelock M, Raj A. Vestibular and balance rehabilitation therapy. Ann Otol Rhinol Laryngol 1993;102(3 Pt 1):198–205

13. Black FO, Angel CR, Pesznecker SC, Gianna C. Outcome analysis of individualized vestibular rehabilitation protocols. Am J Otol 2000;21(4):543–551

14. Hillier SL, McDonnell M. Vestibular rehabilitation for unilateral peripheral vestibular dysfunction. Cochrane Database Syst Rev 2011; (2):CD005397

15. Hillier SL, Hollohan V. Vestibular rehabilitation for unilateral peripheral vestibular dysfunction. Cochrane Database Syst Rev 2007; (4):CD005397

16. Brown KE, Whitney SL, Wrisley DM, Furman JM. Physical therapy outcomes for persons with bilateral vestibular loss. Laryngoscope 2001;111(10):1812–1817

17. Telian SA, Shepard NT, Smith-Wheelock M, Hoberg M. Bilateral vestibular paresis: diagnosis and treatment. Otolaryngol Head Neck Surg 1991;104(1):67–71

18. Herdman SJ, Blatt P, Schubert MC, Tusa RJ. Falls in patients with vestibular deficits. Am J Otol 2000; 21(6):847–851

19. Gillespie MB, Minor LB. Prognosis in bilateral vestibular hypofunction. Laryngoscope 1999;109(1):35–41

20. Porciuncula F, Johnson CC, Glickman LB. The effect of vestibular rehabilitation on adults with bilateral vestibular hypofunction: a systematic review. J Vestib Res 2012;22(5-6):283–298

21. Diaz DS. Management of athletes with postconcussion syndrome. Semin Speech Lang 2014;35(3):204–210

22. Schneider KJ, Meeuwisse WH, Nettel-Aguirre A, et al. Cervicovestibular rehabilitation in sport-related concussion: a randomised controlled trial. Br J Sports Med 2014;48(17):1294–1298

23. Fife TD, Giza C. Posttraumatic vertigo and dizziness. Semin Neurol 2013;33(3):238–243

24. Aligene K, Lin E. Vestibular and balance treatment of the concussed athlete. NeuroRehabilitation 2013;32(3):543–553

25. Gurley JM, Hujsak BD, Kelly JL. Vestibular rehabilitation following mild traumatic brain injury. NeuroRehabilitation 2013;32(3):519–528

26. Leddy JJ, Sandhu H, Sodhi V, Baker JG, Willer B. Rehabilitation of concussion and postconcussion syndrome. Sports Health 2012;4(2):147–154

27. Alsalaheen BA, Whitney SL, Mucha A, Morris LO, Furman JM, Sparto PJ. Exercise prescription patterns in patients treated with vestibular rehabilitation after concussion. Physiother Res Int 2013;18(2):100–108

28. De Kruijk JR, Leffers P, Menheere PP, Meerhoff S, Rutten J, Twijnstra A. Prediction of post-traumatic complaints after mild traumatic brain injury: early symptoms and biochemical markers. J Neurol Neurosurg Psychiatry 2002;73(6):727–732

29. Yang CC, Hua MS, Tu YK, Huang SJ. Early clinical characteristics of patients with persistent post-concussion symptoms: a prospective study. Brain Inj 2009;23(4):299–306

30. Kruger E, Teasell R, Salter K, Foley N, Hellings C. The rehabilitation of patients recovering from brainstem strokes: case studies and clinical considerations. Top Stroke Rehabil 2007;14(5):56–64

31. Balci BD, Akdal G, Yaka E, Angin S. Vestibular rehabilitation in acute central vestibulopathy: a randomized controlled trial. J Vestib Res 2013;23(4-5):259–267

32. Furman JM, Balaban CD, Pollack IF. Vestibular compensation in a patient with a cerebellar infarction. Neurology 1997;48(4):916–920

33. International Classification of Function, Disability, and Health (ICF). Towards a common language for functioning, disability, and health. Geneva, Switzerland: World Health Organization; 2002:9

34. Jacobson GP, Newman CW. The development of the Dizziness Handicap Inventory. Arch Otolaryngol Head Neck Surg 1990;116(4):424–427

35. Powell LE, Myers AM. The Activities-specific Balance Confidence (ABC) Scale. J Gerontol A Biol Sci Med Sci 1995;50A(1):M28–M34

36. Cohen HS, Kimball KT. Development of the vestibular disorders activities of daily living scale. Arch Otolaryngol Head Neck Surg 2000;126(7):881–887

37. Cohen HS, Kimball KT, Adams AS. Application of the vestibular disorders activities of daily living scale. Laryngoscope 2000;110(7):1204–1209

38. Alghwiri AA, Whitney SL, Baker CE, et al. The development and validation of the vestibular activities and participation measure. Arch Phys Med Rehabil 2012;93(10):1822–1831

39. Pavlou M, Lingeswaran A, Davies RA, Gresty MA, Bronstein AM. Simulator based rehabilitation in refractory dizziness. J Neurol 2004;251(8):983–995

40. Watson D, Clark LA, Carey G. Positive and negative affectivity and their relation to anxiety and depressive disorders. J Abnorm Psychol 1988;97(3):346–353

41. Shumway-Cook A, Baldwin M, Polissar NL, Gruber W. Predicting the probability for falls in community-dwelling older adults. Phys Ther 1997;77(8):812–819

42. Shumway-Cook A, Gruber W, Baldwin M, Liao S. The effect of multidimensional exercises on balance, mobility, and fall risk in community-dwelling older adults. Phys Ther 1997;77(1):46–57

43. Wrisley DM, Walker ML, Echternach JL, Strasnick B. Reliability of the dynamic gait index in people with vestibular disorders. Arch Phys Med Rehabil 2003;84(10):1528–1533

44. Wrisley DM, Kumar NA. Functional gait assessment: concurrent, discriminative, and predictive validity in community-dwelling older adults. Phys Ther 2010;90(5):761–773

45. Wrisley DM, Marchetti GF, Kuharsky DK, Whitney SL. Reliability, internal consistency, and validity of data obtained with the functional gait assessment. Phys Ther 2004;84(10):906–918

46. Walker ML, Austin AG, Banke GM, et al. Reference group data for the functional gait assessment. Phys Ther 2007;87(11):1468–1477

47. Shumway-Cook A, Horak FB. Assessing the influence of sensory interaction of balance. Suggestion from the field. Phys Ther 1986;66(10):1548–1550

48. Cohen H, Blatchly CA, Gombash LL. A study of the clinical test of sensory interaction and balance. Phys Ther 1993;73(6):346–351, discussion 351–354

49. Wrisley DM, Whitney SL. The effect of foot position on the modified clinical test of sensory interaction and balance. Arch Phys Med Rehabil 2004;85(2):335–338

50. McCrea M, Guskiewicz KM, Marshall SW, et al. Acute effects and recovery time following concussion in collegiate football players: the NCAA Concussion Study. JAMA 2003;290(19):2556–2563

51. Peterson CL, Ferrara MS, Mrazik M, Piland S, Elliott R. Evaluation of neuropsychological domain scores and postural stability following cerebral concussion in sports. Clin J Sport Med 2003;13(4):230–237

52. Iverson GL, Kaarto ML, Koehle MS. Normative data for the balance error scoring system: implications for brain injury evaluations. Brain Inj 2008;22(2):147–152

53. Broglio SP, Zhu W, Sopiarz K, Park Y. Generalizability theory analysis of balance error scoring system reliability in healthy young adults. J Athl Train 2009;44(5):497–502

54. Dite W, Temple VA. A clinical test of stepping and change of direction to identify multiple falling older adults. Arch Phys Med Rehabil 2002;83(11):1566–1571

55. Whitney SL, Marchetti GF, Morris LO, Sparto PJ. The reliability and validity of the Four Square Step Test for people with balance deficits secondary to a vestibular disorder. Arch Phys Med Rehabil 2007;88(1):99–104

56. Bergquist F, Ludwig M, Dutia MB. Role of the commissural inhibitory system in vestibular compensation in the rat. J Physiol 2008;586(18):4441–4452

57. Kitahara T, Horii A, Kizawa K, Maekawa C, Kubo T. Changes in mitochondrial uncoupling protein expression in the rat vestibular nerve after labyrinthectomy. Neurosci Res 2007;59(3):237–242

58. Sadeghi SG, Minor LB, Cullen KE. Neural correlates of motor learning in the vestibulo-ocular reflex: dynamic regulation of multimodal integration in the macaque vestibular system. J Neurosci 2010;30(30):10158–10168

59. Sadeghi SG, Minor LB, Cullen KE. Multimodal integration after unilateral labyrinthine lesion: single vestibular nuclei neuron responses and implications for postural compensation. J Neurophysiol 2011;105(2):661–673

60. Yakushin SB, Kolesnikova OV, Cohen B, et al. Complementary gain modifications of the cervico-ocular (COR) and angular vestibulo-ocular (aVOR) reflexes after canal plugging. Exp Brain Res 2011;210(3-4):549–560

61. Halmagyi GM, Curthoys IS, Todd MJ, et al. Unilateral vestibular neurectomy in man causes a severe permanent horizontal vestibulo-ocular reflex deficit in response to high-acceleration ampullofugal stimulation. Acta Otolaryngol Suppl 1991;481:411–414

62. Kagerer FA, Contreras-Vidal JL, Stelmach GE. Adaptation to gradual as compared with sudden visuo-motor distortions. Exp Brain Res 1997;115(3):557–561

63. Kilgard MP, Merzenich MM. Order-sensitive plasticity in adult primary auditory cortex. Proc Natl Acad Sci U S A 2002;99(5):3205–3209

64. Black RA, Halmagyi GM, Thurtell MJ, Todd MJ, Curthoys IS. The active head-impulse test in unilateral peripheral vestibulopathy. Arch Neurol 2005;62(2):290–293

65. Weber KP, Aw ST, Todd MJ, McGarvie LA, Curthoys IS, Halmagyi GM. Head impulse test in unilateral vestibular loss: vestibulo-ocular reflex and catch-up saccades. Neurology 2008;70(6):454–463

66. Halmagyi GM, Curthoys IS, Cremer PD, et al. The human horizontal vestibulo-ocular reflex in response to high-acceleration stimulation before and after unilateral vestibular neurectomy. Exp Brain Res 1990;81(3):479–490

67. Halmagyi GM, Curthoys IS. Human compensatory slow eye movements in the absence of vestibular function. In: Graham MD, Kemink JL, eds. The Vestibular System: Neurophysiologic and Clinical Research. New York, NY: Raven Press; 1987:471–479

68. Herdman SJ, Schubert MC, Tusa RJ. Role of central preprogramming in dynamic visual acuity with vestibular loss. Arch Otolaryngol Head Neck Surg 2001;127(10):1205–1210

69. Tian JR, Shubayev I, Demer JL. Dynamic visual acuity during passive and self-generated transient head rotation in normal and unilaterally vestibulopathic humans. Exp Brain Res 2002;142(4):486–495

70. Kasai T, Zee DS. Eye-head coordination in labyrinthine-defective human beings. Brain Res 1978;144(1):123–141

71. Tomlinson RD, Saunders GE, Schwarz DWF. Analysis of human vestibulo-ocular reflex during active head movements. Acta Otolaryngol 1980;90(3-4):184–190

72. Collewijn H, Martins AJ, Steinman RM. Compensatory eye movements during active and passive head movements: fast adaptation to changes in visual magnification. J Physiol 1983;340:259–286

73. Jell RM, Stockwell CW, Turnipseed GT, Guedry FE Jr. The influence of active versus passive head oscillation, and mental set on the human vestibulo-ocular reflex. Aviat Space Environ Med 1988;59(11 Pt 1):1061–1065

74. Demer JL. Mechanisms of human vertical visual-vestibular interaction. J Neurophysiol 1992;68(6):2128–2146

75. Schubert MC, Herdman SJ, Tusa RJ. Vertical dynamic visual acuity in normal subjects and patients with vestibular hypofunction. Otol Neurotol 2002;23(3):372–377

76. Clendaniel RA. The effects of habituation and gaze stability exercises in the treatment of unilateral vestibular hypofunction: a preliminary results. J Neurol Phys Ther 2010;34(2):111–116

77. Ito M. Cerebellar control of the vestibulo-ocular reflex—around the flocculus hypothesis. Annu Rev Neurosci 1982;5:275–296

78. Eggers SD, De Pennington N, Walker MF, Shelhamer M, Zee DS. Short-term adaptation of the VOR: non-retinal-slip error signals and saccade substitution. Ann N Y Acad Sci 2003;1004:94–110

79. Kaga K. Vestibular compensation in infants and children with congenital and acquired vestibular loss in both ears. Int J Pediatr Otorhinolaryngol 1999;49(3):215–224

80. Schubert MC, Das V, Tusa RJ, Herdman SJ. Cervico-ocular reflex in normal subjects and patients with unilateral vestibular hypofunction. Otol Neurotol 2004;25(1):65–71

81. Bronstein AM, Hood JD. Oscillopsia of peripheral vestibular origin. Central and cervical compensatory mechanisms. Acta Otolaryngol 1987;104(3-4):307–314

82. Schubert MC, Hall CD, Das V, Tusa RJ, Herdman SJ. Oculomotor strategies and their effect on reducing gaze position error. Otol Neurotol 2010;31(2):228–231

83. Hafström A, Fransson P-A, Karlberg M, Magnusson M. Idiosyncratic compensation of the subjective visual horizontal and vertical in 60 patients after unilateral vestibular deafferentation. Acta Otolaryngol 2004;124(2):165–171

84. Black FO, Shupert CL, Peterka RJ, Nashner LM. Effects of unilateral loss of vestibular function on the vestibulo-ocular reflex and postural control. Ann Otol Rhinol Laryngol 1989;98(11):884–889

85. Cousins S, Cutfield NJ, Kaski D, et al. Visual dependency and dizziness after vestibular neuritis. PLoS ONE 2014;9(9):e105426

86. Furman JM, Jacob RG. A clinical taxonomy of dizziness and anxiety in the otoneurological setting. J Anxiety Disord 2001;15(1-2):9–26

87. Paquette C, Paquet N, Fung J. Aging affects coordination of rapid head motions with trunk and pelvis movements during standing and walking. Gait Posture 2006;24(1):62–69

88. Bronstein AM. Vision and vertigo: some visual aspects of vestibular disorders. J Neurol 2004;251(4):381–387

89. Sparto PJ, Furman JM, Whitney SL, et al. Vestibular rehabilitation using a wide field of view virtual environment. Conf Proc IEEE Eng Biol Soc. 2004; 7:4836.

90. Viirre E, Sitarz R. Vestibular rehabilitation using visual displays: preliminary study. Laryngoscope 2002; 112(3):500–503

91. Whitney SL, Sparto PJ, Hodges LF, Babu SV, Furman JM, Redfern MS. Responses to a virtual reality grocery store in persons with and without vestibular dysfunction. Cyberpsychol Behav 2006;9(2):152–156

92. Meldrum D, Glennon A, Herdman S, Murray D, McConn-Walsh R. Virtual reality rehabilitation of balance: assessment of the usability of the Nintendo Wii(®) Fit Plus. Disabil Rehabil Assist Technol 2012;7(3):205–210

93. Meldrum D, Herdman S, Moloney R, et al. Effectiveness of conventional versus virtual reality based vestibular rehabilitation in the treatment of dizziness, gait, and balance impairment in adults with unilateral loss: a randomized control trial. BMC Ear Nose Throat Disord 2012;12:3

94. Wang PC, Chang CH, Su MC, et al. Virtual reality rehabilitation for vestibular dysfunction. Otolaryngol Head Neck Surg 2001;145(2, Suppl):158–P159

95. Yardley L, Redfern MS. Psychological factors influencing recovery from balance disorders. J Anxiety Disord 2001;15(1-2):107–119

96. Lacour M, Xerri C, Hugon M. Compensation of postural reactions to fall in the vestibular neurectomized monkey. Role of the reamining labyrinthine afferences. Exp Brain Res 1979;37(3):563–580

97. Igarashi M, Guitierrez O. Analysis of righting reflex in cats with unilateral and bilateral labyrinthectomy. ORL J Otorhinolaryngol Relat Spec 1983;45(5):279–289

98. Xerri C, Zennou Y. Sensory, functional and behavioural substitution processes in vestibular compensation. In: Lacour M, Toupet M, Denise P, Christen Y, eds. Vestibular Compensation: Facts, Theories, and Clinical Perspectives. Paris: Elsevier; 1989:35–38.

99. Zennou-Azogui Y, Xerri C, Harlay F. Visual sensory substitution in vestibular compensation: neuronal substrates in the alert cat. Exp Brain Res 1994;98(3):457–473

100. Zennou-Azogui Y, Xerri C, Harlay F. Visual experience during a sensitive period plays a critical role in vestibular compensation: neuronal substrates within Deiters' nucleus in the alert cat. Restor Neurol Neurosci 1995;7(4):235–246

101. Zennou-Azogui Y, Xerri C, Leonard J, Tighilet B. Vestibular compensation: role of visual motion cues in the recovery of posturo-kinetic functions in the cat. Behav Brain Res 1996;74(1-2):65–77

102. Fetter M, Zee DS, Proctor LR. Effect of lack of vision and of occipital lobectomy upon recovery from unilateral labyrinthectomy in rhesus monkey. J Neurophysiol 1988;59(2):394–407

103. Paige GD. Vestibuloocular reflex and its interactions with visual following mechanisms in the squirrel monkey. II. Response characteristics and plasticity following unilateral inactivation of horizontal canal. J Neurophysiol 1983;49(1):152–168

104. Lisberger SG. The neural basis for motor learning in the vestibulo-ocular reflex in monkeys. Trends Neurosci 1988;11(4):147–152

105. Kapoor N, Ciuffreda KJ. Vision disturbances following traumatic brain injury. Curr Treat Options Neurol 2002;4(4):271–280

21 Implantable Vestibular Devices

Justin S. Golub

■ Introduction

Since the first vestibular implant (VI) prototype was described in 2000,[1] numerous advancements have been made. Clinical trials are now underway in humans and several devices are on their second or third design iteration. While challenges remain, many of the early results are encouraging. Vestibular disorders are common and their incidence will increase as the population ages. Pathologies are diverse and it is likely that only a subset of conditions could be treated with vestibular implantation. The most obvious target disorder is bilateral vestibular hypofunction, where subjects have no vestibulo-ocular reflex (VOR) and any head movement produces visual blurring (oscillopsia). However, several other conditions might be treated as well, such as chronic uncompensated unilateral hypofunction and vertiginous Meniere's attacks.

Medical treatments for chronic or episodic vestibular disorders are often ineffective.[2,3] Most procedural treatments are ablative[4] or unproven.[5] For the hypofunctional disorders, such as uncompensated unilateral loss or bilateral vestibular dysfunction, no treatment exists beyond rehabilitation. These conditions can be severely incapacitating and can impose great economic burdens.[6]

The widespread success of cochlear implantation has led to intense interest in creating an equivalent technology for vestibular pathology. This chapter provides an overview of relevant vestibular physiology, potential VI indications, device design, and early clinical trial results.

■ Relevant Anatomy and Physiology

A detailed description of the anatomy and physiology of the vestibular system is presented in Chapter 5 of this book. In this section, we review anatomy relevant to the field of vestibular implantation. The vestibular system is comprised of five sensory organs. The three semicircular canals lie in what are essentially X, Y, and Z planes. Each canal detects rotation in its respective plane. The canals are named after their relative location in the temporal bone: superior (anterior), horizontal (lateral), and posterior. The remaining two organs, the utricle and saccule, detect horizontal and vertical linear movements, respectively.

The soft membranous labyrinth divides the vestibular system into two compartments. The outer compartment is the perilymphatic space. The inner compartment is the endolymphatic space. Angular acceleration of the head induces movement of fluid in the semicircular canals. This is detected in the ampullae through deflection of hair cell stereocilia. Depending on the direction of fluid movement, either depolarization or hyperpolarization occurs. This signal is then encoded by the primary afferent neurons as either an increase or a decrease in spike rate, respectively.

Within each semicircular canal ampulla, all hair cells are oriented in the same direction. For this reason, each canal encodes motion about one axis (because all hair cells of a particular canal are stimulated equivalently). In comparison, the hair cells of both the utricle and the saccule are oriented in numerous directions. This property is relevant to VI design, and explains why all major VI devices currently focus on semicircular canal implantation.

In the absence of movement, the output from the vestibular organs is not quiescent, but rather has a baseline tonic neural firing rate. A change in motion will either increase or decrease the firing frequency of this resting signal depending on the direction. This is termed *rate encoding*.[1,7]

Each semicircular canal has a contralateral pair that detects motion information in a particular plane. The two horizontal semicircular canals are paired. The left superior (or anterior) semicircular canal is paired with the right posterior semicircular canal. This plane is often abbreviated LARP. The right superior (or anterior) semicircular canal is paired with the left posterior semicircular canal. This plane is abbreviated RALP. The two canals in each pair encode motion within the same plane but in the opposite direction. This system of redundant pairs is called "push–pull," and explains why patients with no vestibular function on one side are usually minimally symptomatic. It also predicts that a unilateral VI should be able to restore vestibular function in a patient with severe bilateral impairment.[8,9,10]

■ Relevant Functions of the Vestibular System

One of the challenges of understanding the vestibular system is that its function is less obvious than that of the auditory system. While not considered a bona fide sense, such as hearing, vestibular perception essentially acts as a "sixth sense." For example, with your eyes closed and sense of touch masked, the vestibular system alone allows you to consciously perceive head movements in space.[11] Pathologic derangement of the vestibular system is dramatic and severe, showcasing its importance. While previous chapters address the function of the vestibular system, a brief discussion of two key functions relevant to vestibular implantation is useful.

The first function is control of balance and posture. This is accomplished through the vestibulospinal tract, comprised of neuronal projections from the brainstem vestibular nuclei to the spinal cord and motor neurons innervating limb muscles. The bodywide system to maintain balance and posture is highly redundant (likely because of its importance) and can be divided into three separate contributing systems: the vestibular system, proprioception, and visual input. Impairment of any of these three systems can perturb balance in challenging situations.

For example, an individual with cataracts may have no difficulty walking until a crack in the pavement causes his/her body to suddenly tilt to one side. Because of the visual impairment, the correlating visual shift in the surroundings may not be appreciated. A fall may then result if the posture derangement is not quickly recognized by the other two systems. Thus, if one system is dysfunctional, then appropriate function of the other two systems becomes paramount. A patient with impairment of the vestibular system may perform adequately until the lights are turned off (impairment of visual input) or until walking on a plush surface, such as soft carpet or sand (impairment of proprioception). Impairment beyond a critical level will cause falls and injury.[12,13] Vestibular implantation might improve balance through restoration of one of these three critical systems.

The second key function of the vestibular system is less obvious, but equally important: stabilization of images when the head is moving. This is accomplished through the vestibulo-ocular reflex (VOR), which is composed of a neural arc from the vestibular nuclei to the extraocular muscles. The VOR prevents visual blurring when the head is moving. Because the head is often in motion (i.e., nearly all situations except quietly sitting or lying), the VOR can be thought of as "image stabilization" for the retina.

The VOR produces compensatory eye movements that are equal and opposite to head movements. One can test the impressive and underappreciated function of the VOR by holding printed text at a comfortable reading distance in front of the face. While keeping the head still, moving the text rapidly to the left and right causes blurring of the words. In contrast, if the text is kept still and the head is rotated at the same rate, the words will be much sharper. This is because head rotation invokes the powerful VOR, which fine-tunes eye movements to maintain alignment of images on the retina. The VOR confers obvious evolutionary advantages, such as keeping an object (e.g., another animal) sharply visible while the head is constantly moving (e.g., while running on a hunt).

Two additional systems help with image stabilization: the smooth pursuit and optokinetic pathways.[14] However, these systems are slower and their inadequacy is demonstrated by the abovementioned example of the moving printed text. Without vestibular input from at least one functioning ear, the VOR is absent. The correlating clinical symptom is oscillopsia, detailed further later.

■ Disease Processes That May Be Treated by a Vestibular Implant

Symptoms from vestibular disease depend more on their time course and sidedness than the underlying condition. In addition, because vestibular implantation replaces the function of the diseased organ rather than reversing the root cause, the underlying disease is less relevant. It is thus useful to organize pathology into six groups based on their timing (acute versus recurrent/episodic versus chronic) and their location (unilateral versus bilateral). Because VI research, at least currently, focuses on disorders peripheral to the vestibular nerve, discussion is limited to peripheral disorders. Central disorders that cause vestibular symptoms are beyond the scope of this chapter. **Table 21.1** provides an overview of this organizational scheme. In the following subsections, we explain how VIs might be employed to treat vestibular pathology based on these categories.

Acute Unilateral Disorders

The cardinal symptom of acute, unilateral vestibular dysfunction is vertigo. This results from the sudden asymmetry in neural output between the two vestibular systems (with the diseased system's output

Table 21.1 Categories of peripheral vestibular disorders* based on time course and sidedness

Time Course	Unilateral	Bilateral
Acute	• Vestibular neuronitis • Labyrinthitis • Trauma (e.g., temporal bone fracture, labyrinthine concussion, perilymphatic fistula, barotrauma)	• Vestibular neuronitis (rare) • Labyrinthitis • Trauma (rare)
Episodic (Recurrent Acute)	• BPPV • *Meniere's disease*	• BPPV (rare) • *Meniere's disease* (rare) • Autoimmune inner ear disease (rare)
Chronic	• *Poor compensation after an acute insult* • *Vestibular schwannoma*	• *Bilateral vestibular hypofunction* or *areflexia*†

BPPV, benign paroxysmal positional vertigo
* Disorders that are potential targets for vestibular implantation are in italics.
† Multiple underlying etiologies, e.g., ototoxicity.

typically reduced compared with the contralateral system's). The brain interprets the mismatch as vertigo, the illusory perception of spinning. Underlying etiologies of acute, unilateral disease include trauma as well as inflammatory/infectious causes, such as vestibular neuronitis or labyrinthitis.[15,16]

The affected vestibular system may recover or, perhaps more commonly, the brain may compensate for the permanent asymmetry. As a result, the fulminant acute symptoms of vertigo are transient. In rare cases, the vestibular system may not compensate, resulting in subtler chronic symptoms. Vestibular implantation may be indicated for these chronic unilateral disorders, as discussed later in this chapter.

Episodic (Recurrent Acute) Unilateral Disorders

In diseases with recurrent episodes, the brain cannot compensate. Vertigo is then experienced anew with every attack. The most common example is benign paroxysmal positional vertigo (BPPV). Because medical (and more rarely surgical) treatment is straightforward and effective,[17,18] vestibular implantation would likely not be relevant.

Meniere's disease is the second most common cause of recurrent vertigo. Symptoms include a tetrad of fluctuating sensorineural hearing loss, tinnitus, vertigo attacks, and aural fullness. Patients are often incapacitated by the unpredictable vertigo episodes. Meniere's disease is also relatively common, with a prevalence of ~ 43 per 100,000.[19,20,21]

Treating Meniere's has been challenging due to the poorly understood root cause. It has been theorized that acute ruptures in the membranous labyrinth cause mixing of perilymph and endolymph. This reduces the endolymphatic potential, blocking neural transmission. The acute unilateral loss of

tonic vestibular output then results in vertigo, manifested by an "attack."[22]

While the initial management for Meniere's disease is medical, ~ 15% of patients do not respond. The only nonablative procedures are endolymphatic sac surgery and myringotomy with the Meniett device, both of which may have limited long-term efficacy.[19,20,23] Intratympanic steroids have also been used but more controlled data are needed.[24] The remaining interventions are all destructive, including intratympanic gentamicin, vestibular nerve section, and labyrinthectomy. These ablative techniques carry risks, including hearing loss and chronic unsteadiness due to poor central compensation.[19,20,21]

Because vertigo in Meniere's disease is thought to be triggered by a sudden unilateral loss of tonic vestibular output, attacks could potentially be aborted by a vestibular "pacemaker." This type of device would simply provide the absent vestibular output by electrically stimulating the vestibular nerve. Patients would turn on the device only during the onset of a vertigo attack. Details of a pacemaker-based VI are further discussed later in the chapter.

Chronic Unilateral Disorders

Central compensation is a phenomenon that allows the brain to acclimate to asymmetric vestibular input. Because of compensation, disorders that begin with an acute phase of vertigo ordinarily cease to be symptomatic with time. Even when a fixed deficit persists, patients are usually unaffected because only one functioning ear is required to maintain adequate vestibular function, as previously explained. Chronic unilateral vestibular deficits are thus typically asymptomatic. In fact, slowly progressive unilateral disorders that lack an acute phase (such as a vestibular schwannoma) may not ever produce obvious vestibular symptoms. These well-compensated conditions would not benefit from vestibular implantation.

Rarely, however, central compensation may not appropriately follow an acute insult. Vestibular neuronitis, for example, is a relatively common acute unilateral vestibular disorder. Although most patients become well compensated, the incidence of vestibular neuronitis is high enough that there may be a relatively high prevalence of people with poorly compensated unilateral deficits. In these cases, the brain is unable to acclimate to the asymmetric vestibular output. Vestibular implantation may be able to help restore normal vestibular output from the diseased side, restoring the bilateral symmetry, and obviating the need for compensation. Restoring normal levels of vestibular output could involve either increasing the gain or increasing the tonic output from the affected nerve. This might be achieved through either a pacemaker-based VI or a sensor-based implant. In the case of a pacemaker VI, tonic supplementary electrical stimulation would elevate the resting discharge rate of the ipsilateral vestibular nerve. This might assist in the restoration of ipsilateral modulation, either through inhibition from the contralateral vestibular nucleus or through intact residual input from the affected ear.

Acute Bilateral Disorders

Acute bilateral vestibular disorders are extraordinarily rare. When they are associated with trauma, there are usually a myriad to other more serious injuries. A discussion is outside the scope of this chapter.

Episodic (Recurrent Acute) Bilateral Disorders

Recurrent episodic bilateral disorders are also rare. In bilateral Meniere's disease, ablative procedures, such as intratympanic gentamicin and labyrinthectomy, are far higher risk because of the potential for eventual bilateral vestibular hypofunction. This is a crippling disorder for which there is no current treatment. Unilateral vestibular implantation might be able to manage bilateral Meniere's disease. During an attack in the implanted ear, the device could provide the missing tonic vestibular output (as explained previously). If the attack occurs in the contralateral ear, the device could decrease the tonic vestibular output in the implanted ear to match that of the other side. In both cases, symmetry between the two ears is restored, aborting attack symptoms.

Moreover, a sensor-based VI could provide a treatment for bilateral vestibular hypofunction (detailed in the following section). This could poten-

tially allow chemical labyrinthectomy to be used as a destructive cure for Meniere's attacks, followed by functional restoration with vestibular (or combined vestibulocochlear) implantation.

Chronic Bilateral Disorders

In chronic bilateral vestibular disease, there is inadequate vestibular function. Symptoms present in two ways. First, absence of the vestibulo-ocular reflex (VOR) causes oscillopsia. Without the VOR, images cannot be kept stable on the retina during head movement. Thus "visual bobbing" and reduced visual acuity occur, even during basic activities like walking. Second, impairment of the vestibulospinal system causes balance and postural instability as well as disequilibrium. While the propriopceptive and visual symptoms are also involved in balance, falls may occur if either of these additional systems is impaired. Unfortunately such scenarios are common, such as walking on soft or uneven surfaces (impaired proprioception) or in dim lighting (impaired vision).

Bilateral vestibular disease has a variety of causes, including hair cell loss caused by ototoxicity (e.g., aminoglycosides, cisplatin) and presbystasis (idiopathic age-related decline of vestibular function). Regardless, acquired bilateral vestibular hypofunction results in the same debilitating symptoms no matter what the underlying etiology. This entity represents one of the most obvious targets of a sensor-based VI, as no therapies exist beyond vestibular rehabilitation. A sensor-based VI could restore vestibular function, including the VOR, and the vestibulospinal contribution to balance. The term *anastasis* is proposed as the vestibular analog of *anacusis* to describe this debilitating and important end-stage condition more succinctly than the variety of other terms currently used.

■ Design and Function of Vestibular Implants

The goal of vestibular implantation is to restore vestibular functionality and/or reduce symptoms through electrical stimulation of the vestibular nerve. It has been known since the 1960s that stimulation of the vestibular nerve can induce the VOR, thus providing the basis for the field of vestibular neurostimulation.[25,26] At the present, VIs can be divided into two types of designs. The first design would serve as a complete prosthetic vestibular system, replacing the diseased motion-sensing end-organs with angular gyroscopes and linear accelerometers. A schematic of such a design is illustrated in **Fig. 21.1a**. The three components would be motion sensors, a signal processor, and a nerve stimulator.[27] This design is equivalent to the microphone, speech processor, and nerve stimulator (receiver/stimulator) of a cochlear implant. This device is referred to as a *sensor-based vestibular implant.*

The second design is simpler and eschews a motion sensor. This type of device would use a pre-programmed signal to replace absent tonic activity from vestibular afferents (**Fig. 21.1b**). In some cases, the signal could instead attempt to supplement afferent input to increase VOR gain by providing an elevated baseline around which the remaining depressed natural input could modulate central neurons (**Fig. 21.1c**). This device is referred to as a *pacemaker-based vestibular implant.*[28]

In both design types, the stimulator component creates a biphasic charge-balanced pulsatile current delivered to branches of the vestibular nerve at their end-organ terminals. Each electrode array is implanted into an end-organ, and each array may contain multiple electrodes. The stimulation signal may be modulated (modified) by varying the amplitude of the current (μA) or the frequency of the pulse (pulse rate, Hz). Increasing either variable will result in increased velocity input to the central nervous system, resulting in higher slow-phase velocity eye movements (a component of the VOR, explained later). Conversely, lowering these parameters would produce the reverse effect.[1]

Unlike the auditory system, which contains only a single organ (the organ of Corti), the vestibular system contains five sensory organs. This makes prosthetic implantation of the vestibular system more complicated than cochlear implantation.

Each of the three semicircular canals encodes rotational motion in only one axis. Stimulating a single canal results in stereotyped eye movements in a corresponding axis. The utricle and saccule, however, each encode motion in multiple directions because their hair cells are oriented in multiple directions. Stimulating the utricle or saccule does not result in predictable eye movements.[29,30,31,32,33] For this reason, current VI designs are semicircular canal prostheses only.[10]

Sensor-Based Vestibular Implant

When symptoms result from not being able to detect motion, a sensor-based VI is needed. The model condition is bilateral vestibular dysfunction, usually due to dysfunction of the vestibular mechanosensory

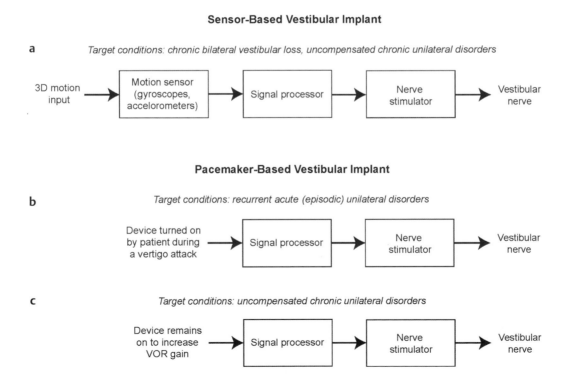

Fig. 21.1 Schematics of various vestibular implant designs. Several recent devices additionally incorporate an integrated cochlear implant for concomitant sensorineural hearing loss (not pictured). **(a)** Sensor-based device that would restore the VOR and the ability to perceive 3D movement. **(b)** Pacemaker-based device that would be turned on during the onset of acute vertigo attacks in recurrent conditions such as Meniere's disease. Turning on the stimulus would theoretically abort the attack. **(c)** Pacemaker-based device that would be chronically kept on to increase VOR gain in uncompensated chronic unilateral disorders. Used with permission from Waltzman SB, Roland JT Jr. Cochlear Implants. 3rd ed. New York, NY: Thieme; 2014.

hair cells. Electromechanical components that detect a change in motion, such as angular gyroscopes and linear accelerometers, would replace the nonfunctioning semicircular canals and (possibly) the utricle and saccule.

Another disorder that could theoretically benefit from this type of implant design is uncompensated chronic unilateral disorders. In this situation, the pathologically low vestibular output would be amplified to equal that of the contralateral side. This might be accomplished with either a sensor-based or pacemaker-based device.

During rest, a sensor-based VI would output a constant-rate, baseline pulsatile stimulation equivalent to the resting rate of a healthy vestibular system. With head acceleration in a particular plane, the signal would be modulated (varied) appropriately and specifically. For example, if the head were rotated in the plane of the horizontal semicircular canal, the motion would be specifically detected by an angular gyroscope in this same plane, sending a signal to the horizontal canal electrode. In one direction, the signal would be increased; likewise, in the opposite direction, the signal would be decreased.

The normal bilateral vestibular systems convey redundant information since each vestibular end-organ has a contralateral paired organ that detects motion in the same plane, but the opposite direction. Because of this push–pull redundancy, unilateral vestibular implantation theoretically should be capable of restoring motion detection in all planes/directions in patients with bilateral pathology.[9,10] One technical issue, however, is due to the relatively low level of the baseline vestibular output. There is "unlimited" room to increase the frequency of the signal, but limited room to decrease before zero is reached. A possible solution to increase this dynamic range is to set the baseline signal at an artificially high level. This might still allow ample room to up-modulate the signal but also provide more room to down-modulate.[10,34] Simultaneously modulating both the current (amplitude) and the rate (frequency) of the signal may also increase dynamic range.[35]

Pacemaker-Based Vestibular Implant

A pacemaker-based VI contains no motion-sensing components and would not restore the sense of motion in patients with bilateral pathology. Rather, the goal of such devices is to alter the output of a diseased side to either neutralize acute vertiginous symptoms or to increase the gain in uncompensated unilateral vestibular hypofunction.

Medically refractory Meniere's disease is one possible target of a vestibular pacemaker. As previously alluded to, it is theorized that during attacks, the diseased system becomes suddenly hypofunctional,

with an abnormally low baseline signal.[22] The acute asymmetry between the diseased side and the normal contralateral side produces vertigo. The unique feature of Meniere's disease is that the attacks are self-limited (< 12 hours). As a result, the brain never learns to compensate for the asymmetry as it would after a vestibular neuronitis. With each Meniere's attack, vertigo manifests anew.

To fix this problem, an implant could simply "pace" the vestibular nerve of the affected ear during acute attacks. The processor would be preprogrammed with a "map" of signal intensities. This map would be created during the asymptomatic period by stimulating the patient at a range of intensities. Stimulation would cause transient vertigo similar to a Meniere's attack (but, theoretically, opposite in direction). The map would contain intensity levels ranging from, for example, 1 to 10, where 1 is the threshold for detection and 10 is of greater intensity than the worst Meniere's attack the patient has ever experienced. During the onset of an attack, the patient would turn up the map setting, starting from 1 until the vertigo stopped or was minimized.[28] After the attack, the pacing output would be turned off.

In bilateral Meniere's disease, the pacing would be chronic in the implanted ear, driving that side at higher rates than the natural baseline. Attacks in either ear could then be treated by increasing or decreasing the pacing intensity, depending on which ear is affected in a particular attack.

The other potential application of a pacemaker-based VI would be to increase the gain in uncompensated chronic unilateral vestibular hypofunction. In this condition, the pacing signal would augment the pathologically low vestibular output. This supplemental signal might increase the gain of the system overall by providing an elevated baseline around which the residual natural inputs could still provide motion-based modulation.

Because vestibular physiology nearly or completely recovers between Meniere's attacks,[19,20] it would be important for a pacemaker-based VI for Meniere's disease to preserve native vestibular function postoperatively. Similarly, in subjects with serviceable hearing, postoperative preservation of native auditory function would be desired. This is analogous to the goal of Hybrid, or electroacoustic, cochlear implant that supplements residual auditory hearing with electric hearing using minimally traumatic electrodes and surgical techniques. Function-preserving VI surgery would benefit from the same techniques and principles already learned from electroacoustic cochlear implants[36] and surgical plugging of semicircular canals.[37,38,39]

Preservation of native vestibular function would be made easier by placing ultranarrow electrodes in the perilymphatic space without distorting the membranous labyrinth. The electrode also would need only enter a small segment of the perilymphatic space, since the ampullary nerve terminals are anatomically confined to the ampulla. (This is in contrast to the cochlea, which contains nerve terminals along the entire length of the organ's multiple turns.) Local current spread would then activate the adjacent ampullary nerve terminals.[28] Admittedly, one of the challenges of such a shallow insertion may be ensuring no postoperative electrode migration.

History of Vestibular Implant Prototypes

The first VI prototype was reported in 2000 by Merfeld, Gong, and colleagues at the Massachusetts Eye and Ear Infirmary. This early sensor-based device has been implanted only in animals. It contained a single piezoelectric vibrating gyroscope that acted as a rotational sensor about one axis. The gyroscope was integrated into a circuit board and was connected to a single array with three electrodes. The array was implanted into a single semicircular canal adjacent to the ampulla. The circuitry of the device (**Fig. 21.2a**) was attached to the top of the animal's head. Using this device, the VOR was partially restored in both monkeys[8,34,40,41] and guinea pigs.[1,9,42] Efforts are more recently focused on a newer version with the ability to sense motion in three axes, rather than one (**Fig. 21.2b**).[43]

Several years later, Della Santina and colleagues at Johns Hopkins developed an integrated sensor-based VI with three rotational sensors, called the Multichannel Vestibular Prosthesis 1 (MVP1).[44] A newer device, the MVP2, contains three rotational sensors (via one single-axis gyroscope and one dual-axis gyroscope) and a tri-axis linear accelerometer (**Fig. 21.3**). Several evolutionary improvements in miniaturization and power consumption make the newer device more suitable for in vivo testing and surgical implantation. The integrated circuit board, which includes the motion sensors, is less than 3 cm in its largest dimension. This size should allow a footprint similar to that of a commercially available cochlear implant receiver/stimulator. The device contains three electrode arrays, one for each semicircular canal. Each array contains three electrodes (two additional electrodes serve as grounds). Three-dimensional reconstructions of rhesus monkey labyrinths were used to help design the electrode array. The eventual goal of the device is to be totally implanted, requiring only periodic transcutaneous charging of an implanted battery.[45]

Vestibular testing of the MVP2 was performed in a rhesus monkey with drug-induced bilateral vestibular deficiency. Partial restoration of the VOR was achieved in all three semicircular canals.[45] There was

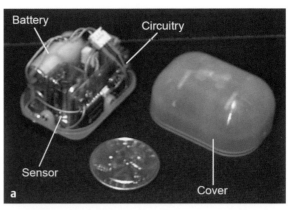

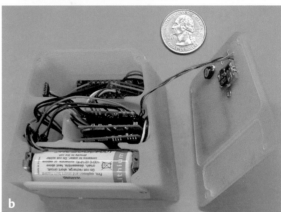

Fig. 21.2 (a) Circuitry of the first vestibular implant prototype, which was developed at Harvard in the late 1990s. The circuit board contained one gyroscope to sense rotation in a single axis. Not pictured is the electrode array, which was inserted into one semicircular canal. A cover encloses the electronics. Used with permission from Gong W, Merfeld DM. Prototype neural semicircular canal prosthesis using patterned electrical stimulation. Ann Biomed Eng 2000;28(5):572–581. (b) A newer generation of the Harvard device. Three sensors can detect rotation in three axes. The electrode array is not pictured. This research device has been implanted only in animals. Courtesy of Daniel Merfeld, PhD.

a small 5- to 10-dB drop in hearing in four implanted monkeys.[46] More extensive testing with the first-generation device has been performed in both monkeys[47] and chinchillas.[10,35,44,48,49,50,51,52,53]

Future research is focused on increasing the evoked VOR gain, lowering response latency, and improving axis alignment via current steering and virtual electrodes. Reduced power consumption for sensor-based implants is also needed. Motion sensors are relatively energy hungry compared with cochlear implants. However, with the rapid improvements in consumer electronics, which incorporate similar motion-sensing technology in smartphones, a totally implantable sensor-based VI incorporating an internal rechargeable battery might soon exceed a full day of use.[45,54]

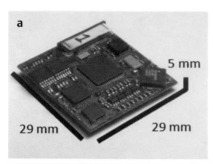

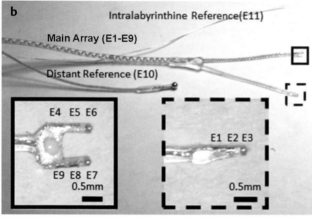

Fig. 21.3 Johns Hopkins Multichannel Vestibular Implant 2 (MVP2). **(a)** Circuit board, featuring reduced dimensions from the earlier MVP1 device. Three rotational sensors are integrated (including one single-axis gyroscope and one dual-axis gyroscope) as well as one tri-axis linear accelerometer. **(b)** Electrode array. Pictured above, the main array bifurcates into an array for the superior and horizontal semicircular canals (*solid boxes*; note second bifurcation), and an array for the posterior semicircular canal (*dashed boxes*). Three electrodes are thus employed for each of the three semicircular canals. Also pictured above are two ground (reference) electrodes. This device version has not been implanted in humans. Used with permission from Chiang B, Fridman GY, Dai C, Rahman MA, Della Santina CC. Design and performance of a multichannel vestibular prosthesis that restores semicircular canal sensation in rhesus monkey. IEEE Trans Neural Syst Rehabil Eng 2011;19(5):588–598.

Rubinstein, Phillips, and colleagues at the University of Washington (UW) recently developed an implant in conjunction with Cochlear Ltd. This device has been implanted in several human subjects, as detailed in the next section. The UW device is based on the widely used Nucleus Freedom system (**Fig. 21.4**). As of this writing, the current clinical device functions as a pacemaker-based VI. However, an external multiaxis gyroscope intended to be attached to an osseointegrated abutment has restored VOR in monkeys with bilateral vestibular hypofunction. The receiver/stimulator contains a trifurcating array of nine electrodes, each with three distal electrodes. The electrodes are implanted 2.5 mm into the perilymphatic space of each semicircular canal, adjacent to the ampullary nerve terminals.

The external signal processor can be programmed to allow a patient-specific pacing algorithm. For example, in a Meniere's patient, a map can be programmed with settings from 1 to 10, where 10 is an intensity exceeding that of a severe vertigo attack.

The UW device was designed to potentially allow preservation of native auditory and vestibular function. Each electrode is 150 µA wide, narrower than that of an electroacoustic (Hybrid) implant, and narrow enough to theoretically avoid compression of the membranous labyrinth. In eight implanted monkeys, completely preserved hearing was achieved in five, a transient mild loss in one, and moderate to severe losses in two.[55]

Finally, a device designed by a group in Geneva, Switzerland, and Maastricht, The Netherlands, is based on a Med El cochlear implant (**Fig. 21.5**). This device is actually a vestibulocochlear implant, consisting of a standard intracochlear array as well as three arrays for each of the three semicircular canals. This device has been implanted in humans, and has been able to partly restore the VOR (detailed later).[56]

Vestibulocochlear Implants

Because of the overlap in vestibular and auditory dysfunction, combined vestibulocochlear implants have been investigated. This type of device may be especially relevant in developing countries, where more frequent aminoglycoside use results in a higher rate of bilateral vestibular impairment and also severe-to-profound hearing loss. In addition, a relatively common mitochondrial mutation in Asian individuals renders this population even more susceptible to combined auditory and vestibular insult.

Treating patients with combined impairments may result in fewer regulatory hurdles for the first clinical trials. For example, there is smaller incremental risk in placing vestibular electrodes in a patient who is already receiving a cochlear implant (CI). Performing a CI also obviates the concern of iatrogenic hearing loss from a labyrinthotomy.[57] The growing interest in placing CIs for single-sided deafness opens the door to potentially implanting a simultaneous pacemaker-based prosthesis in patients with unilateral Meniere's disease.

Vestibular Implant Clinical Trials

As of this writing, VI clinical trials are underway with the pacemaker-based UW/Cochlear device, and the sensor-based Geneva-Maastricht/Med-El device.

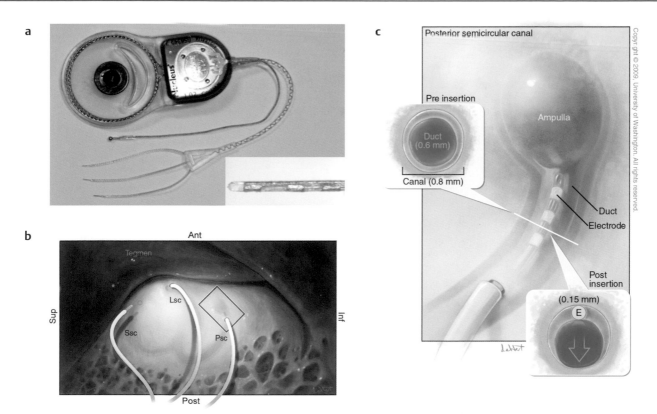

Fig. 21.4 University of Washington/Nucleus Vestibular Implant, first generation. This device has been in human clinical trials. **(a)** Cochlear Nucleus Freedom-based receiver/stimulator with trifurcating electrode array and ground electrode. The case serves as a second ground. Each of the three arrays contains three electrodes. The inset depicts the distal portion of an array, containing three platinum electrodes. **(b)** Illustration of surgical view after electrode insertion. Each array is placed into the perilymphatic space of a semicircular canal. The tip of the array should be located adjacent to the ampulla. **(c)** Enlargement of the box in *(b)*, showing an inserted electrode array correctly located in the semicircular canal perilymphatic space. The narrow width of the electrode should, in theory, minimally distort the membranous labyrinth (duct). Used with permission from Rubinstein JT, Bierer S, Kaneko C, et al. Implantation of the semicircular canals with preservation of hearing and rotational sensitivity: a vestibular neurostimulator suitable for clinical research. Otol Neurotol 2012;33(5):789–796.

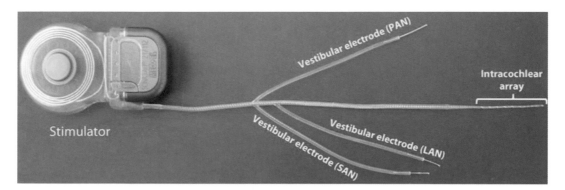

Fig. 21.5 The Geneva/Maastricht/Med El Vestibulocochlear Implant. This device, based on the Sonata receiver/stimulator, has been in human clinical trials. Three vestibular arrays are inserted into each of the three semicircular canals. A fourth array is inserted into the cochlea to treat concomitant sensorineural hearing loss. PAN = posterior ampullary nerve, LAN = lateral ampullary nerve, SAN = superior ampullary nerve. Used with permission from Perez Fornos A, Guinand N, van de Berg R, et al. Artificial balance: restoration of the vestibulo-ocular reflex in humans with a prototype vestibular neuroprosthesis. Front Neurol 2014;5:66.

The UW site is conducting a Food and Drug Administration (FDA) feasibility study on the safety of its device and its physiologic function. Results have been published on four patients with AAO-HNS definite Meniere's disease refractory to medical therapy. The expected eye movements were seen with activation of some of the semicircular canal electrodes. Out-of-plane movements were seen as well, particularly with the superior and posterior canal electrodes. This was likely due to current spread, a topic further addressed later.[58,59]

Slow-phase eye velocity (the slow eye movement portion of nystagmus that is caused by vestibular output) increased as predicted with increasing current amplitude. Interestingly, increasing the pulse frequency had less of an effect. This was surprising, since the natural physiologic encoding is through pulse frequency variation. Eye velocities were also variable between both patients and canals, illustrating the challenge and importance of precise electrode placement.[60] Over time, the eye velocities tended to decrease for a given stimulation level. This latter observation was unexpected, since it was not seen in monkeys implanted with the same device.[61] While a variety of explanations are proposed, the cause is unclear.[58,59]

Subjects experienced perceptual vertigo in-plane with their eye movements. For example, when the horizontal canal was stimulated, the subjects felt as if they were rotating in the horizontal plane. In general, the perception increased as current amplitude and eye velocities increased.[58,59]

While the device was designed to attempt preservation of the residual native vestibular and auditory function, most of this function was lost. It is possible that this was due to implanting an end-stage diseased ear, since function was preserved with the same device in healthy monkeys.[28] For example, the hydropic (i.e., expanded) endolymphatic space may have compressed the perilymphatic space. Electrode insertion into the perilymphatic space may then have resulted in tears in the membranous labyrinth, causing mixture of fluids and resulting hair cell damage.[58,59] A newer version of the UW device that contains an additional cochlear implant electrode array is currently under investigation.

Efficacy for treating Meniere's attacks was not a primary goal of this feasibility study. Anecdotally, one of the subjects believed he had a single vertigo attack, for which activating the device was helpful in symptom reduction.[59]

At least seven patients have been implanted by the Geneva-Maastricht group using a sensor-based Med-El vestibulocochlear implant. Patients had both bilateral vestibular hypofunction as well as profound deafness in the implanted ear. The primary goal of the studies to date has been to assess VOR restoration. With the device off, the patients had minimal eye movements during sinusoidal oscillation in a rotatory chair, confirming their hypofunctional state. When the sensor-based device was turned on, partial restoration of the VOR was observed (**Fig. 21.6**). Similar to a natural VOR, the evoked VOR varied with the rotatory chair oscillation frequency, with higher gains occurring at higher frequencies. Several other evoked VOR parameters were also similar to that of a natural VOR. Future studies will assess postural control and function in activities of daily living.[56,62,63]

As of this writing, a device from the Johns Hopkins team just received FDA approval for a clinical trial. This device was developed by Labyrinth Devices LLC in collaboration with Med-El, based on technology developed at the Johns Hopkins Vestibular NeuroEngineering Laboratory and licensed from the Johns Hopkins School of Medicine.[64]

■ Basic Topics in Vestibular Implantation

Evoked Vestibulo-ocular Reflex (EVOR) and Evoked Compound Action Potential (ECAP)

While electrical stimulation of the cochlear nerve produces only an auditory percept, stimulation of the vestibular nerve produces both a vestibular percept and a physically observable nystagmus.[25] This is due to activation of the vestibulo-ocular reflex (VOR). The term *evoked VOR (EVOR)* is used to refer to the electrically induced reflex. The ability to measure an EVOR aids with optimizing intraoperative electrode placement and testing postoperative device function. In clinical use, sensor-based VIs would improve image stabilization during movement by replacing the missing physiologic VOR with an EVOR.

Unlike cochlear implants, where relatively long electrode arrays are placed deeply into the end-organ, vestibular implantation involves both shallower insertion and implantation of multiple semicircular canals. Electrode insertion may thus be a greater technical challenge. One technique to confirm appropriate placement is to measure the EVOR intraoperatively immediately after electrode insertion.[34,42] For example, a robust horizontal nystagmus after stimulation of the horizontal canal electrode would suggest correct insertion.

Another method to confirm electrode placement intraoperatively is to measure an electrically evoked compound action potential (ECAP). This response occurs after stimulation of the vestibular nerve, just as it occurs after stimulation of the cochlear nerve. ECAP and EVOR have also been observed to correlate.[60]

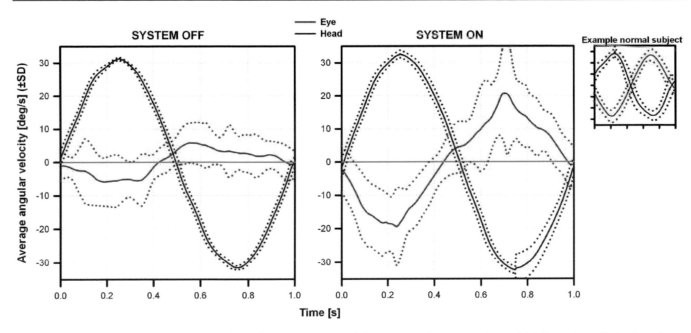

Fig. 21.6 A sensor-based vestibular implant allows restoration of the VOR in a human patient with bilateral vestibular hypofunction. When the vestibular implant is off ("SYSTEM OFF"), there are minimal eye movements (*red tracing*) in response to head movements (*blue tracing*). When the vestibular implant is turned on ("SYSTEM ON"), the eye movements are nearly equal/opposite to the head movements, showing improvement of the VOR. In the upper right, a control subject with a normal VOR is shown for comparison. Used with permission from Pelizzone M, Fornos AP, Guinand N, et al. First functional rehabilitation via vestibular implants. Cochlear Implants Int 2014;15(Suppl 1):S62–64.

Postoperatively, EVOR has been measured in numerous VI animal studies as a technique to assess appropriate device function. For example, sinusoidal modulation of pulse frequency has resulted in sinusoidal eye movements.[28,42] Appropriate EVORs have recently been measured in human trial subjects with both VIs[58,59] and vestibulocochlear implants.[56,65]

Current Spread and Canal Specificity

Specificity of stimulation from the electrode array is important for optimizing the signal. If current spreads to neighboring structures, side effects will result. Stimulation of the superior canal ampulla when the horizontal canal electrode is activated, for example, will result in unwanted vertical eye movements and the perception of motion in the wrong plane.[10,66]

Current spread to the cochlea would cause undesired auditory perception, while current spread to the facial nerve would cause facial movement. In a study of four rhesus monkeys implanted with the MVP2 VI, ABR hearing thresholds increased ~ 5 dB during electrical stimulation.[46] In one of four humans implanted with the UW/Cochlear VI, auditory percepts were rare, with a high-pitched tone heard during stimulation of the horizontal canal at two high frequencies during a single testing session. Facial movements were not seen in the first human study[58,59] and were observed in monkeys only at high currents (unpublished results).

Current focusing and steering are two technologies that may be able to help overcome these problems by channeling current toward the appropriate ampulla.[52,67] Using high-frequency pulses, for example, causes less current spread than using low-frequency pulses.[42,68] Bipolar simulation also produces less spread than monopolar stimulation. Finally, adaptation is a central mechanism that may help correct for misalignments due to spread to adjacent ampullae.[34,40,48]

Adaptation versus Habituation

Adaptation occurs when the central nervous system appropriately adjusts to a change in neural input. *Plasticity* describes the ability to retain this adaptive state.[69] *Habituation* is a process where repeated exposure to a sensory stimulus causes a decline in the response. Adaptation is a complex, dynamic process, whereas habituation is a simple tendency toward zero. The impressive capacity for adaptation was demonstrated in a classic study where the direction of the VOR was reversed in human subjects whose vision was optically flipped.[70]

When a VI is initially turned on, any suprathreshold stimulation of the vestibular nerve will result in evoked eye movements (EVOR). At first, this may occur even when the stimulation intensity is designed to mimic the missing normal resting output from the vestibular system. In this situation, the eye movements (and accompanying perception of spinning) are undesired. Within hours, however, the central nervous system will adapt to this acute stimulus, and the nystagmus will cease.[34,40] Rapid adaptation will also occur to stimulation pulse rates more than double that of an animal's normal physiologic baseline.[9]

One concern is that with chronic vestibular nerve stimulation, the brain will habituate, rather than adapt, to the signal. If this were to occur, any stimulation over baseline would also decay, and the EVOR desired during head movement would eventually cease. Fortunately, several animal studies suggest that there is central adaptation, but not habituation, to VIs. For example, monkeys that were exposed to continuous tonic VI stimulation for more than 3 months were still able to have robust EVORs in response to modulation of the baseline signal during head rotation. This occurred despite complete adaptation (i.e., lack of EVOR) from the tonic baseline stimulation.[34]

Another important finding is that after adaptation to baseline stimulation occurs, turning the device off for the first time leads to acute nystagmus (in the opposite direction from that of activation). Such "after-effects" are another characteristic of adaptation, but not habituation.[9,34] Furthermore, the evoked nystagmus upon switching the device on or off will also fatigue to zero. In a guinea pig study, the EVOR decayed to 20% of the original value after only three on–off cycles. Acclimation to either device state (on or off) may represent a form of *dual-state adaptation*.[42] This finding has important consequences because VI users may need to abruptly deactivate their device in several situations, e.g., showering, sleeping, changing batteries. Evoked nystagmus and accompanying vertigo would clearly be undesirable, and could lead to injuries. It is unclear whether humans implanted with a VI may benefit from periodically turning the device on and off to maintain dual-state adaptation. If so, this could be integrated into perioperative VI rehabilitation programs.

The central vestibular system has the ability to adapt to EVOR gain. In monkeys, when the device was intentionally set to understimulate and thus result in a low gain, the gain increased over time. However, the increase was modest and did not reach normal levels.[34]

Finally, adaptation has been shown to minimize effects of current spread beyond the desired canal ampulla. In the same study, undesired vertical EVOR resulting from horizontal canal stimulation eventually disappeared.[34] More impressively, intentional simulation of the posterior canal during yaw rotation can result in adjustment of the EVOR to the appropriate horizontal direction.[40]

■ Future Efforts and Regenerative Therapies

Similar to when cochlear implants emerged 40 years ago, the field of vestibular implantation is in its early stages. Early studies are promising; however, further research is certainly needed. While recapitulation of the EVOR has been repeatedly demonstrated in both animals and humans, the gain in sensor-based implants needs to be optimized. Even if a subnormal gain were tolerated in early generation implants through central plasticity, improvements in signal processing should attempt to approach more physiologic capabilities.

Research is also needed to create a totally implantable VI. Similar efforts are underway in CI research. A totally implantable VI may be more feasible, however, since a gyroscope would be easier to internalize than a microphone. Improving battery longevity from efforts in the consumer electronics and automotive industries may also trickle down to help the field of vestibular implantation.

Finally, miniaturization of device components could allow reduced fabrication costs and easier development of a totally implanted prosthesis. For example, a microelectromechanical system (MEMS)-based prototype with three gyroscopes and three linear and angular accelerometers integrated on a 5×5 mm ultrathin silicone wafer has been developed, allowing "balance on a chip."[27] Refinement and miniaturization of electrode design[71] may also allow reduced current spread and preservation of native vestibular function.

Despite all these potential advances, it may prove impossible to achieve completely normal vestibular physiology with an artificial device. Hair cell regeneration is a field that employs manipulation at the cellular level to replace lost function with biologic, rather than electronic, technologies. As of this writing, a phase 2 clinical trial is underway using gene therapy to treat severe-to-profound sensorineural hearing loss. While not the primary endpoint, vestibular function is one of the measures being utilized in the trial.[72]

Even if successful hair cell regeneration proves to be decades away, a nearer-term goal may be to combine the two technologies. For example, it is known that vestibular neurons will slowly degenerate following hair cell death.[73] This could potentially reduce implant efficacy. Degenerative effects may be even more pronounced than with cochlear implantation because Scarpa's ganglion lies farther away from the vestibular end-organs than the spiral ganglion lies from the cochlea.[12] An electrode array that elutes neurotrophic growth factors may help solve this problem.

■ Conclusion

Vestibular implantation has recently made the critical transition from preclinical to early human clinical trials. Early data have shown that sensor-based prostheses can subtotally restore the VOR in patients with severe bilateral vestibular hypofunction. Primate studies suggest that implantation of the vestibular system may allow preservation of vestibular and auditory function, which could ultimately broaden implant candidacy. These advances will hopefully expand the surgical armamentarium of otologist/neurotologists in the near future. Most importantly, procedural treatment of vestibular disorders may soon shift from ablative procedures to ones that preserve and restore function.

References

1. Gong W, Merfeld DM. Prototype neural semicircular canal prosthesis using patterned electrical stimulation. Ann Biomed Eng 2000;28(5):572–581

2. van Sonsbeek S, Pullens B, van Benthem PP. Positive pressure therapy for Ménière's disease or syndrome. Cochrane Database Syst Rev 2015;3:CD008419

3. Thirlwall AS, Kundu S. Diuretics for Ménière's disease or syndrome. Cochrane Database Syst Rev 2006;(3):CD003599

4. Pullens B, van Benthem PP. Intratympanic gentamicin for Ménière's disease or syndrome. Cochrane Database Syst Rev 2011;(3):CD008234

5. Pullens B, Verschuur HP, van Benthem PP. Surgery for Ménière's disease. Cochrane Database Syst Rev 2013;2:CD005395

6. Sun DQ, Ward BK, Semenov YR, Carey JP, Della Santina CC. Bilateral Vestibular Deficiency: Quality of Life and Economic Implications. JAMA Otolaryngol Head Neck Surg 2014;140(6):527–534

7. Goldberg JM, Fernandez C. Physiology of peripheral neurons innervating semicircular canals of the squirrel monkey. I. Resting discharge and response to constant angular accelerations. J Neurophysiol 1971;34(4):635–660

8. Gong W, Haburcakova C, Merfeld DM. Vestibulo-ocular responses evoked via bilateral electrical stimulation of the lateral semicircular canals. IEEE Trans Biomed Eng 2008;55(11):2608–2619

9. Gong W, Merfeld DM. System design and performance of a unilateral horizontal semicircular canal prosthesis. IEEE Trans Biomed Eng 2002;49(2):175–181

10. Della Santina CC, Migliaccio AA, Patel AH. A multichannel semicircular canal neural prosthesis using electrical stimulation to restore 3-d vestibular sensation. IEEE Trans Biomed Eng 2007;54(6 Pt 1):1016–1030

11. Mardirossian V, Karmali F, Merfeld D. Thresholds for human perception of roll tilt motion: patterns of variability based on visual, vestibular, and mixed cues. Otol Neurotol 2014;35(5):857–860

12. Wall C III, Merfeld DM, Rauch SD, Black FO. Vestibular prostheses: the engineering and biomedical issues. J Vestib Res 2002-2003;12(2-3):95–113

13. White JA. Laboratory tests of vestibular and balance functioning. In: Hughes GB, Pensak ML, eds. Clinical Otology. 3rd ed. New York, NY: Thieme; 2007

14. Carey JP, Della Santina CP. Principles of applied vestibular physiology. In: Cummings CW, Flint PW, Haughey BH, et al., eds. Cummings Otolaryngology—Head & Neck Surgery. 4th ed. Philadelphia, PA: Elsevier; 2005:3115–3159

15. Lempert T, Neuhauser H. Epidemiology of vertigo, migraine and vestibular migraine. J Neurol 2009;256(3):333–338

16. Neuhauser HK, Radtke A, von Brevern M, Lezius F, Feldmann M, Lempert T. Burden of dizziness and vertigo in the community. Arch Intern Med 2008;168(19):2118–2124

17. Bhattacharyya N, Baugh RF, Orvidas L, et al; American Academy of Otolaryngology-Head and Neck Surgery Foundation. Clinical practice guideline: benign paroxysmal positional vertigo. Otolaryngol Head Neck Surg 2008;139(5, Suppl 4):S47–S81

18. Epley JM. The canalith repositioning procedure: for treatment of benign paroxysmal positional vertigo. Otolaryngol Head Neck Surg 1992;107(3):399–404

19. Gates GA. Ménière's disease review 2005. J Am Acad Audiol 2006;17(1):16–26

20. Thorp MA, James AL. Prosper Ménière. Lancet 2005;366(9503):2137–2139

21. Van de Heyning PH, Wuyts F, Boudewyns A. Surgical treatment of Meniere's disease. Curr Opin Neurol 2005;18(1):23–28

22. Schuknecht HF. Ménière's disease, pathogenesis and pathology. Am J Otolaryngol 1982;3(5):349–352

23. Boudewyns AN, Wuyts FL, Hoppenbrouwers M, et al. Meniett therapy: rescue treatment in severe drug-resistant Ménière's disease? Acta Otolaryngol 2005;125(12):1283–1289

24. Phillips JS, Westerberg B. Intratympanic steroids for Ménière's disease or syndrome. Cochrane Database Syst Rev 2011; (7):CD008514

25. Cohen B, Suzuki JI. Eye movements induced by ampullary nerve stimulation. Am J Physiol 1963;204:347–351

26. Suzuki JI, Cohen B, Bender MB. Compensatory eye movements induced by vertical semicircular canal stimulation. Exp Neurol 1964;9:137–160

27. Shkel AM, Zeng FG. An electronic prosthesis mimicking the dynamic vestibular function. Audiol Neurootol 2006;11(2):113–122

28. Rubinstein JT, Bierer S, Kaneko C, et al. Implantation of the semicircular canals with preservation of hearing and rotational sensitivity: a vestibular neurostimulator suitable for clinical research. Otol Neurotol 2012;33(5):789–796

29. Goto F, Meng H, Bai R, et al. Eye movements evoked by the selective stimulation of the utricular nerve in cats. Auris Nasus Larynx 2003;30(4):341–348

30. Goto F, Meng H, Bai R, et al. Eye movements evoked by selective saccular nerve stimulation in cats. Auris Nasus Larynx 2004;31(3):220–225

31. Curthoys IS. Eye movements produced by utricular and saccular stimulation. Aviat Space Environ Med 1987;58(9 Pt 2):A192–A197

32. Curthoys IS, Oman CM. Dimensions of the horizontal semicircular duct, ampulla and utricle in rat and guinea pig. Acta Otolaryngol 1986;101(1-2):1–10

33. Fluur E, Mellström A. The otolith organs and their influence on oculomotor movements. Exp Neurol 1971; 30(1):139–147

34. Merfeld DM, Haburcakova C, Gong W, Lewis RF. Chronic vestibulo-ocular reflexes evoked by a vestibular prosthesis. IEEE Trans Biomed Eng 2007;54(6 Pt 1): 1005–1015

35. Davidovics NS, Fridman GY, Della Santina CC. Comodulation of stimulus rate and current from elevated baselines expands head motion encoding range of the vestibular prosthesis. Exp Brain Res 2012; 218(3):389–400

36. Gantz BJ, Turner C, Gfeller KE, Lowder MW. Preservation of hearing in cochlear implant surgery: advantages of combined electrical and acoustical speech processing. Laryngoscope 2005;115(5):796–802

37. Agrawal SK, Parnes LS. Transmastoid superior semicircular canal occlusion. Otol Neurotol 2008; 29(3):363–367

38. Beyea JA, Agrawal SK, Parnes LS. Transmastoid semicircular canal occlusion: a safe and highly effective treatment for benign paroxysmal positional vertigo and superior canal dehiscence. Laryngoscope 2012;122(8):1862–1866

39. Ward BK, Agrawal Y, Nguyen E, et al. Hearing outcomes after surgical plugging of the superior semicircular canal by a middle cranial fossa approach. Otol Neurotol 2012;33(8):1386–1391

40. Lewis RF, Gong W, Ramsey M, Minor L, Boyle R, Merfeld DM. Vestibular adaptation studied with a prosthetic semicircular canal. J Vestib Res 2002-2003; 12(2-3):87–94

41. Lewis RF, Haburcakova C, Gong W, Makary C, Merfeld DM. Vestibuloocular reflex adaptation investigated with chronic motion-modulated electrical stimulation of semicircular canal afferents. J Neurophysiol 2010;103(2):1066–1079

42. Merfeld DM, Gong W, Morrissey J, Saginaw M, Haburcakova C, Lewis RF. Acclimation to chronic constant-rate peripheral stimulation provided by a vestibular prosthesis. IEEE Trans Biomed Eng 2006;53(11):2362–2372

43. Lewis RF, Haburcakova C, Gong W, et al. Vestibular prosthesis tested in rhesus monkeys. Conference proceedings: Annual International Conference of the IEEE Engineering in Medicine and Biology Society. IEEE Engineering in Medicine and Biology Society 2011; 2277–2279.

44. Della Santina C, Migliaccio A, Patel A. Electrical stimulation to restore vestibular function development of a 3-D vestibular prosthesis. Conf Proc IEEE Eng Med Biol Soc 2005;7:7380–7385

45. Chiang B, Fridman GY, Dai C, Rahman MA, Della Santina CC. Design and performance of a multichannel vestibular prosthesis that restores semicircular canal sensation in rhesus monkey. IEEE Trans Neural Syst Rehabil Eng 2011;19(5):588–598

46. Dai C, Fridman GY, Della Santina CC. Effects of vestibular prosthesis electrode implantation and stimulation on hearing in rhesus monkeys. Hear Res 2011;277(1-2):204–210

47. Dai C, Fridman GY, Davidovics NS, Chiang B, Ahn JH, Della Santina CC. Restoration of 3D vestibular sensation in rhesus monkeys using a multichannel vestibular prosthesis. Hear Res 2011;281(1-2):74–83

48. Dai C, Fridman GY, Chiang B, et al. Cross-axis adaptation improves 3D vestibulo-ocular reflex alignment during chronic stimulation via a head-mounted multichannel vestibular prosthesis. Exp Brain Res 2011; 210(3-4):595–606

49. Sun DQ, Rahman MA, Fridman G, Dai C, Chiang B, Della Santina CC. Chronic stimulation of the semicircular canals using a multichannel vestibular prosthesis: effects on locomotion and angular vestibulo-ocular reflex in chinchillas. Conference Proceedings 2011;3519–3523

50. Hayden R, Sawyer S, Frey E, Mori S, Migliaccio AA, Della Santina CC. Virtual labyrinth model of vestibular afferent excitation via implanted electrodes: validation and application to design of a multichannel vestibular prosthesis. Exp Brain Res 2011;210(3-4):623–640

51. Davidovics NS, Fridman GY, Chiang B, Della Santina CC. Effects of biphasic current pulse frequency, amplitude, duration, and interphase gap on eye movement responses to prosthetic electrical stimulation of the vestibular nerve. IEEE Trans Neural Syst Rehabil Eng 2011;19(1):84–94

52. Fridman GY, Davidovics NS, Dai C, Migliaccio AA, Della Santina CC. Vestibulo-ocular reflex responses to a multichannel vestibular prosthesis incorporating a 3D coordinate transformation for correction of misalignment. J Assoc Res Otolaryngol 2010;11(3):367–381

53. Tang S, Melvin T-A, Della Santina CC. Effects of semicircular canal electrode implantation on hearing in chinchillas. Acta Otolaryngol 2009;129(5):481–486

54. Rahman MA, Dai C, Fridman GY, et al. Restoring the 3D vestibulo-ocular reflex via electrical stimulation: The Johns Hopkins multichannel vestibular prosthesis project. IEEE Engineering in Medicine and Biology Society. Conference 2011;3142–3145

55. Bierer SM, Ling L, Nie K, et al. Auditory outcomes following implantation and electrical stimulation of the semicircular canals. Hear Res 2012;287(1-2):51–56

56. Perez Fornos A, Guinand N, van de Berg R, et al. Artificial balance: restoration of the vestibulo-ocular reflex in humans with a prototype vestibular neuroprosthesis. Front Neurol 2014;5:66

57. Lu T, Djalilian H, Zeng FG, Chen H, Sun X. An integrated vestibular-cochlear prosthesis for restoring balance and hearing. IEEE Engineering in Medicine and Biology Society. Conference. 2011;1319–1322.

58. Phillips C, Ling L, Oxford T, et al. Longitudinal performance of an implantable vestibular prosthesis. Hear Res 2015;322:200–211

59. Golub JS, Ling L, Nie K, et al. Prosthetic implantation of the human vestibular system. Otol Neurotol 2014;35(1):136–147

60. Nie K, Bierer SM, Ling L, Oxford T, Rubinstein JT, Phillips JO. Characterization of the electrically evoked compound action potential of the vestibular nerve. Otol Neurotol 2011;32(1):88–97

61. Phillips JO, Shepherd SJ, Nowack AL, et al. Longitudinal performance of a vestibular prosthesis as assessed by electrically evoked compound action potential recording. Conf Proc IEEE Eng Med Biol Soc 2012;2012:6128–6131

62. Pelizzone M, Fornos AP, Guinand N, et al. First functional rehabilitation via vestibular implants. Cochlear Implants Int 2014;15(Suppl 1):S62–S64

63. van de Berg R, Guinand N, Nguyen TA, et al. The vestibular implant: frequency-dependency of the electrically evoked vestibulo-ocular reflex in humans. Front Syst Neurosci 2014;8:255

64. Personal communication, Charley Della Santina, PhD, MD.

65. Guyot JP, Sigrist A, Pelizzone M, Kos MI. Adaptation to steady-state electrical stimulation of the vestibular system in humans. Ann Otol Rhinol Laryngol 2011;120(3):143–149

66. Weinberg MS, Wall C, Robertsson J, O'Neil E, Sienko K, Fields R. Tilt determination in MEMS inertial vestibular prosthesis. J Biomech Eng 2006;128(6):943–956

67. Bonham BH, Litvak LM. Current focusing and steering: modeling, physiology, and psychophysics. Hear Res 2008;242(1-2):141–153

68. Rubinstein JT, Spelman FA. Analytical theory for extracellular electrical stimulation of nerve with focal electrodes. I. Passive unmyelinated axon. Biophys J 1988;54(6):975–981

69. Jones GM. Posture. In: Kandel ER, Schwartz JH, Jessell TM, eds. Principles of Neural Science. New York, NY: McGraw-Hill; 2000

70. Gonshor A, Jones GM. Proceedings: Changes of human vestibulo-ocular response induced by vision-reversal during head rotation. J Physiol 1973;234(2):102P–103P

71. Poppendieck W, Sossalla A, Krob MO, et al. Development, manufacturing and application of double-sided flexible implantable microelectrodes. Biomed Microdevices 2014;16(6):837–850

72. Clinicaltrials.gov. identifier NCT02132130, https://clinicaltrials.gov/ct2/show/NCT02132130?term=CGF166&rank=1

73. Schuknecht HF. Behavior of the vestibular nerve following labyrinthectomy. Ann Otol Rhinol Laryngol Suppl 1982;97:16–32

Appendix: Frequently Asked Questions with Answers

Q1: In the medical treatment of Meniere's disease, is there anything else useful other than a low-salt, no-caffeine, no-alcohol diet and diuretics?

Yes, some patients will also respond to the use of a more centrally acting calcium channel blocker called nimodipine. We prescribe 30 mg twice a day, which has helped numerous patients who have otherwise not had benefit from medical management. In addition, some people believe that lipoflavonoids may have some benefits as well, and lipoflavonoids are certainly an option that can be used with few side effects. In addition, sometimes the cost of nimodipine can be prohibitive. In those cases, we have tried other calcium channel blockers, such as amlodipine besylate (Norvasc, Pfizer, New York, NY) 5 mg once a day. However, the results do not seem to be as good as when we are able to use nimodipine (Aimidopine, Bayer, West Hartford, CT). Certainly, there are other medications, as elucidated in Chapter 7 of this book, but these are my personal preferences.

Q2: Is benign paroxysmal positional vertigo (BPPV) more prevalent in patients with Meniere's disease?

Yes. The incidence of BPPV in the general population is less than the incidence in patients with Meniere's disease. This is probably due to repeated trauma to the vestibular system causing otoconia to become displaced. The symptoms of BPPV in a Meniere's patient are the same as those in the general public and certainly are different from the typical dizzy spell that the patient has with Meniere's disease. It is important to differentiate the two, as obviously the treatment is completely different.

Q3: Why would anyone want to consider an endolymphatic shunt operation for the treatment of Meniere's disease?

Unlike a lot of surgical procedures for Meniere's disease, endolymphatic shunt is the one surgical option that does preserve the vestibular system. This is important because, although most patients will compensate for the loss of one unilateral vestibular system, there are many patients who have professions or hobbies where the loss of one vestibular system may hinder their ability to perform such activities. These include occupations like construction worker, roofer, fireman, or driver, and hobbies like rock climbing, skiing, and horseback riding. So, although the chance of controlling Meniere's disease is less with this procedure than with those that destroy the balance system, the fact that it preserves the vestibular system is a very significant plus for many patients.

Q4: Why would you choose a vestibular nerve section over an intratympanic gentamicin treatment if you were going to perform a vestibular destructive procedure?

There is a significant risk of hearing loss associated with gentamicin injections. The hearing loss normally ranges from 20 to 30%, although there have been reports of very minimal risk from a few centers. In our own experience, we have not, as of yet, had any appreciable hearing loss after vestibular nerve section. The control rate of vertigo spells is also significantly higher with the vestibular nerve section, ~ 95%, versus ~ 80% with intratympanic gentamicin injections. Thus, although it is an intracranial procedure, a number of patients choose nerve section over gentamicin injections.

Q5: Do you recommend the Meniett device?

We have had a number of patients who have tried the Meniett device. The beauty of the Meniett device procedure is that it is relatively minor, that is, a myringotomy with a tube insertion followed by the use of the Meniett device. However, many of our patients have not experienced the dramatic results reported in published data. In fact, most of our patients have not been helped by the device. Also, early on, the cost of the device precluded many of our patients from being able to use this technology, and even now it is still difficult for patients to get insurance companies to cover the device, which is really expensive.

Q6: What do you recommend for controlling acute vertiginous episodes?

Just about any of the known medications are useful. Personally, we tend to use either sublingual lorazepam (Ativan, Biovail Pharmaceuticals, Bridgewater, NJ) or diazepam (Valium, Roche Laboratories, Nutley, NJ) by mouth as needed. Either one tends to work well. Phenergan (promethazine hydrochloride, Baxter Healthcare Corporation, Deerfield, IL) is another good choice. We do not have as much success with meclizine for acute attacks. However, in our experience, the medication that seems to work the least is Zofran (ondansetron hydrochloride, Glaxo Smith-Kline, Research Triangle Park, NC). Although Zofran seems to be very good for controlling nausea and vomiting in patients receiving chemotherapy and for other reasons, it did not seem to have any significant effect on acute vertigo.

Q7: If surgical treatment "cures" the vestibular attacks, will I still get other symptoms of Meniere's disease?

Yes. Although we have many methods at hand for treating recurrent vertigo, patients often will still complain of episodic ear fullness, which may or may not be coupled with hearing loss and tinnitus. The reason for this is that the surgical treatment doesn't treat the cause of the Meniere's disease so much as it takes away the ability of the vestibular system to deliver its information to the brain to cause the dizzy spell.

Q8: Do you know what causes Meniere's disease?

In essence, Meniere's disease should probably be called a syndrome rather than a "disease," because there are many causes of Meniere's symptoms, causes that can range from allergy to immunologic disorders to migraines and so forth. Thus, it is often better to actually find or determine what the cause of the spells is and then treat accordingly.

Q9: I had BPPV successfully treated once, and now my symptoms seem to have returned. Is this possible?

Indeed, BPPV comes back in approximately 30% of patients. The treatment is still the same. At times, patients may learn to do maneuvers on their own to help clear the loose otoconia. Otherwise, repeated vestibular therapy is certainly indicated and should be just as useful in recurrent episodes as it was with the initial episode.

Q10: Is it possible for the otoconia BPPV to go from one canal to the other?

Yes, it is. Indeed, this has happened on several occasions, and it is indicated by the changing directions of the nystagmus and is able to be treated accordingly with the proper change in positioning movements.

Q11: I was diagnosed with vestibular neuronitis, but I am still having problems with my equilibrium. How long will this last?

In vestibular neuronitis, the acute phase will usually last anywhere from 24 to 72 hours. After this time period, patients still complain of dizziness; however, when questioned thoroughly, they reveal they are experiencing more of a disequilibrium or feeling that they are sort of drunk rather than the true spinning vertigo. In most patients, the average recovery time is about 6 weeks, maybe a little longer. Yet with the use of vestibular rehab therapy, the amount of recovery time decreases dramatically and allows the patients to get back to work and on with their lives very quickly.

Q12: I have episodic dizzy spells and my doctor made the diagnosis of Meniere's disease and started treatment without doing any other tests. Is this advisable?

No. Meniere's disease is a diagnosis of exclusion. Many other disorders can mimic Meniere's disease. At the very least, magnetic resonance imaging (MRI) with gadolinium should be obtained. Eliminating a diagnosis like multiple sclerosis, acoustic neuroma, or repeated transient ischemic attacks is indeed essential before arriving at the diagnosis of Meniere's disease.

Q13: What is the best way to treat a unilateral hypoactive vestibular system or complete paralysis (unilateral paralysis) of the vestibular system?

Vestibular rehab therapy is essential in helping patients obtain optimal compensation for their loss.

Q14: Do perilymphatic fistulas (PLFs) really exist?

Yes. Perilymphatic fistulas do exist. Indeed, there is almost always a reason or significant event that one can point to as the cause. Events like trauma to the ear, whether blunt or concussive, barotrauma from diving, or unpressurized plane travel are causes.

Q15: What would be the best treatment for an acoustic neuroma to minimize damage to the vestibular system?

Depending on the size of the tumor, there are three options for treatment: observation, with repeated MRI scans; surgical excision; and Gamma Knife radiation. If the tumor is small and can be observed and is not growing, then observation is the best choice; it is the least invasive management and is also the treatment with no significant complications. However, if the tumor does start to grow, there is risk of having some vestibular complaints or hearing loss. If the patient has no complaints at the time and it is a small tumor, observation is certainly a reasonable approach to management. Surgical excision will cause a significant vestibular response, with severe dizziness usually lasting a few days. Then there will be a complete unilateral loss of the vestibular system, which will cause problems with equilibrium. The use of vestibular rehab therapy will, on average, take the patient about 6 weeks before he or she will be back to most activities. However, once there is loss of vestibular nerve, there are certain things that the patient will always notice that will be difficult. These will include quick movements, which may cause a little bit of a wobble. Getting up in the middle of the night, if it is totally dark, will usually result in balance trouble, and the patient may stumble or fall. It would be advisable to use a nightlight in these situations. As for Gamma Knife, the effects of the radiation are usually seen over extended periods of time, and thus an acute dizzy phase is not usually as prevalent as with surgery. In fact, most patients do not have a significant "dizzy spell." Over time, there is loss of vestibular function, but it happens slowly, and in most cases patients compensate and do not notice any appreciable difference.

Certainly, one would also have to take into account the effects on hearing and facial nerve function in making a final decision of which treatment to pursue.

Q16: What is vascular loop compression syndrome?

This is a normal anatomic variant where an artery presses into the vestibular nerve, which at times may cause vestibular complaints. The most common or reliable complaint is that patients have significant difficulty walking up and down the aisles of large stores or being passengers in cars because objects moving by them induce significant symptoms. This diagnosis can sometimes be made with magnetic resonance angiogram. The treatment that I usually use for something of this nature is a Klonopin (clonazepam, Roche Laboratories, Nutley, NJ) and Baclofen (Watson Labs, Corona, California) combination. Usually my treatment of choice is 0.5 mg of Klonopin taken twice a day.

Q17: Is there such a thing as mal de debarquement syndrome?

Yes. Mal de debarquement syndrome is a feeling that the patient is still on a boat, even though he or she is not. Treatment with Klonopin 0.5 mg twice a day is usually the treatment of choice.

Q18: Are electronystagmography (ENG) and computerized posturography really necessary?

Although some clinicians feel that the information from an ENG is not very useful, I respectfully disagree. ENG can tell us whether the patient has a unilateral weakness or not. It can discern whether there is a central pathology that may be causing the patient's symptoms. It may tell us which balance problems the patient has, or it may confirm difficult positional vertigo cases, especially those with cervical ocular vertigo. All this information is useful not only in the medical/surgical management of patients but also to our vestibular rehab therapists who treat these patients. The bottom line is, the tests provide vital information on our patients that is useful in their treatment.

Q19: Why get an audiogram?

When patients have vestibular complaints, even if they feel their hearing is normal, there are many times that we find discrepancies, such as a small conductive loss or a unilateral low- or high-frequency loss that the patient was unaware of but that points us to a specific diagnosis.

Q20: Loud noises tend to make me feel dizzy— is this indeed possible?

Yes. This is commonly known as the Tullio phenomenon. It could be associated with superior semicircular canal dehiscence, which is seen on computed tomography imaging.

Index

Note: Page numbers followed by f and t indicate figures and tables, respectively.

227